NICKEL
AND THE SKIN
Absorption, Immunology,
Epidemiology, and Metallurgy

DERMATOLOGY: CLINICAL & BASIC SCIENCE SERIES
Series Editor Howard I. Maibach, M.D.

Published Titles:

Pesticide Dermatoses
Homero Penagos, Michael O'Malley, and Howard I. Maibach

Hand Eczema, Second Edition
Torkil Menné and Howard I. Maibach

Dermatologic Botany
Javier Avalos and Howard I. Maibach

Dry Skin and Moisturizers: Chemistry and Function
Marie Loden and Howard I. Maibach

Skin Reactions to Drugs
Kirsti Kauppinen, Kristiina Alanko, Matti Hannuksela, and Howard I. Maibach

Contact Urticaria Syndrome
Smita Amin, Arto Lahti, and Howard I. Maibach

Bioengineering of the Skin: Skin Surface, Imaging, and Analysis
Klaus P. Wilhelm, Peter Elsner, Enzo Berardesca, and Howard I. Maibach

Bioengineering of the Skin: Methods and Instrumentation
Enzo Berardesca, Peter Elsner, Klaus P. Wilhelm, and Howard I. Maibach

Bioengineering of the Skin: Cutaneous Blood Flow and Erythema
Enzo Berardesca, Peter Elsner, and Howard I. Maibach

Bioengineering of the Skin: Water and the Stratum Corneum
Peter Elsner, Enzo Berardesca, and Howard I. Maibach

Human Papillomavirus Infections in Dermatovenereology
Gerd Gross and Geo von Krogh

The Irritant Contact Dermatitis Syndrome
Pieter van der Valk, Pieter Coenrads, and Howard I. Maibach

Dermatologic Research Techniques
Howard I. Maibach

Skin Cancer: Mechanisms and Human Relevance
Hasan Mukhtar

Skin Cancer: Mechanisms and Human Relevance
Hasan Mukhtar

Protective Gloves for Occupational Use
Gunh Mellström, J.E. Walhberg, and Howard I. Maibach

Pigmentation and Pigmentary Disorders
Norman Levine

Nickel and the Skin: Immunology and Toxicology
Howard I. Maibach and Torkil Menné

Bioengineering of the Skin: Skin Biomechanics
Peter Elsner, Enzo Berardesca, Klaus-P. Wilhelm, and Howard I. Maibach

Nickel and the Skin: Absorption, Immunology, Epidemiology, and Metallurgy
Jurij J. Hostýneck and Howard I. Maibach

DERMATOLOGY: CLINICAL & BASIC SCIENCE SERIES

NICKEL AND THE SKIN

Absorption, Immunology, Epidemiology, and Metallurgy

Edited by
Jurij J. Hostýnek
Howard I. Maibach

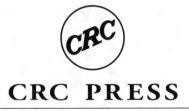

CRC PRESS

Boca Raton   London   New York   Washington, D.C.

Library of Congress Cataloging-in-Publication Data

Nickel and the skin : absorption, immunology, epidemiology, and metallurgy / edited by
Jurij J. Hostynek and Howard I. Maibach.
     p. ; cm. -- (Dermatology : clinical & basic science series)
  Includes bibliographical references and index.
  ISBN 0-8493-1072-5 (alk. paper)
    1. Contact dermatitis. 2. Nickel--Toxicology. 3. Nickel--Immunology. I. Hostynek,
Jurij J. II. Maibach, Howard I. (Howard Ira) III. Dermatology (CRC Press)
    [DNLM: 1. Dermatitis, Allergic Contact--etiology. 2. Nickel--adverse effects. 3.
Nickel--immunology. WR 175 N6317 2002]
  RL244 .N534 2002
  616.97′3--dc21
                                                         2002017440

Chapter 3, "Oxidative Properties of the Skin: A Determinant for Nickel Diffusion," and Chapter 6, "Diagnostic Testing for Nickel Allergic Hypersensitivity: Patch Testing versus Lymphocyte Transformation Test," were originally published in *Exogenous Dermatology*. With permission from S. Karger, Basel.

Visit the CRC Press Web site at www.crcpress.com

© 2002 by CRC Press LLC

No claim to original U.S. Government works
International Standard Book Number 0-8493-1072-5
Library of Congress Card Number 2002017440
Printed in the United States of America 1 2 3 4 5 6 7 8 9 0
Printed on acid-free paper

Ad majorem Dei gloriam,
si hoc licet dicere in opusculo.

Series Preface

Our goal in creating the *Dermatology: Clinical & Basic Science Series* is to present the insights of experts on emerging applied and experimental techniques and theoretical concepts that are, or will be, at the vanguard of dermatology. These books cover new and exciting multidisciplinary areas of cutaneous research; and we want them to be the books every physician will use to become acquainted with new methodologies in skin research. These books can be given to graduate students and postdoctoral fellows when they are looking for guidance to start a new line of research.

The series consists of books that are edited by experts and that consist of chapters written by the leaders in a particular field. The books are richly illustrated and contain comprehensive bibliographies. Each chapter provides substantial background material relevant to the particular subject. These books contain detailed tricks of the trade and information regarding where the methods presented can be safely applied. In addition, information on where to buy equipment and helpful Web sites for solving both practical and theoretical problems are included.

We are working with these goals in mind. As the books become available, the efforts put in by the publisher, book editors, and the individual authors will contribute to the further development of dermatology research and clinical practice. The extent to which we achieve this goal will be determined by the utility of these books.

Howard I. Maibach, M.D.

Preface

From the viewpoint of immunotoxicology, hazards associated with nickel primarily derive from its type-IV immunogenic properties, as it consistently ranks as the premier anthropogenic allergen among the general population in industrialized countries. Thus, immunology of nickel represents the major part of reviews addressing human health aspects of the metal. A comprehensive discussion of nickel immunology invariably presents a composite picture consisting of diverse environmental, physiological, and chemical components, and in 1989 a first such mosaic was composed by Maibach and Menné in their book, *Nickel and the Skin: Immunology and Toxicology*, published by CRC Press.

Since then much insight was gained into diverse aspects of nickel's action in the human organism, mainly concerning the skin and the immune system, and a synoptic presentation of the subject from a somewhat different viewpoint now appears in order. Impetus for this new undertaking came from the Nickel Producers Environmental Research Association (NiPERA), and for most of the chapters Katherine Reagan, toxicologist in that organization, collaborated as author.

Subjects that are part of this review deal with the initial event of nickel-containing objects coming in contact with the skin and the formation of soluble, skin-diffusible salts, the phenomenon of skin penetration, induction and elicitation of allergic reactions, diagnosis, tolerance, and epidemiology. The biochemistry of nickel interacting with the organism is discussed by Baldassarré Santucci and collaborators, who had investigated and discussed that aspect in several earlier publications. Finally, the metallurgy of nickel and its interaction with other metals in alloys are addressed by Messrs. Flint and Cutler of the Nickel Development Institute.

Partial support for the book project was provided by NiPERA.

Editors

Jurij J. Hostýnek, Ph.D., currently serves as president of Euromerican Technology Resources, Inc., a Lafayette, California-based company that provides contract research and consulting services to the chemical, personal-care, and health-care industries. He is also an associate specialist at the University of California, San Francisco (UCSF) School of Medicine.

Dr. Hostýnek earned his Ph.D. in physical organic chemistry at the University of Basel, Switzerland, and conducted postdoctoral research at the University of California, Berkeley. He has published in the fields of physical organic chemistry, toxicology, dermatology, immunology, quantitative structure activity relationships (QSAR), and percutaneous absorption of organic and metallic compounds, and holds U.S. patents in metallurgy, organic synthesis, and cell biology. His current fields of research at UCSF include QSAR, skin permeation, and allergic sensitization potential of chemicals.

Howard Maibach, M.D., is a professor of dermatology at the University of California, San Francisco, and has been a leading contributor to experimental research in dermatopharmacology, and to clinical research on contact dermatitis, contact urticaria, and other skin conditions. His work on pesticides includes clinical research on glyphosate, chlorothalonil, sodium hypochlorite, norflurazon, diethyl toluamide, and isothiazolin compounds. His experimental work includes research on the local lymph node assay, and the evaluation of the percutaneous absorption of atrazine, boron-containing pesticides, phenoxy herbicides, acetochlor, glyphosate, and many other compounds.

Contributors

Emanuela Camera
Polo Dermatologico IFO San Gallicano
Rome, Italy

C. Peter Cutler
Nickel Development Institute
The Holloway, Alvechurch
Birmingham, U.K.

G. Norman Flint
Nickel Development Institute
The Holloway, Alvechurch
Birmingham, U.K.

Jurij J. Hostýnek
Euromerican Technology Resources, Inc.
Lafayette, CA
and
UCSF School of Medicine
Department of Dermatology
San Francisco, CA

Howard I. Maibach
UCSF School of Medicine
Department of Dermatology
San Francisco, CA

Mauro Picardo
Polo Dermatologico IFO San Gallicano
Rome, Italy

Katherine E. Reagan
NiPERA
Durham, NC

Baldassarré Santucci
Polo Dermatologico IFO San Gallicano
Rome, Italy

Contents

Chapter 1 Aspects of Nickel Allergy: Epidemiology, Etiology,
Immune Reactions, Prevention, and Therapy......................................1

Jurij J. Hostýnek

Chapter 2 Nickel Allergic Hypersensitivity: Prevalence and Incidence
by Country, Gender, Age, and Occupation...39

Jurij J. Hostýnek, Katherine E. Reagan, and Howard I. Maibach

Chapter 3 Oxidative Properties of the Skin: A Determinant
for Nickel Diffusion..83

Jurij J. Hostýnek, Katherine E. Reagan, and Howard I. Maibach

Chapter 4 Release of Nickel Ion from the Metal and Its Alloys
as Cause of Nickel Allergy...99

Jurij J. Hostýnek, Katherine E. Reagan, and Howard I. Maibach

Chapter 5 Skin Absorption of Nickel and Methods
to Quantify Penetration...147

Jurij J. Hostýnek, Katherine E. Reagan, and Howard I. Maibach

Chapter 6 Diagnostic Testing for Nickel Allergic Hypersensitivity:
Patch Testing versus Lymphocyte Transformation Test..................167

Jurij J. Hostýnek, Katherine E. Reagan, and Howard I. Maibach

Chapter 7 Orally Induced Tolerance to Nickel: The Role of Oral
Exposure (Orthodontic Devices) in Preventing Sensitization.........185

Jurij J. Hostýnek, Katherine E. Reagan, and Howard I. Maibach

Chapter 8 Biochemical Aspects of Nickel Hypersensitivity:
Factors Determining Allergenic Action...201

Baldassarré Santucci, Emanuela Camera, and Mauro Picardo

Chapter 9 Nickel Metal and Alloys 219

G. Norman Flint and C. Peter Cutler

Glossary of Terms...239

Index 243

1 Aspects of Nickel Allergy: Epidemiology, Etiology, Immune Reactions, Prevention, and Therapy

Jurij J. Hostýnek

CONTENTS

Abstract 2
1.1 Introduction 2
1.2 Epidemiology 3
1.3 Prognosis 5
1.4 Etiology 6
    1.4.1 Exposure 6
    1.4.2 Skin Penetration 6
1.5 The Immune Response to Nickel 7
    1.5.1 Divergent Immune Response 7
    1.5.2 Immediate-Type Hypersensitivity 10
    1.5.3 Delayed-Type Hypersensitivity 12
    1.5.4 Asymptomatic or Silent ACD 13
    1.5.5 Methods of Diagnosis and Instrumentation 14
    1.5.6 Immunotoxicity 15
    1.5.7 The Immunogenic Forms of Nickel 16
1.6 Prevention 16
    1.6.1 Prevention through Workroom Exposure Monitoring 17
    1.6.2 Prevention through Personal Hygiene 17
    1.6.3 Use of Gloves 18
    1.6.4 Protective Creams 18
        1.6.4.1 Barrier Creams 18
        1.6.4.2 Passive Protective Creams 18
        1.6.4.3 Active Protective Creams 19
    1.6.5 Prevention through Metal Plating 20
    1.6.6 Prevention through Regulation 21
1.7 Therapy 22
    1.7.1 Topical Therapy 22
    1.7.2 Systemic Therapy 23

1

1.8   Conclusions 24
Abbreviations 25
References 25

ABSTRACT

Nickel is an allergen causing type I and type IV hypersensitivity, mediated by reagins and allergen-specific T lymphocytes. Expressing in a wide range of cutaneous eruptions following dermal or systemic exposure, nickel has acquired the distinction of being the most frequent cause of hypersensitivity, occupationally as well as among the general population. In synoptic form the many effects that nickel has on the organism are presented, to provide a comprehensive picture of the aspects of that metal with many biologically noxious but metallurgically indispensable character-istics. This chapter reviews the epidemiology, the prognosis for occupational and nonoccupational nickel allergic hypersensitivity (NAH), the many types of exposure, the resulting immune responses, its immunotoxicity, and rate of diffusion through the skin. Alternatives toward prevention and remediation, topical and systemic, for this pervasive and increasing form of morbidity resulting from multiple types of exposure are discussed. Merits and limitations of preventive measures in industry and private life are considered, as well as the effectiveness of topical and systemic therapy in treating nickel allergic hypersensitivity.

1.1 INTRODUCTION

Since its introduction and with its ever-expanding application in metallurgy, nickel has gradually become the premier etiologic and contributing factor of allergy — either of the immediate, antibody-mediated or the delayed, cell-medi-ated type, or sometimes of both types in the same individual — as a consequence of exposure through skin, mucous membranes, diet, inhalation, or implants (Hostýnek, 1999). Magnusson-Kligman has classified nickel as an allergen of moderate potency in the human maximization test by use of the repeated insult patch test protocol (Kligman, 1966), ranking it as a medium-level hazard. Risk of developing nickel allergic hypersensitivity (NAH), however, is high in indus-tries such as metal refining and nickel plating, as well as in the general population. In the general population the risk is due to nickel's ubiquitous occurrence in tools and articles of everyday use — leading to frequent, intimate, and potentially long-term exposure — and to nickel's ready oxidation by the skin's exudates, which promote its diffusion through the skin barrier (Hostýnek et al., 2001b). Recent regulation of permissible nickel levels in consumer products intended for intimate and prolonged skin contact issued in the European Community now appears to reverse the trend, at least among the youngest generation (Johansen et al., 2000; Veien et al., 2001). The pernicious effects that nickel can have on the organism are magnified by depot formation in the stratum corneum (SC) and the cumulative effect of different routes of entry. The numerous reports widely disseminated in specialized journals on the adverse effects that nickel can have on the human organism, whether comprehensive and systematic, or anecdotal, address aspects of exposure, epidemiology, methods for prevention, and cure. This chapter presents a comprehensive overview of the most important aspects of causes, effects, prognosis, and remediation for this serious and growing public health problem as they have been discussed in the recent literature.

1.2 EPIDEMIOLOGY

In the overall category of contact allergens (natural or man-made), metals and their compounds represent a small minority (De Groot, 2000). Nickel, however, has been confirmed in recent epidemiological studies as the most prevalent chemical contact allergen among the general population of the industrialized world (Dickel et al., 1998; Johansen et al., 2000; Marks et al., 1998; Sertoli et al., 1999; Uter et al., 1998; Veien et al., 2001). Results from studies of unselected populations show overall percentages of NAH of 13% (age group 20 to 29) (Peltonen, 1979) and 12% (age group 15 to 34) (Nielsen and Menné, 1992). Among first-year female university students in Finland, 39% were patch-test positive to nickel (Mattila et al., 2001). What started mainly as an occupational hazard in the metal-working industry in the late nineteenth and early twentieth centuries (Blaschko, 1889; Bulmer and Mackenzie, 1926) has become, since World War II, an affliction of the general population, especially due to fashion and lifestyle trends. Positive results from patients in dermatology clinics exceed 40% among women (Young et al., 1988; Massone et al., 1991). The highest incidence is seen among women in the age group 21 to 30 (Lim et al., 1992; Brasch and Geier, 1997; Brasch et al., 1998; Dickel et al., 1998). Results from a Spanish patch-test program involving 964 consecutive dermatology patients complaining of intolerance to metals identify 607 (63%) females as positive to nickel sulfate, versus 20 (2%) of the men (Romaguera et al., 1988). A survey of allergic contact dermatitis (ACD) among 448 German metalworkers places nickel in first place as the allergen, with 20% of cases (Diepgen and Coenraads, 1999). In an analysis of hand eczema cases in Singapore, nickel was seen as the premier allergen in both the occupational (8% of 217) and nonoccupational (13% of 504) cohorts (Goh, 1989).

Longitudinal surveys also indicate an increase in NAH due to habits such as intimate skin contact with metal objects and practices such as skin piercing (Angelini and Veña, 1989; Kiec-Swierczynska, 1990; Kiec-Swierczynska, 1996; Mattila et al., 2001). A study in an American dermatology clinic correlating body piercing with incidence of nickel allergy in men showed that the number of body piercings had a positive bearing on NAH (Ehrlich et al., 2001). In some dermatological clinics the incidence of NAH appears to increase over time, most markedly among women, which is attributed mainly to the wearing of nickel-containing alloys in costume jewelry.

In Denmark, from 1985–86 (1232 tested) to 1997–98 (1267 tested), NAH in dermatology patients increased from 18.3% to 20.0% in women, and from 4.2% to 4.9% in men (Johansen et al., 2000). That study, however, noted a significant decrease, from 24.8% to 9.2%, in NAH among the youngest age group (0 to 18), attributable to the nickel-exposure regulation that became law in that country in

1991. In a retrospective study of patients with NAH seen in dermatological practice by Veien et al., also in Denmark, the comparison was made between the number of cases before (1986–1989) and after (1996–1999) implementation of limits that regulate nickel exposure. A significant reduction in the number of cases was seen in the female age group under 20. Incidence went from 22.1% (n = 702) in the earlier period to 16.7% (n = 324) (p < 0.05) in the postregulatory period (Veien et al., 2001).

Among Finnish female students surveyed by skin patch testing from 1985 to 1995, the prevalence of nickel allergy rose from 13 to 39% (n = 188), while among males the rate remained constant at 3% (n = 96) (Mattila et al., 2001). Among the female cohort tested there in 1995, the practice of skin piercing was seen in 167 individuals (89%). In a cohort of over 4000 patients in Finnish patch-test clinics tested with the dental screening series, nickel was identified as the premier allergen, with 14.6% positive reactions, although a number of the patients were symptomless. The authors conclude that only a minority of the cases registered may be attributable to dental materials, and NAH may be attributable to different etiologies not readily characterized (Kanerva et al., 2001). Since the risk of disabling hypersensitivity and the resulting economic impact have been recognized, environmental and occupational controls have been instituted in the U.S. Such limitations are effective because they can be more easily enforced in an industrial environment (Anon., 2001). In industrial environments, inhalation of nickel aerosols from the mist in plating operations and of arc-welding fumes constitute the highest risk factor in worker exposure, potentially resulting in asthma since respiratory absorption is on the order of 50% of inhaled nickel. Occupational exposure to nickel salts and dust also occurs in spraying and in the production of storage batteries (Block and Yeung, 1982; Brooks, 1977; Keskinen et al., 1980; Menné and Maibach, 1987; Shirakawa et al., 1990; Sunderman et al., 1986). Aside from NAH and contact urticaria syndrome (CUS), long-term occupational exposure also carries the risk of cancer in the respiratory organs, the GI tract, and the kidneys (Costa et al., 1981; Doll et al., 1970; Flessel et al., 1980). Dermatitis, pneumoconiosis (due to elemental Ni), central nervous-system damage (soluble Ni compounds), and lung cancer (insoluble Ni compounds) are among the critical effects listed in the latest edition of the Threshold Limit Values and Biological Exposure Indices developed by the American Conference of Governmental Industrial Hygienists, addressing various classes of nickel compounds (Anon., 2001).

In the workplace the trend in exposure and resulting incidence of sensitization appears to decrease, possibly due to regulated limits, particularly in the high-risk nickel-producing and -using industries (Symanski et al., 1998). Data evaluated from ten nickel-producing and -using industries, which include over 20,000 measurements made internationally from 1973 to 1995, lead to the conclusion exposure to nickel aerosols, the most hazardous route of exposure, is reduced both in primary production of nickel (mining, milling, smelting, or refining) and in the manufacture of nickel alloys overall. Significant declining trends were recorded in mining, smelting, and refining activities (−7 to −9% per year), and only in milling did total nickel exposures show a significantly positive trend (+4% per year) (Symanski et al., 2001; Symanski et al., 2000).

1.3 PROGNOSIS

While a specific contact allergen can usually be identified by skin patch testing, and the affected patient may avoid further exposure, the cause for NAH is multifactorial; total avoidance of the allergen in the workplace and in private life is difficult or impossible. Once an individual is sensitized, the outlook for remission from NAH may be poor due to the omnipresence of nickel in all aspects of daily life: in metal tools, food, urban air, and numerous objects of daily use (Bennett, 1984; Boyle and Robinson, 1988; Creason et al., 1975; Fisher, 1986; Hogan et al., 1990b; Shah et al., 1996; Shah et al., 1998). Cases of pompholyx (vesicular hand eczema) due to systemic sensitization to nickel are alleged to have a particularly poor prognosis (Christensen, 1982a). Prognosis may be poor for metalworkers, as they may remain symptomatic over many years. Of 52 occupational cases of nickel dermatitis followed longitudinally, 42 (81%) still suffered from the condition over an average of 56.5 months after the initial diagnosis (Harrison, 1979). Chia and Goh saw 77% total clearance in occupational contact dermatitis cases from all causes, but 75% of patients with metal allergy (Ni and Co) had persistent dermatitis despite job change and efforts to avoid any further contact with the metals (Chia and Goh, 1991). An international survey by dermatologists on the prognosis of occupational CD of the hands revealed that 75% of patients required a job change; they designated NAH as the most serious condition after chromate allergy (Hogan et al., 1990a). Review of several studies addressing chronic occupational hand dermatitis (of both the irritant and allergic type) found that in most cases a job change did not improve the prognosis (Hogan et al., 1990c). While cement dermatitis is the most frequent manifestation of occupational chromate allergy among construction workers, incidence of such chromate allergy is now diminishing thanks to controls in work exposure; in certain European countries legislation limits the content of water-soluble chromate in dry cement to a maximum of 2 mg/kg (2 ppm) and addition of ferrous sulfate to cement mix reduces hexavalent chromium ion, its most skin-diffusible form, to trivalent chromium (Avnstorp, 1989; Zachariae et al., 1996). Nickel, in contrast, is as ubiquitous at home as it is in most workplaces, and avoidance is harder to implement. Workers have the best outlook for remission by continuing on the job and making a systematic effort to avoid the allergen, e.g., by modifying the work routine (Hogan et al., 1990b).

The literature noted above must be interpreted with caution, as there have been no adequately validated algorithms to separate the roles of endogenous factors, irritation, and nickel exposure. It appears that far fewer workers require job changes today compared to a generation ago, possibly due in part to increasing awareness of irritant and endogenous factors, and to improvements in therapy. Quantification of exposure and serial-dilution patch testing may provide new insights into this complex issue.

The fact that occupational skin diseases are the most common non–trauma-related category of occupational illnesses is vividly illustrated by "Proposed National Strategies for the Prevention of Leading Work-Related Diseases and Injuries, Part 2" (NIOSH, 1988), a document that has been reinforced by the comprehensive position statement resulting from the American Academy of Dermatology–sponsored

National Conference on Environmental Hazards to the Skin in 1992 (AAD, 1992). Both irritant and allergic contact dermatitis are considered priority research areas as outlined in the National Occupational Research Agenda introduced in 1996 by NIOSH (NIOSH, 1996).

The consensus among several authors who examined the prognosis in nickel contact dermastitis is that the best outlook for that condition is strict (as may be practical) avoidance of contact with the metal, in private life as well as in the workplace (Kalimo et al., 1997). The untoward effects of exposure to nickel motivate a review of the etiology of nickel hypersensitivity and an outline of possible strategies towards prevention and relief of NAH.

1.4   ETIOLOGY

1.4.1   EXPOSURE

Naturally occurring nickel compounds (ores and minerals) are not immunogenic, due to their lack of solubility and the dilution in natural deposits. Concentration of the metal through its smelting and machining and in anthropogenic salts — and particularly the wide use of the metal in alloys (tools) (Lidén et al., 1998), jewelry (Lidén, 1992; Romaguera et al., 1988), orthopedic implants, dental alloys (Bumgardner and Lucas, 1995; Veien et al., 1994), coins (Bang Pedersen et al., 1974; Gilboa et al., 1988; Gollhausen and Ring, 1991; Kanerva et al., 1998; Räsänen and Tuomi, 1992), and household utensils (Christensen and Möller, 1978) — have come to represent a potential hazard that requires appropriate risk-benefit assessment.

1.4.2   SKIN PENETRATION

Literature on induction and challenge of NAH describes the quantitative release of nickel ion from the metal and its alloys in various corrosive media (Bumgardner and Lucas, 1994; Haudrechy et al., 1997; Kanerva et al., 1994b; Park and Shearer, 1983) and the diffusion of water-soluble nickel salts — such as sulfate and chloride — through animal or human skin, *in vitro* and *in vivo*. The results from skin-penetration studies show that nickel ion is a minimal penetrant, with diffusion constants Kp on the order of 10^{-7} to 10^{-4} cm/h (Emilson et al., 1993; Fullerton et al., 1988a; Fullerton et al., 1986; Samitz and Katz, 1976; Tanojo et al., 2001), a rate that is typical for other transition-metal ions. Such slow rates of diffusion are difficult to reconcile with the notoriously facile elicitation, let alone induction of hypersensitivity, in skin that comes in contact with nickel in its metallic form, phenomena responsible for most of the hypersensitivity problems attributed to the metal. In the endeavor to address the apparent paradox and explain the ready absorption of metallic nickel coming in contact with the skin, we sought to provide evidence that nickel readily ionizes in the microenvironment of the skin, and by transiting the SC reaches the guardian dendritic cells residing in the epidermis. Evidence at hand so far points to ready dissolution (oxidation) of finely divided nickel metal kept in occluded contact with human skin *in vivo*, under formation of lipophilic and potentially more diffusible nickel soaps (fatty acid derivatives) with skin exudates (Hostýnek et al., 2001a). When nickel reacts with strong inorganic acids such as hydrochloric or nitric, the metal is oxidized to Ni (II) and forms salts that are readily soluble in water. With weak organic acids, ranging from acetic to longer-chain fatty acids such as octanoic or lauric as they occur in the skin (Schurer and Elias, 1991; Weerheim and Ponec, 2001; Wertz, 1992), however, the metal forms so-called soaps, in which nickel ion only partially dissociates from the acid moiety; the longer the acid chain, the less dissociated, less water-soluble, and more lipophilic the soap. The amount of nickel ion diffusing is small, to be sure, but appears to proceed at a continuous rate, in contrast with inorganic nickel salts (sulfate, chloride), which essentially form deposits in the outermost layers of the SC (Hostýnek et al., 2001b).

1.5 THE IMMUNE RESPONSE TO NICKEL

1.5.1 DIVERGENT IMMUNE RESPONSE

Remarkable in the etiology of immunological reactivity of metals is the observation that most metals that cause a delayed-type reaction (ACD) can also induce immunologic contact urticaria (ICU) (Hostýnek, 1997). Nickel, which belongs to that category, is capable of evoking multiple (dual) responses in the human immune system, sometimes in the same subject. Dermatitis and urticaria, the primary manifestations of NAH, are observed in the area of contact as well as at distant sites. Also, systemic allergic reaction (SAR) to nickel may express both as ICU and ACD (Dearman and Kimber, 1992; Guimaraens et al., 1994; Harvell et al., 1994; Kimber and Dearman, 1994; McKenzie and Aitken, 1967; Tosti et al., 1986; van Loveren et al., 1983). The different manifestations of NAH are presented in Table 1.1.

Allergic contact dermatitis of the delayed type is mediated by allergen-specific T lymphocytes and expressed as a wide range of cutaneous and mucous-membrane eruptions following dermal contact, oral or systemic exposure to a hapten, a type IV allergic reaction in the Coombs-Gell classification (Coombs and Gell, 1975).

Immunologic contact urticaria, immediate-type hypersensitivity involving antibody, most notably results in respiratory allergy but can also manifest in separate stages collectively described as contact urticaria syndrome (Lahti and Maibach, 1993), a type I reaction after Coombs-Gell (Katchen and Maibach, 1991): local or generalized urticaria; urticaria with extracutaneous reactions such as asthma, rhinoconjunctivitis, and gastrointestinal (GI) involvement; and ultimately anaphylaxis.

The difference in clinical manifestation of immediate and delayed-type hypersensitivity is attributed to the preferential activation of different subpopulations of T helper cells (Th), Th1 and Th2 (Mosmann and Coffman, 1989; Mosmann et al., 1991; Dearman and Kimber, 1992; Dearman et al., 1992). Activation of Th1 cells results in secretion of soluble cytokines that promote the cell-mediated response (e.g., IL-2, interferon-γ); activated Th2 cells, on the other hand, secrete IL-3 and IL-10, promoting antibody-mediated, immediate-type hypersensitivity. In man, T cell clones secrete both Th1- and Th2-type cytokines; this nonexclusive activation of T cells can lead to the release of a mixture of biological response modifiers, causing both IgE production (from Th2) and the development of contact sensitivity (from

TABLE 1.1
Dual (ICU and ACD) Allergic Reactions to Nickel — Table of Authors

Immunologic Contact Urticaria	Allergic Contact Dermatitis[a]	Systemic Allergic Reactions	Allergic Contact Stomatitis
Stoddard, 1960	Stoddard, 1960	Gaul, 1967	van Loon et al., 1984
McKenzie and Aitken, 1967	Holti, 1974	Watt and Baumann, 1968	Mobacken et al., 1984
Fisher, 1969	Marzulli and Maibach, 1976	Fisher, 1969	Fisher, 1987
Wahlberg and Skog, 1971	Warin and Smith, 1982	Barranco and Solomon, 1973	van Joost et al., 1988
Forman and Alexander, 1972	Legiec, 1984a	Fisher, 1974[b]	Temesvári and Racz, 1988
McConnell et al., 1973	Legiec, 1984b	Levantine, 1974[b]	Hildebrand et al., 1989b
Holti, 1974	Grandjean, 1984	Elves et al., 1975	Romaguera et al., 1989
Eversole, 1979	Weston and Weston, 1984	Fisher, 1977	Hensten-Pettersen, 1989
Veien et al., 1979	Dooms-Goossens et al., 1986	Lacroix et al., 1979	Stenman and Bergman, 1989
Osmundsen, 1980 Keskinen, 1980	Tosti et al., 1986	Meneghini and Angelini, 1979	Guerra et al., 1993
Niordson, 1981	Valsecchi and Cainelli, 1987	Christensen et al., 1981[b]	Estlander et al., 1993
Block and Yeung, 1982	Menné et al., 1989	Romaguera and Grimalt, 1981	Vilaplana et al., 1994
Warin and Smith, 1982	Weismann and Menné, 1989	Block and Yeung, 1982[b]	Veien, 1994 #1376
Fisher et al., 1982	Hildebrand et al., 1989a	Kaaber et al., 1983	Fernández-Redondo et al., 1998
Malo et al., 1982	Nethercott and Holness, 1990	Peters et al., 1984	
Novey et al., 1983	Schubert, 1990	Blanco-Dalmau et al., 1984	
Dolovich et al., 1984	Veien and Menné, 1990	Tosti et al., 1986	
Nieboer et al., 1984	Hogan et al., 1990a	Menné and Maibach, 1987a	
Malo, 1985 Tosti et al., 1986	Hogan et al., 1990b	Temesvári and Racz, 1988[b]	
Jones et al., 1986	Gollhausen and Ring, 1991	Wilson and Gould, 1989[b]	
Valsecchi and Cainelli, 1987	Vilaplana et al., 1994	Veien, 1989	
Shirakawa et al., 1987	Shirakawa et al., 1992	Wilkinson, 1989[b]	

TABLE 1.1 (CONTINUED)
Dual (ICU and ACD) Allergic Reactions to Nickel — Table of Authors

Immunologic Contact Urticaria	Allergic Contact Dermatitis[a]	Systemic Allergic Reactions	Allergic Contact Stomatitis
Shirakawa et al., 1990	Hensten-Pettersen, 1992	Hensten-Pettersen, 1989[b]	
Shirakawa et al., 1992	Abeck et al., 1993	Nielsen et al., 1990	
Motolese et al., 1992	Estlander et al., 1993	Hensten-Pettersen, 1992[b]	
Abeck et al., 1993	Basketter et al., 1993	Trombelli et al., 1992[b]	
Bezzon, 1993	Menné, 1994[b]	Guimaraens et al., 1994[b]	
Estlander et al., 1993	Sosroseno, 1995	Menné et al., 1994b	
Kusaka, 1993	Richter, 1996	Veien et al., 1994[b]	
	Savolainen, 1996	Richter, 1996[b]	
	Slaweta and Kiec-Swierczynska, 1998	Kerosuo et al., 1997[b]	
	Meding, 2000	Hensten-Pettersen, 1998[b]	
	Wataha, 2000	Giménez-Arnau et al., 2000	
		Richter, 2001[b]	

[a] Review articles only.
[b] SAR due to orthodontic or orthopedic implant.
Note: Entries do not differentiate between induction and elicitation of allergy.

Th1) (Paliard et al., 1988), with a predominance of Th2 by peripheral blood cells as demonstrated by Borg (Borg et al., 2000).

Another subpopulation of T cells, the Th0 cells, produce both Th1 and Th2 type cytokines (Probst, 1995; Hentschel, 1996). Derived from nickel-specific T cells, Th1 cytokines predominate among peripheral blood clones, while Th2 or Th0 cytokine profiles are found among skin-derived clones (Hentschel, 1996; Werfel, 1997).

While organic compounds infrequently cause both immediate-type reactions (anaphylactoid or immunologic contact urticaria reactions) and delayed-type reactions (cell-mediated or contact allergy), dual immune response appears more common for metals and metallic compounds, some being reactive toward protein and, hence, resulting in a complete antigen that triggers both IgE production and cellular immune reactions. The production of Th1 and Th2 cytokines was demonstrated from nickel-specific T lymphocyte clones isolated from peripheral blood of NAH patients (Ring and Thewes, 1999).

Immunogenic effects that result from exposure to metals can be attributed to the same factors that determine their toxicological and biological effects. Metal ions in general, and certainly those belonging to the transition group of elements such as nickel, contain a partially filled d-shell and oxidize readily to highly electropositive cations. While they have ionic radii too small to be antigenic, they can act as haptens interacting with tissue protein. They form bonds that range from the fully ionized to the fully chelated, and have the ability to modify the native protein configuration, which is recognized as nonself by hapten-specific T cells in the host immune system. Sinigaglia demonstrated experimentally that nickel specifically reacts with the histidine residue in the native peptide, which as a result is no longer recognized by the peptide-specific T-cell clone and leads to allergic reactions of both type I and type II (Sinigaglia, 1994).

The compartmentalization of hypersensitivity into distinct types as originally defined by Coombs and Gell (1975) thus no longer appears adequate; distinctions become less and less clear, particularly between type I and type IV responses. References to the dual forms of NAH and its manifestations are listed in Table 1.1.

1.5.2 IMMEDIATE-TYPE HYPERSENSITIVITY

Type I (mostly IgE-) antibody-mediated hypersensitivity, manifest in asthma, hay fever, generalized urticaria, or anaphylactoid reactions setting in within minutes or hours following (re-)exposure, for a long time has been primarily attributed to large-molecular weight xenobiotics — proteins and polysaccharides of animal, vegetable, or microbial origin. Their absorption may occur through the GI or respiratory tract, as well as intact or damaged skin. Also the oral mucosa can be the port of antigen entry; immediate contact stomatitis or stomatitides is then the resulting reaction, manifest as erythema, edema, and vesicle formation with ulceration, mediated by IgE mast-cell mechanisms (Eversole, 1979). These signs are collectively described as (immunological) CUS (von Krogh and Maibach, 1982) or ICU (Amin and Maibach, 1997; Katchen and Maibach, 1991). CUS results from allergen-IgE-mast-cell interaction with release of vasoactive amines (e.g., histamine). Appearance of symptoms in organs other than at the site of contact on the skin is common. Only recently have small molecules — fragrances, medicinals, pesticides, preservatives, and finally also metals — moved into the scope of the immunologist, dermatologist, allergologist, and occupational-health specialist, as awareness of the multiple effects that xenobiotics can have on the immune system is rapidly expanding. Exposure to a significant number of metals is now recognized to cause hypersensitivity reactions of the immediate type; for most of those metals specific IgE immunoglobulins have been identified, to the metal itself or to the metal-protein conjugate (Hostýnek, 1997).

Upon skin challenge the contact urticant penetrates the epidermis and reacts with preformed, specific IgE molecules encountered on the surface of basophils and mast-cell membranes, causing subsequent release of histamine and other cell-bound mediators of inflammation. The presence of immediate hypersensitivity to nickel can be determined in vitro or in vivo by several diagnostic methods (Table 1.3), such as the radioallergosorbent test (RAST), which identifies the presence of IgE antibodies against specific causative agents in the patient's serum, or in vivo by the skin-prick test, which assesses immediate-type allergy in the patient's skin.

Particularly in the industrial setting, volatilization of metals and their compounds presents a respiratory occupational risk leading to type I hypersensitivity (Table 1.2). In contrast to dusts generated in mining and construction, highly dispersible and

TABLE 1.2

Immediate Type Allergy Due to Nickel

Etiology	Symptoms	Diagnostic Test	Reference
Systemic; surgery	Anaphylaxix, urticaria, pruritus	Prick	Stoddart and Durh, 1960
Prosthesis	Urticaria, pruritus	Patch disc, scratch, passive transfer	McKenzie and Aitken, 1967
4 NAH patients	4 Patients	Prick	Wahlberg and Skog, 1971
Metal plating	Dyspnea	Scratch, RAST, provocation	McConnell et al., 1973
NAH patients	Erythema	Provocation, RAST (IgG, IgM)	Veien et al., 1979
Metal polishing	Eczema, urticaria	Patch, prick	Osmundsen, 1980
Welding	Asthma	Provocation	Keskinen et al., 1980
Welding	Rhinitis, eczema	Provocation	Niordson, 1981
Metal polishing	Asthma, rash	Provocation, prick	Block and Yeung, 1982
Metal plating	Asthma, urticaria	Provocation, RAST, prick	Malo et al., 1982
Systemic	Bronchospasm, pruritus	Provocation, patch	Fisher et al., 1982
NAH patients	Urticaria	Patch	Warin and Smith, 1982
Metal plating	Asthma	Provocation, RAST	Novey et al., 1983
Metal plating	Asthma	RAST (IgG)	Nieboer et al., 1984
Metal plating	Asthma	RAST (IgE, IgG), provocation	Dolovich et al., 1984
Metal plating	Asthma	Provocation	Malo et al., 1985
Systemic	Urticaria	Prick, passive transfer	Tosti et al., 1986
Jewelry	Urticaria, eczema	Patch	Valseccchi and Cainelli, 1987
NAH patients	Asthma	Provocation, RAST	Shirakawa et al., 1990
NAH patients	Dermatitis	Prick, RAST	Motolese et al., 1992
Oral	Urticaria, eczema	Provocation, patch	Bezzon, 1993
Oral	Angioedema, eczema, urticaria	Provocation, prick, patch	Abeck et al., 1993
Metal grinding	Rhinitis, urticaria	Provocation, scratch, RAST	Estlander et al., 1993

respirable aerosols are formed during smelting and pyrometallurgical processes (Roshchin, 1971). Of particular concern in the industrial environment is the potential for anaphylactic vascular shock caused by inhalation of contact urticaria-generating nickel and its derivatives (Lahti, 1992; Lahti and Maibach, 1992).

Nickel-reactive IgE antibodies as well as elevated levels of the IgG, IgA and IgM types have been confirmed in sera of asthmatics exposed to emissions (e.g., welding fumes) containing the metal (Dolovich et al., 1984; Malo et al., 1982; Nieboer et al., 1984; Novey et al., 1983; Shirakawa et al., 1987; Shirakawa et al., 1990; Shirakawa et al., 1992) eliciting both immediate and late-phase reactions. Also, Prausnitz Kustner tests have been used to confirm the presence of antibody in sensitized patients (Table 1.2). Primary induction of ICU leading to SAR may also occur through the oral mucosa, the respiratory tract, or the GI tract. Positive skin patch test reactions are also seen in NAH patients sensitized through inhalation, since primed IgE is also located on epidermal LCs, inducing type IV reactions and eczematous skin lesions (Najem and Hull, 1989).

1.5.3 DELAYED-TYPE HYPERSENSITIVITY

As a first event, ACD is triggered by an encounter between an epidermal Langerhans cell (LC) and a hapten-carrier complex, i.e., between a xenobiotic agent (most often an electrophilic or electron-seeking organic compound) and a native, electron-rich group or nucleophile (e.g., a protein), which have formed a stable covalent bond by sharing an electron pair. Formation of covalent bonds is not possible between metal ions bearing an electric charge and electron-rich protein groups, however. The hapten-carrier adduct there results from the electrostatic interaction between species of opposite charges or formation of coordination compounds where unoccupied orbitals in the metal are filled with electron pairs from the donor, electron-rich atoms such as sulfur, oxygen, or nitrogen (Dupuis and Benezra, 1982).

Nickel is an example of such an electrophilic agent avidly seeking to combine with free electrons available in nucleophilic groups such as aminoacid residues in native proteins; it is a transition metal with partially filled electron orbitals that readily form complexes (coordination compounds) with ligands that have electron pairs available for sharing — four such pairs in the case of nickel, in a square, planar, tetra-coordinated arrangement. Nickel and similar electrophilic metals form chelate rings, which distort native structures and result in relatively stable antigenic hapten-carrier complexes that are recognized as nonself by the immune system. Lymphocytes activated by the encounter with such an antigen move through the blood and lymphatic circulation, potentially resulting in a generalized response even though contact with the antigen occurred only locally, e.g., on a limited area of the skin. SAR may include generalized eruptions or flare-ups in the skin, often as a consequence of oral, respiratory, parenteral, or implantation exposure (Veien, 1991; Menné et al., 1994).

Occurrence of dermatitis in NAH patients at sites other than those of direct contact with nickel-containing materials led to coining the terms *secondary eruption*, eruption attributed to ingested nickel (Christensen and Möller, 1975), or *endogenous dermatitis* (Ricciardi et al., 2001). Such endogenous, nickel-induced secondary dermatitis can be elicited in NAH patients upon oral challenge with nickel sulfate (Ricciardi et al., 2001).

Over the past 25 years, considerable effort has been made to replace the use of traditional materials such as nickel (and mercury) in dental restorative work. However, introduction of various substitute metal-based materials has proceeded without the necessary corollary knowledge of their irritant and allergenic potential. Reports of contact stomatitis (contact allergy of the oral mucous membrane), lichen planus (Mobacken, 1984), and asymptomatic contact hypersensitivity (dental alloy contact dermatitis) are increasingly being linked with oral exposure to materials such as nickel used in dental fillings, orthodontic appliances, or dentures (van Loon, 1984; Fisher, 1986; van Joost, 1988; Haberman, 1993; Vilaplana, 1994). Such reactions, collectively referred to as allergic stomatitides, can be either immediate contact stomatitis or systemic anaphylactic stomatitis (immediate, type I reactions), or contact stomatitis (delayed, type II reactions). Nickel is most often involved in the etiology of the latter.

1.5.4 Asymptomatic or Silent ACD

Patients with NAH can also be asymptomatic (described as silent or subclinical allergy), nonreacting to skin patch testing. It is taken to be an indication of atopy by Möller (Möller and Svensson, 1986), but that is disputed by Todd et al., who base their conclusions on nickel reactivity of NAH patients and atopics without signs of NAH (Todd et al., 1989). Möller would suggest false-negative test reactions for such apparent nonreactivity. In evaluating patients with a history of metal intolerance but who are negative to nickel patch tests, Seidenari et al. (1996a; 1996b) modified standard testing methods in order to enhance the reaction to nickel, which otherwise would give false-negative readouts, by 24-h occlusion or pretreatment with sodium lauryl sulfate (SLS) of the test area prior to patch application. Also, reactions were read with echographic scanning and image analysis for improved (objective) sensitivity in detecting dermal edema (Levin and Maibach, 2000). Of 28 volunteers with a history of intolerance to jewelry but negative skin patch test with nickel sulfate, 9 were patch-test positive at SLS-pretreated sites and 8 under occlusion. When Lisby et al. (1999a; 1999b) investigated T-cell reactivity toward nickel sulfate *in vitro* from patch-test-negative (nonallergic) individuals in the lymphocyte-proliferation test, nickel induced dose-dependent proliferation of peripheral blood mononuclear cells from 16 of the 18 individuals tested, a specific activation by primed T cells with a T-cell receptor responding to nickel-modified peptides. Investigating differences in cytokine release in nickel-allergic and nonallergic individuals, Lisby et al. also found that functional capabilities of T-cell populations were similar in both groups. The authors conclude that as to T-cell reactivity, no qualitative differences exist between Ni-allergic individuals and nonallergics. In the former, stimulation of the immune system apparently is not sufficiently high under standard skin-test conditions to elicit a clinical reaction. *In vitro*, nickel-inducible T cell activation occurs in non-allergics as well as in allergics.

Self-described sensitive-skin reactants — people with exaggerated response to exogenous stimulants and a history of jewelry and cosmetics intolerance, but no overt signs of hypersensitivity (Amin et al., 1998; Maibach, 2000) — were enrolled in a standard skin patch test program (GIRDCA test series) by Francomano et al.; 57.6% showed positive response to nickel sulfate, compared with 10.2% in a control group without history of skin diseases. The authors concluded that perceived sensitive skin is an indication of subclinical ACD that responds to skin-patch challenge (Francomano et al., 2000).

An additional element of uncertainty in distinguishing between negative and false-negative, or positive and false-positive skin patch test results is the potential for reaction to cobalt, rather than to nickel, leading to a false-positive result due to cobalt allergy. Nickel compounds are normally contaminated with cobalt because the two metals are naturally associated and difficult to separate quantitatively. During skin patch testing for nickel or cobalt dermatitis, it is difficult to obtain reagents in which one metal compound is totally free of the other (Lammintausta et al., 1985; Pirilä and Kajanne, 1965).

1.5.5 METHODS OF DIAGNOSIS AND INSTRUMENTATION

Diagnosis of nickel-induced hypersensitivity can proceed on the basis of several different allergology tests, as indicated by the patient's signs or symptoms (Table 1.3). Since the beginning of the industrial age, incidence of immune reactions to nickel has shifted from a predominantly occupational hazard among men, leading to type I respiratory problems due to inhalation of nickel containing dusts and aerosols (metal grinding, electroplating), to the more broadly based, type IV allergy presenting as dermatitis or eczema, encountered increasingly among females and acquired through intimate contact with garment accessories and jewelry. While epidemiology among the general population shows that sensitization among men has remained fairly constant, moving between 2 and 4%, among women it now can exceed 20%.

Since nickel belongs to the group of xenobiotics that can induce dual (or multiple) response in the immune system, the allergologist testing patients for NAH is well advised to broaden the spectrum of tests to encompass both type I and type II allergy, regardless of obvious clinical presentation; a link exists between cell-mediated and humoral immunity, and both forms can occur in the same patient (Table 1.1). Nickel-specific IgE antibody was also seen to mediate late-phase reactions, which

---

TABLE 1.3
Diagnostic Methods for (Nickel-Induced) Allergic Diseases

Disease	Diagnostic test
Type I	
Asthma	Skin: prick (open/closed); patch (open/closed); scratch; intradermal
Urticaria	IgE (RAST)
Rhinitis	Precipitation (Ouchterlony)
Conjunctivitis	Hemagglutinin, passive transfer (P.-K.)
Pompholyx	Provocation: nasal; bronchial; oral; conjunctival
	Peroral
Type IV	
Dermatitis	Open patch, closed patch, lymphocyte transformation, macrophage migration
Eczema	inhibition
Stomatitides	Oral provocation
Granuloma	

only begin 3 to 4 h following challenge (Malo et al., 1985; Estlander et al., 1993). Holti (1974) reports also seeing Arthus-type hypersensitivity to nickel salts, besides types I and II. The various types of diagnostic tests for type I and type II hypersensitivity to nickel are presented in Table 1.3.

Bioengineering methods have brought objectivity to the process of assessing physiological and pathological conditions of the skin, e.g., evaluation of the intensity of reactions in predictive testing for allergenicity potential of xenobiotics, such as nickel, or investigation of therapeutic efficacy of antiinflammatories, where subtle nuances in skin reaction may be difficult to ascertain (Berardesca et al., 1995). Utility and efficacy of such instrumental methods has been evaluated during investigation of the efficacy of topical corticosteroids to alleviate nickel dermatitis experimentally elicited in volunteers: laser Doppler flowmetry to evaluate intensity of inflammatory reaction, colorimetry to assess the blanching action, echography to evaluate edema and inflammation. Levin and Maibach thereby critically reviewed procedures and results obtained by a number of researchers, identifying respective limitations in the different detection methods, and suggested potential for improvement in the several experimental designs. Transepidermal water loss is not a method sensitive enough to evaluate allergic responses in the skin. Visual scoring is to be preferred over laser Doppler flowmetry on low-density reactions, with reflectance spectroscopy being equivalent to the visual score. While colorimetry measures a blanching effect, it does not assess the decrease in edema which is due to corticosteroids (CS). While it is assumed that echography will detect a relative decrease in inflammation and edema and allow evaluation of the CS efficacy tested, it is not sensitive enough to detect the effect of low-potency CS. The instrument did not discern the (subtle) difference between hydrocortisone acetate and untreated skin. The routine occlusion on CS application is criticized because it produces artifacts in skin reactivity, and open application is advocated instead for objective evaluation of CS efficacy. Finally, the authors advocate a combined approach using visual score, echography, colorimetric, and blood-flow measurements to achieve a more accurate clinical picture (Levin and Maibach, 2000).

1.5.6 IMMUNOTOXICITY

Besides being an allergen, nickel also exhibits immunomodulatory, if not immunotoxicity, effects as noted in several experiments conducted in humans and in rodents. It was linked to a decrease in the number of T lymphocytes in humans (Eggleston, 1984). Nickel sulfate causes a dose- and time-dependent inhibition of human keratinocyte growth and viability in culture, with a concomitant increase in inflammatory cytokine release such as interleukin-1 and activation of lipoxygenase in leukocytes (Guéniche et al., 1993).

Nickel chloride dosed intraperitoneally in mice affected antibody response and phagocytosis in host-resistance assays against experimental infections (Laschi-Loquerie et al., 1987) and inhalatory exposure of mice to various nickel compounds led to suspected immunodysfunction (Haley et al., 1990). That nickel will significantly alter the functioning of host defense mechanisms was demonstrated in rabbits: alveolar macrophages are reduced in number and lose activity, primary antibody production is reduced, and lysozyme levels and activity are significantly decreased (Lundborg and Camner, 1984; Waters et al., 1975). Such immunosuppressant effects were reflected in enhanced mortality upon challenge of animal models with infectious microorganisms (Graham et al., 1978; Dooms-Goossens, 1986).

1.5.7 THE IMMUNOGENIC FORMS OF NICKEL

Evidence is growing that points to the actual immunogenic form of nickel as the trivalent ion, Ni III, rather than Ni II of the conventional view. *De novo* sensitization with Ni II in animal experiments has proven difficult, or has even failed (Cornacoff et al., 1984; Ishii et al., 1993; Möller, 1984; van Hoogstraten et al., 1991; Wahlberg, 1989). Furthermore, in classifying immunogenic potency by the human Repeat Insult Patch Test, Kligman's score for nickel ion was only 48% positives, making the metal a moderate (class III) sensitizer (Kligman, 1966). In humans, NAH develops more readily on exposure of irritated skin than from application on intact, normal skin; also the minimum eliciting concentration in NAH subjects is lower when the condition of the skin has been compromised by pretreatment with SLS (Allenby and Basketter, 1993; Allenby and Goodwin, 1983; Nielsen et al., 1999). Building on these observations in humans and from experiments in animals, Artik et al. (1999) hypothesize that the immunogenic activity of nickel is enhanced when Ni II is oxidized to the more reactive Ni III (or Ni IV) by endogenous reactive oxygen species in the form of hydrogen peroxide or hypochlorite occurring in inflamed skin. In animal and cell line tests Artik et al. observed that Ni II only sensitizes naive T cells following bio-oxidation to Ni III or Ni IV, but not Ni II as such.

Nickel is the premier allergen among the general population, and ranks among the top occupational sensitizers. The incidence of NAH as gauged in the general population by skin patch testing is high. Together with the potential chronicity of this disorder, its effect on the quality of life of those afflicted, and the economic impact this conveys are sufficient indications that a search for prevention or alleviation of this problem is justified. Several avenues appear open toward reduction, if not prevention, of this condition of public-health importance.

1.6 PREVENTION

Induction of NAH can be prevented by using a multi-tier approach toward reducing, if not avoiding, nickel exposure. Important reduction of occupational exposure and thus sensitization has been demonstrated in the nickel-producing and -processing industry on a worldwide basis (Symanski et al., 1998; Symanski et al., 2000; Symanski et al., 2001). Education and personal protective equipment for the workforce are important first steps toward that goal; appropriate engineering for implementing environmental controls, particularly as they apply to air quality, is another step toward risk reduction, in particular since inhalation is a prime route of NAH induction (Block and Yeung, 1982; Menné and Maibach, 1987; Sunderman et al., 1986) and possibly of cancer if such exposure continues on a sustained basis (Doll et al., 1970; Flessel et al., 1980; Costa et al., 1981).

That prevention among the general population is feasible is demonstrated by the positive effect regulation has had in Denmark. Recent epidemiology from that country shows a flexure in the otherwise ascending prevalence curve of NAH, specifically among the youngest female age group as noted by Johansen et al. (2000) and Veien et al. (2001). Apparently, observance of maximum permissible nickel release, especially in ear studs and jewelry, now has yielded a measurable benefit among the youngest population. Induction of tolerance to nickel by (early) low-level exposure, e.g., through application of nickel-containing orthodontic appliances in early life, has been convincingly demonstrated (Kerosuo et al., 1996; van Hoogstraten et al., 1991; van Hoogstraten et al., 1989; von der Burg et al., 1986). Such materials are corroded in the oral environment, releasing low levels of nickel over an extended period.

1.6.1 PREVENTION THROUGH WORKROOM EXPOSURE MONITORING

Workroom surveillance and health monitoring for exposure to hazardous materials is recommended as an important step in preventive strategy. It is possible to effectively monitor exposure to heavy metals such as nickel through refined analytical techniques that detect sub–part per billion levels in tape strips taken from exposed skin of personnel. That noninvasive method makes pharmacokinetic studies possible that provide detailed mechanistic insights into skin diffusion by chemical agents. Corneocyte layers are removed sequentially from one spot on the skin with adhesive tape until the skin has a shiny appearance, typically 20 to 30 strips, depending on the anatomical site. Subsequent metal analysis of the strips by inductively coupled plasma mass spectroscopy yields a depth profile of the metal or other xenobiotics in the uppermost SC layers. This method has been used to investigate skin penetration (and depot formation) by chemicals (Rougier et al., 1987; Hostýnek, 2001a; Hostýnek, 2001b; Weerheim, 2001).

1.6.2 PREVENTION THROUGH PERSONAL HYGIENE

The best and simplest prophylactic practice to prevent nickel ACD due to exposure to the metal is cleansing of the skin with sequestering agents that were demonstrated to immobilize the allergen. In contrast to many organic compounds such as agrochemicals or pesticides, nickel is slow to diffuse through the SC (Fullerton et al., 1988a; Fullerton and Hoelgaard, 1988b; Tanojo et al., 2001). Traces of the metal on the skin or in the superficial layers of the SC can be removed with an aqueous combination of surfactant and a complexing agent. Decontamination of the skin surface thus appears as an expeditious and effective preventive measure in the case of suspected contact, without the need to change the work routine through use of protective wear. Establishing an efficient cleansing routine in operations where handling of nickel metal or nickel compounds is necessary for personnel who cannot avoid exposure therefore appears prudent and effective, such a routine to be followed at work as well as postshift at home. Consistent hygiene practice can not only reduce the risk of eliciting reactions in those sensitized, but may also prevent induction of NAH.

Healy et al. evaluated a number of (conventional) chemicals for their ability to sequester surface nickel, described earlier by Gawkrodger et al. (1995). The authors evaluated the stability of the complexes formed, potentially in competition with nickel complexes in the skin, and their complexing efficacy in function of pH. Also investigated were the ancillary aspects of safety from the point of skin diffusivity of the chemicals or complexes and their relative cytotoxicity in cell culture. Ethylenediamine tetraacetic acid di-sodium salt and L-histidine seem to best fit the prerequisites for effectively preventing NAH following skin contact with the allergen (Healy et al., 1998).

1.6.3   USE OF GLOVES

Gloves offer a sense of protection and security thanks to their obvious nature as a barrier between potentially injurious chemicals and the skin. Among the advantages of using gloves is the protection they give in wet work and in the handling of aqueous corrosive agents such as acids, alkalis, and detergents, or dyes and foods. Reluctance to comply with recommended wear due to discomfort, the macerating effect on the skin, or their interference with work operations must be overcome with adequate motivation. Made of natural latex or synthetic polymers, gloves can also offer a false sense of safety, however, because they sometimes contribute problems of their own, depending on the terms of use. Constituent materials may lead to irritation or allergy (Heese et al., 1991). Allergy to latex especially is a widely recognized and discussed problem. Latex proteins can induce asthma and eczema (Cormio et al., 1993; Estlander et al., 1994; Hamann, 1993; Seaton et al., 1988). Gloves made of synthetic rubber or plastic contain potential allergens such as thiuram, dithiocarbamate, or mercaptobenzothiazole derivates (Conde-Salazar et al., 1993; Estlander et al., 1995; Hanson and Ågrup, 1993; Kanerva et al., 1994a; Kwangsukstith and Maibach, 1995; Wrangsjö and Meding, 1994). Leather gloves may contain dichromate from the tanning process. An additional element of risk in the use of gloves is the effect of occlusion, whereby maceration of the skin enhances penetration of an opportunistic chemical (nickel), inadvertently contaminating the skin prior to the donning of gloves. Occluding gloves can be made safer and cause less discomfort if used in combination with inner cotton gloves.

Choice of glove material for protection in occupations that require handling of nickel salts, such as electroforming operations, must be selective since it was demonstrated that nickel is absorbed through rubber gloves (Wall, 1980). No such absorption occurred through PVC material.

1.6.4   PROTECTIVE CREAMS

1.6.4.1   Barrier Creams

Creams without chemically active ingredients (passive creams) and those formulated with chelating or oxidizing agents to inactivate nickel (active creams) are designed to act as barriers to block the allergenic effects of nickel in sensitive patients.

1.6.4.2   Passive Protective Creams

Formulated without active ingredients, the passive type of cream is designed to block permeation of the SC. In broader terms, lipophilic (water-repellent) barriers are based on propylene glycol, petrolatum, or anhydrous lanolin. Hydrophilic components in "anti-solvent" (oil- or solvent-repellent) creams or gels are cellulose esters, glycerin, ethanol, or water.

The effectiveness of barrier creams to prevent skin contact with noxious chemicals has met with some skepticism (Lachapelle, 1995; Orchard, 1984). In some instances, workers using barrier creams may appear to have higher prevalence of occupational contact dermatitis than those not using a cream (Varigos and Dunt, 1981).

Critical investigations of the benefits of commercial barrier creams intended for protection from both lipophilic and hydrophilic agents elicited qualified support, indicating shortcomings in performance (or manufacturer's information) and reflecting the importance of exposure parameters, such as duration of use (Frosch et al., 1993b; Frosch et al., 1993a; Pigatto et al., 1992; Zhai and Maibach, 1996). Since chemical agents fall into several distinct categories exhibiting a myriad of different properties, no one cream can be formulated that: (a) will be toxicologically safe and well tolerated on the skin, and (b) will constitute a universally effective barrier against diffusion. Minor prerequisites would be: (c) a cosmetically acceptable form (spreadability), (d) formation of a continuous, shear- and wash-off-resistant film, and (e) ease of skin cleansing. An educated choice is necessary in selecting the appropriate cream for a particular chemical exposure.

1.6.4.3 Active Protective Creams

Barrier materials designed for active protection of the SC mostly contain "binding agents" that render nickel inactive by reacting with it. Those are mainly chelating agents: 5-chloro-7-iodoquinolin-8-ol or clioquinol, ethylenediamine tetraacetic acid, H_4EDTA or its metal salts, tetraethylthiuramdisulfide (TETD, Antabuse®, disulfiram) and diethyldithiocarbamate (DDC) (Gawkrodger et al., 1995). Antioxidants, intended to prevent the oxygen-dependent dissolution of metallic nickel on skin contact (Memon et al., 1994), are also used. Such "neutralizing" creams have had mixed success under real-life conditions. Objectively, a film of 20 to 50 μm of such a cream can contain only a limited amount of active ingredient per square centimeter of skin surface, which soon is exhausted, particularly under conditions of occupational exposure.

Chelators form soluble, stable complexes with heavy metal ions which no longer are antigenic, as tested on triethylenediamine tetraacetic acid (Rostenberg and Perkins, 1951). In an *in vivo* study with nickel-sensitive subjects, Kurtin and Orentreich confirmed that, using Na_2 H_2EDTA, chelation of nickel deprives it of its sensitizing ability (Kurtin and Orentreich, 1954).

The protective effect of barrier gels can be measured *in vitro* by determining the degree of nickel penetration in diffusion cells; another test based on a colorimetric method can be also used to evaluate the binding efficacy of sequestrants (Zhai and Maibach, 1996).

In vivo tests evaluate the elicitation of patch test reactions in hypersensitive patients while they apply protective creams. Of the antioxidants and chelators they studied, Memon et al. found clioquinol at 10% to be the most effective inhibitor of nickel-provoked hypersensitivity reactions in all 29 NAH subjects challenged.

Challenge with nickel-containing coins coated with creams containing EDTA (15%), ascorbic acid as reducing agent (20%), and α-tocopherol (10%), also intended to reduce nickel ion, showed only partial success (Memon et al., 1994). When van Ketel and Bruynzeel evaluated the chelating agent diethyldithiocarbamate in 10% concentration, however, they noted no statistical difference in protection when they challenged the skin of NAH patients with and without protection (van Ketel and Bruynzeel, 1982).

EDTA and derivatives show different efficacy in sequestering nickel ion (Gawk-rodger et al., 1995). In practice, alkali and earth alkali salts of EDTA or combinations of the two have been evaluated. *In vitro*, a cream with 2% Na_2H_2EDTA and 4% $CaNa_2EDTA$ was found to be more effective than other EDTA derivatives for rapid binding of nickel ion. A preparation with 1.8% Na_2H_2EDTA and 5.4% $CaNa_2EDTA$ had the greatest such capacity (Resl and Sykora, 1965).

The clinical efficacy of chelators was evaluated by Bracun et al. (1999) on NAH patients, incorporating the chemicals in oil-in-water and water-in-oil emulsions and applying them on the skin of patients prior to occlusive elicitation tests. Pretreatment with levels of 10% diethylenetriamine (DTPA) and 10% EDTA, both as oil-in-water emulsions, showed best efficacy, completely inhibiting allergic response to 1% nickel sulfate; they were 93% effective on application of 2.5% of the allergen in petrolatum. Against the background of earlier test results with the same or similar compounds, these results underscore the importance of the vehicle formulation. The same research group confirmed the results with DTPA in a randomized double-blind study, including other heavy metals to check for a broader efficacy of the creams. The skin of 27 of 28 patients pretreated with the active cream was negative to 2.5% nickel sulfate, and 30 of 32 to 5% of the salt in petrolatum. Similar results were registered with cobalt and copper salt challenge; however, not with palladium or dichromate salts (Wöhrl et al., 2001).

In an *in vitro* barrier study with human skin by Fullerton and Menné (1995), a layer of various EDTA barrier gels prevented the diffusion of nickel from superim-posed nickel alloys into the skin, but: (a) the gels appeared to promote the release of nickel from the alloys, and (b) nickel was immobilized in the superficial layers of the skin. In using such a protective barrier it appears critical that the barrier material be removed following exposure. *In vivo* application of a carboxyvinyl polymer gel (Carbopol®) containing 10% $CaNa_2$-EDTA on the skin beneath a nickel disc prevented the allergic contact response in all hypersensitive patients tested.

In summary, efforts to incorporate chelators inactivating nickel ion or inhibiting its diffusion have had only limited success. A potential downside effect inherent in the vehicle is its impact on the skin's barrier function per se, potentially increasing its permeability.

1.6.5 PREVENTION THROUGH METAL PLATING

Surface plating and anti-corrosive techniques would appear to be an effective step toward protecting the skin from direct contact with nickel, because the allergen is present in so many objects of everyday use (Cavelier et al., 1985; Ingber et al., 1997; Lidén et al., 1996; Lidén et al., 1998).

Systemic exposure to nickel through items such as earring studs appears to be one of the more common etiological factors among women (Lidén et al., 1996). Even though earrings are often gold-plated, the nickel interliner beneath the gold plating can become exposed with use. Scanning electron microscopy and x-ray microanalysis of the surface of both used or unused gold-plated jewelry, for instance, reveals that the gold surface can be defective, allowing the underlying nickel to be corroded and released on skin contact (Ishikawaya et al., 1997). Fisher (1989) concluded that if skin contact is intimate and long enough, nickel from the base in gold-plated jewelry will penetrate the gold layer, resulting in surface nickel concentrations that approximate those of metallic nickel itself.

An in-depth investigation correlated plating and elicitation potential for those sensitized to nickel. Cavelier et al. (1985) studied the merits of plating to prevent contact with nickel-containing alloys in items of everyday use, such as metal fasteners on clothing items. Analysis by x-ray energy dispersion and the DMG spot test was performed for nickel on 57 metal clothing objects; reactivity was then tested in 22 NAH patients by skin contact with items and patch testing with nickel-plated discs of gold-copper-cadmium and chromium. Positive reactions were recorded to all items if the materials contained any level of nickel at all. Cavelier concluded that nickel-containing objects can be plated effectively only with chromium, a metal more electronegative than nickel, if such plating is heavier than 1 µm; at lighter plating, due to (unavoidable) fissures in the surface layer, chromium will act as a pile, resulting in dissolution of the passivated chromium, and thus remove the anticorrosive layer. Effective plating of nickel-containing alloys is possible by application of highly electropositive (noble) metals, e.g., gold, silver, platinum, or palladium, and only if plating is heavier than 5 µm because a continuous layer of the overlay, free of fissures, cannot be assumed in lighter coatings. In continuation of that earlier work, Cavelier et al. (1988) searched for a metallurgical answer toward providing tolerance to nickel-containing objects by appropriate coatings. While not providing a guarantee of tolerance, an optimal solution is seen by interposing a 5 µm layer of copper between the nickel alloy and a 0.5 µm surface coat of chrome. The authors concluded that ultimately tolerance to such materials greatly depends on the degree of individual nickel sensitivity (Cavelier et al., 1989).

1.6.6 Prevention through Regulation

In response to the ascending trend of NAH in the general population, dermatologists have investigated release of nickel from metal objects, defined threshold of sensitization anticipated in the average individual, and proposed regulation that would minimize at least elicitation, if not induction, of NAH. A standard was elaborated that would limit nickel released from commonplace metal items to less than 0.5 $mg/cm^2/week$ (Menné et al., 1987; Menné and Rasmussen, 1990). After verification that such a threshold is appropriate, a standard analytical methodology that includes a modification of the dimethylglyoxime test to ascertain observance of these limits was adopted by the European Union in the European Nickel Directive in 1994 (EU, 1994). This is intended to reduce the prevalence of sensitization (primary prevention) and recurring dermatitis in the sensitized population (secondary prevention). In

Denmark, the Nickel Directive already became law in 1989. The directive states that nickel may not be used: (a) in earring-post assemblies used during epithelization unless they are homogenous and in which the concentration of nickel is less than 0.05%; (b) in products intended to come into direct and prolonged contact with the skin, such as earrings, necklaces, watch straps, or zippers, if the nickel release is greater than 0.5 mg/cm^2/week; and (c) in coated products under (b), unless the coating is sufficient to ensure that nickel release will not exceed 0.5 mg/cm^2/week after 2 years of normal use.

This threshold of 0.5 mg/cm^2/week will avoid ACD in most sensitized subjects, although some nickel-allergic individuals may still be expected to react even to levels of 0.05 mg/cm^2/week (Fischer et al., 1984; Gawkrodger, 1996).

That such regulation has its desired effect becomes evident in the latest statistics on NAH from Denmark. Epidemiology from that country shows that, counter to the unremitting increase of NAH in most populations, among the youngest female age group in Denmark prevalence of nickel sensitivity is on the decline (Johansen et al., 2000; Veien et al., 2001).

The new European Dangerous Preparations Directive requires that household products and personal-care preparations containing skin sensitizers of more than 0.1% feature a warning label cautioning the sensitized consumer of the risk of eliciting an allergic reaction on contact with the skin. An earlier directive required such labeling in the presence of 1% sensitizer with the intent of preventing induction of sensitivity. Neither of the two regulations takes threshold levels or degree of allergen release into consideration, a shortcoming that hopefully will be rectified upon intervention by the scientific community (Roggeband et al., 2001).

1.7 THERAPY

1.7.1 TOPICAL THERAPY

While *in vitro* DDC gave indications that it would detoxify nickel ion (Resl and Sykora, 1965), its application in ointments for the suppression of patch test reactions in nickel-sensitive patients proved ineffective (Samitz and Pomerantz, 1958; van Ketel and Bruynzeel, 1982). To test the prophylactic effect of cream formulations, Fisher and Rystedt (1990) incorporated nickel ion as a dilution series in the preparations and applied the creams under occlusion to the skin of NAH patients. As an alternative treatment, nickel was applied over the cream-pretreated skin. While some formulations increased test reactivity due to an irritative effect, a surprising result was the (partial) effectiveness of polyethylene glycol (PEG) as base in that it had a strong inhibitory effect in both application modes. The authors hypothesize that PEG may have augmented the skin's barrier properties by interacting with the SC. CS formulations also had a suppressive effect, most likely due to their antiinflammatory action. Acceleration in the healing process of nickel ACD was demonstrated by application of an essentially unmedicated, hydrating cream after inducing nickel ACD reactions on the skin of volunteers. Experimentally elicited dermatitis was followed by treatment with the object cream over four days. Recovery as measured by transepidermal water loss (TEWL) demonstrated a marked improvement of the cream-treated test spots as compared to untreated skin. Recovery was complete to baseline TEWL values after five days, whereas the TEWL values were still unchanged for cream-untreated skin. The clinical scores, however, remained unchanged after five days (de Paepe et al., 2001).

In a review of 36 cases of women with pompholyx-type eczema due to NAH, Christensen (1982b) noted that topical application of CS brought only partial relief. Inherent risk in the topical use of CS is acquisition of (often undiagnosed) allergies due to components used in formulating the cream (Dooms-Goossens, 1988).

1.7.2 SYSTEMIC THERAPY

In cases of extremely hypersensitive patients, an alternative therapeutic approach to using antiinflammatory topical corticoids is the systemic administration of chelating agents such as tetraethylthiuramdisulfide (TETD, Antabuse, disulfiram), DDC, or triethylenetetramine. It only yields limited success, however; the dermatitis is not completely suppressed or resumes after cessation of treatment. Eleven patients whose NAH status was confirmed by oral nickel dosing were given 100 mg TETD tablets orally over 2 months. In some of the patients dermatitis cleared, but skin flares reappeared when treatment was discontinued (Kaaber et al., 1979). A similar course and outcome of chelation therapy with a daily oral dose of 200 mg disulfiram over 8 weeks was reported by Christensen. Although in 11 patients with pompholyx the condition resolved and 8 showed partial improvement, relapse occurred in all patients within weeks after treatment was discontinued (Christensen and Kristensen, 1982). TETD and DDC given orally brought relief in nickel dermatitis only as long as dosing continued (Menné and Kaaber, 1978). TETD given orally caused a measurable rise in serum and urinary nickel levels, suggesting that preexisting nickel deposits are mobilized and excreted by chelation (Christensen, 1982b; Christensen and Kristensen, 1982; Kaaber et al., 1979; Menné et al., 1980). Chelating drugs given systemically were reported to produce toxic side effects, however (Spruit et al., 1978). TETD caused lassitude in patients (Kaaber et al., 1979) and hepatotoxicity (Kaaber et al., 1987).

Following up on reports that PUVA therapy was successful in the treatment of ACD (Bruynzeel et al., 1982; Kalimo et al., 1983; Volden et al., 1978), Kalimo et al. investigated the merits of such treatment on nickel dermatitis. Five NAH patients were given oral methoxypsoralen, followed by whole-body UVA irradiation. Lymphocyte stimulation was monitored prior to UVA treatment, during PUVA therapy, and 1 year thereafter. Dermatosis of the patients cleared to varying degrees during radiation treatment, in one case ending with complete remission. Sensitivity of blood lymphocytes to nickel remained unchanged or even increased as measured by the lymphocyte transformation tests, however. This leads to the conclusion that nickel-specific, suppressive immune-regulative mechanisms had not been activated, because systemic sensitivity to nickel remained undiminished (Kalimo et al., 1989).

The scope of desensitization through oral (sublingual) therapy using increasing doses of nickel sulfate in glycerin was tested by Morris in a program with 39 intradermally confirmed NAH patients. Degree of reactivity was first established by intradermal testing with a dilution series of nickel sulfate. According to the readout, nickel sulfate solutions ranging from 0.008 to 0.2% nickel were given to the patients sublingually three times a day. Periodic intradermal tests to verify degree of sensitivity showed increasing tolerance, and the sublingual dose was increased accordingly. At the end of treatment, averaging 16 months, all in the cohort tested showed at least partially improved tolerance for nickel, expressed as decreased intradermal reactivity. Four patients registered unlimited tolerance for the allergen (Morris, 1998).

1.8 CONCLUSIONS

The action of nickel ion in the human organism presents the medical practitioner and cell biologist with several paradoxes. A large part of the general population tests positive to skin patch testing with nickel sulfate, but clinical relevance is questionable since large numbers of those tested who are positives remain asymptomatic, i.e., show no overt signs of NAH. Conversely, many of those who complain of metal intolerance test negative on skin patch testing. Epidemiological data on NAH, therefore, indicating a steady increase in most countries, may be flawed by uncertainty due to frequent false positive and false negative readings of (mostly nickel sulfate) skin patch test reactions, contamination of patch test materials with traces of cobalt, and the incidence of nonreactants in population and clinical studies. The clinical relevance of NAH statistics therefore may not be as dire as the numbers imply.

Recent data on the prevalence of NAH give indications of public-health benefits resulting from regulations, which in some countries seek to limit the release of nickel ion from articles intended for prolonged and intimate skin contact. Warnings required by the European Dangerous Preparations Directive for the presence of skin sensitizers, however, appear to be unwarranted as presently formulated.

Data acquired in our laboratory offer an explanation for the observed facile elicitation of NAH reactions upon skin contact with nickel-releasing objects. Diffusion of lipophilic derivatives resulting from contact of the metal with free fatty acids present on the skin appear to follow different pathways from those observed for simple inorganic nickel salts. Prognosis for NAH status remains poor, in the workplace as well as among the general population.

Experimental evidence points to nickel trivalent ion as the actual immunogenic species, generated by active oxygen in endogenous peroxide or hypochlorite formed in the process of tissue inflammation.

Prevention, particularly in the nickel-manufacturing and -utilization industries, appears to be effective because industry-wide statistics of NAH indicate a decline in the total number of cases recorded; the only exceptions are nickel-milling operations.

Protection through the use of gloves and barrier creams may introduce new sources of allergens, potentially leading to an increase in skin problems; nevertheless, additional quantitative data is welcomed.

Most types of plating leave a number of avenues open for nickel to diffuse to the surface of metal objects, which defeats the intent of preventing release of the allergen. The benefits of topical or systemic therapies often are only partial or temporary, and systemic chelation especially brings the risk of toxic side effects.

ABBREVIATIONS

ACD allergic contact dermatitis
CS corticosteroids
DMG dimethyl glyoxime
CUS contact urticaria syndrome
ICU immunological contact urticaria
LC Langerhans cells
NAH nickel allergic hypersensitivity
SAR systemic allergic reactions
SC stratum corneum
SLS sodium lauryl sulfate

REFERENCES

AAD, Position Statement, National Conference on Environmental Hazards to the Skin, Washington, D.C., 1992.

Abeck, D. et al., Chronic urticaria due to nickel intake, *Acta Derm. Venereol.*, 73, 438–439, 1993.

ADA Council on Dental Materials, Instruments, and Equipment, Biological effects of nickel-containing dental alloys, *J. Am. Dent. Assoc.*, 104, 501, 1982.

Adams, R.M., Contact dermatitis due to irritation and allergic sensitization, in *Occupational Skin Disease*, Grune & Stratton, New York, 1983a, pp. 1–26.

Adams, R.M., Metals, in *Occupational Skin Disease*, Grune & Stratton, New York, 1983b, pp. 204–237.

Allenby, C.F. and Goodwin, B.F., Influence of detergent washing powders on minimal eliciting patch test concentrations of nickel and chromium, *Contact Dermatitis*, 9, 491–499, 1983.

Allenby, C.F. and Basketter, D.A., An arm immersion model of compromised skin. II. Influence on minimal eliciting patch test concentrations of nickel, *Contact Dermatitis*, 28, 129–133, 1993.

Amin, S. and Maibach H.I., Immunologic contact urticaria syndrome, in *Contact Urticaria Syndrome*, Amin, S., Lahti, A., and Maibach, H.I., Eds., CRC Press, Boca Raton, FL, 1997, pp. 11–26.

Amin, S., Engasser, P., and Maibach, H.I., Sensitive skin: what is it?, in *Textbook of Cosmetic Dermatology*, Baran, R. and Maibach, H.I., Eds., Martin Dunitz, Ltd., London, 1998, pp. 343–349.

Angelini, G. and Veña, G.A., Allergia da contatto al nickel: considerazioni su vecchie e nuove acquisizioni, *Bollettino di Dermatologia Allergologica e Professionale*, 4, 5–14, 1989.

Anon., Nickel, in Threshold Limit Values for Chemical Substances and Physical Agents, American Conference of Governmental Industrial Hygienists, Cincinnati, 2001, p. 38.

Artik, S. et al., Nickel allergy in mice: enhanced sensitization capacity of nickel at higher oxidation states, *J. Immunol.*, 163, 1143–1152, 1999.

Avnstorp, C., Prevalence of cement eczema in Denmark before and since addition of ferrous sulfate to Danish cement, *Acta Derm. Venereol. (Stockh.)*, 69, 151–155, 1989.

Bang Pedersen, N. et al., Release of nickel from silver coins, *Acta Derm. Venereol. (Stockh.)*, 54, 231–234, 1974.

Barranco, V.P. and Solomon, H., Eczematous dermatitis caused by internal exposure to nickel, *South. Med. J.*, 66, 447–448, 1973.

Basketter D.A. et al., Nickel, cobalt, and chromium in consumer products: a role in allergic contact dermatitis?, *Contact Dermatitis*, 28, 15–25, 1993.

Bennett, B.G., Environmental nickel pathways to man, in Nickel in the Human Environment: Proceedings of a Joint Symposium Held at the International Agency for Research on Cancer, Lyon, France, 8–11 March 1983, Sunderman, F.W. and Aitio, A., Eds., Oxford University Press, New York, 1984, pp. 487–495.

Berardesca, E. et al., Eds., *Bioengineering of the Skin: Methods and Instrumentation*, CRC Press, Boca Raton, FL, 1995.

Bezzon, O.L., Allergic sensitivity to several base metals: a clinical report, *J. Prosth. Dent.*, 69, 243–244, 1993.

Blanco-Dalmau, L., Carrasquillo-Alberty, H., and Silva-Parra, J., A study of nickel allergy, *J. Prosth. Dent.*, 52, 116–119, 1984.

Blaschko A., Die Berufsdermatosen der Arbeiter, Ein Beitrag zur Gewerbehygiene (I), *Deutsche Medizinische Wochenschrift*, 15, 925–927, 1889.

Block, G.T. and Yeung, M., Asthma induced by nickel, *JAMA*, 247, 1600–1602, 1982.

Borg, L. et al., Nickel-induced cytokine production from mononuclear cells in nickel-sensitive individuals and controls, *Arch. Dermatol. Res.*, 292, 285–291, 2000.

Boyle, R.W. and Robinson, H.A., Nickel in the natural environment, in *Nickel and Its Role in Biology*, Sigel, H. and Sigel, A, Eds., Marcel Dekker, New York, 1988, p. 17.

Bracun, R. et al., Wirksamkeit von Diethylentetramin-pentaacetat und anderen Chelatoren in der Praevention Nickel-induzierter Kontaktekzeme, *Dermatosen*, 47, 8–12, 1999.

Brasch, J. and Geier, J., Patch test results in schoolchildren, Results from the Information Network of Departments (IVDK) and the German Contact Dermatitis Research Group (DKG), *Contact Dermatitis*, 37, 286–293, 1997.

Brasch, J., Geier, J., and Schnuch, A., Differentiated contact allergy lists serve in quality improvement, *Hautarzt, Zeitschrift fur Dermatologie, Venerologie und Verwandte Gebiete*, 49, 184–191, 1998.

Brooks, S.M., Bronchial asthma of occupational origin: a review, *Scand. J. Work Environ. Health*, 3, 53–72, 1977.

Bruynzeel, D.P., Boork, W.J., and van Koteel, W.G., Oral psoralen photochemotherapy of allergic contact dermatitis of the hands, *Dermatosen*, 30, 16–20, 1982.

Bulmer, F.M.R. and Mackenzie, E.A., Studies in the control and treatment of nickel rash, *J. Ind. Hyg.*, 8, 517–527, 1926.

Bumgardner, J.D. and Lucas, L.C., Corrosion and cell culture evaluations of nickel-chromium dental castings, *J. Appl. Biomat.*, 5, 203–213, 1994.

Bumgardner, J.D. and Lucas, L.C., Cellular response to metallic ions released from nickel-chromium dental alloys, *J. Dent. Res.*, 74, 1521–1527, 1995.

Cavelier, C., Foussereau, J., and Massin, M., Nickel allergy: analysis of metal clothing objects and patch testing to metal samples, *Contact Dermatitis*, 12, 65–75, 1985.

Cavelier, C. et al., Nickel allergy: tolerance to metallic surface-plated samples in nickel-sensitive humans and guinea pigs, *Contact Dermatitis*, 19, 358–361, 1988.

Cavelier, C. et al., Allergy to nickel or cobalt: tolerance to nickel and cobalt samples in man and in the guinea pig allergic or sensitized to these metals, *Contact Dermatitis*, 21, 72–78, 1989.

Chia, S.E. and Goh, C.L., Prognosis of occupational dermatitis in Singapore workers, *Am. J. Contact Dermat.*, 2, 105–109, 1991.

Christensen, O.B. and Möller, H., External and internal exposure to the antigen in the hand eczema of nickel allergy, *Contact Dermatitis*, 1, 136–141, 1975.

Christensen, O.B. and Möller, H., Release of nickel from cooking utensils, *Contact Dermatitis*, 4, 343–346, 1978.

Christensen, O.B. et al., Micromorphology and specificity of orally induced flare-up reactions in nickel-sensitive patients, *Acta Derm. Venereol.*, 61, 505–510, 1981.

Christensen, O.B., Prognosis in nickel allergy and hand eczema, *Contact Dermatitis*, 8, 7–15, 1982a.

Christensen, O.B., Disulfiram treatment of three patients with nickel dermatitis, *Contact Dermatitis*, 6, 105–108, 1982b.

Christensen, O.B. and Kristensen, M., Treatment with disulfiram in chronic nickel hand dermatitis, *Contact Dermatitis*, 8, 59–63, 1982.

Conde-Salazar, L. et al., Type IV allergy to rubber additives, *J. Am. Acad. Dermatol.*, 29, 176–180, 1993.

Coombs, R.R.A. and Gell, P.G.H., Classification of allergic reactions responsible for hypersensitivity and clinical disease, in *Clinical Apects of Immunology*, Gell, P.G.H., Coombs, R.R.P., and Lachman, J., Eds., Plenum, New York, 1975, pp. 261–280.

Cormio, L. et al., Toxicity and immediate allergenicity of latex gloves, *Clin. Exp. Allergy*, 23, 618–623, 1993.

Cornacoff, J.B., House, R.V., and Dean, J.H., Comparison of a radioisotopic incorporation method and the mouse ear swelling test, MEST, for contact sensitivity to weak sensitizers, *Fund. Appl. Toxicol.*, 10, 40–44, 1984.

Costa, M. et al., Phagocytosis, cellular distribution, and carcinogenic activity of particulate nickel compounds in tissue culture, *Canc. Res.*, 41, 2868–2876, 1981.

Creason, J.P. et al., Trace elements in hair, as related to exposure in metropolitan New York, *Clin. Chem.*, 21, 603–612, 1975.

De Groot, A.C., Patch testing concentrations and vehicles for testing contact allergens, in *Handbook of Occupational Dermatology*, Kanerva, L. et al., Eds., Springer, New York, 2000, pp. 1257–1276.

de Paepe, K. et al., Beneficial effects of a skin tolerance-tested moisturizing cream on the barrier function in experimentally-elicited irritant and allergic contact dermatitis, *Contact Dermatitis*, 44, 337–343, 2001.

Dearman, J. and Kimber, I., Divergent immune responses to respiratory and contact chemical allergens: antibody elicited by phthalic anhydride and oxazolone, *Clin. Exp. Allergy*, 22, 241–250, 1992.

Dearman, R.J. et al., Differential ability of occupational chemical contact and respiratory allergens to cause immediate and delayed dermal hypersensitivity reactions in mice, *Int. Arch. Allergy Immunol.*, 97, 315–321, 1992.

Dickel, H. et al., Patch testing with a standard series, *Dermatosen*, 46, 234–243, 1998.

Diepgen, T.L. and Coenraads, P.J., The epidemiology of occupational contact dermatitis, *Int. Arch. Occup. Environ. Health*, 72, 496–506, 1999.

Doll, R., Morgan, L.G., and Speizer, F.E., Cancers of the lung and nasal sinuses in nickel workers, *Br. J. Cancer*, 24, 623–632, 1970.

Dolovich, J., Evans, S.L., and Nieboer, E., Occupational asthma from nickel sensitivity: I. Human serum albumin in the antigenic determinant, *Br. J. Ind. Med.*, 41, 51–55, 1984.

Dooms-Goossens, A. et al., Contact dermatitis caused by airborne agents: a review and case reports, *J. Am. Acad. Dermatol.*, 15: 1–10, 1986.

Dooms-Goossens, A., Identification of undetected corticosteroid allergy, *Contact Dermatitis*, 18, 124–129, 1988.

Dupuis, G. and Benezra, C., *Contact Dermatitis to Simple Chemicals*, Marcel Dekker, New York, 1982.

Eggleston, D.W., Effect of dental amalgam and nickel alloys on T-lymphocytes: preliminary report, *J. Prosth. Dentistry*, 51, 617–623, 1984.

Ehrlich, A., Kucenic, M., and Belsito, D.V., Role of body piercing in the induction of metal allergies, *Am. J. Contact Dermat.*, 12, 151–155, 2001.

Elves, M.W. et al., Incidence of metal sensitivity in patients with total joint replacements, *Br. J. Dermatol.*, 4, 376–378, 1975.

Emilson, A., Lindberg, M., and Forslind, B., The temperature effect on in vitro penetration of sodium lauryl sulfate and nickel chloride through human skin, *Acta Derm. Venereol.*, 73, 203–207, 1993.

España, A. et al., Chronic urticaria after implantation of 2 nickel-containing dental prosthesis in a nickel-allergic patient, *Contact Dermatitis*, 21, 204–206, 1989.

Estlander, T. et al., Immediate and delayed allergy to nickel with contact urticaria, rhinitis, asthma and contact dermatitis, *Clin. Exp. Allergy*, 23, 306–310, 1993.

Estlander, T., Jolanki, R., and Kanerva, L., Allergic contact dermatitis from rubber and plastic gloves, in *Protective Gloves for Occupational Use*, Mellstrom, G.A., Wahlberg, J.E., and Maibach, H.I., Eds., CRC Press, Boca Raton, FL, 1994, pp. 221–239.

Estlander, T., Kanerva, L., and Jolanki, R., Rubber additive sensitization from synthetic rubber gloves and boots, *Allergologie*, 18, 470, 1995.

EU, Nickel, *Official Journal of the European Communities*, 22 July 1994 (L 188)/1–2 nickel.

Eversole, L.R., Allergic stomatitides, *J. Oral. Med.*, 34, 93–102, 1979.

Fernández-Redondo, V., Gomez-Centeno, P., and Toribio, J., Chronic urticaria from a dental bridge, *Contact Dermatitis*, 38, 178–179, 1998.

Fischer, T. et al., Nickel release from ear piercing kits and earrings, *Contact Dermatitis*, 10, 39–42, 1984.

Fisher, A.A., "Internal" allergic contact dermatitis, *Cutis*, 5, 407–410, 1969.

Fisher, A.A., Contact stomatitis, glossitis, and cheilitis, *Otolaryngologic Clin. North Am.*, 7, 827–843, 1974.

Fisher, A.A., Allergic dermatitis presumably due to metallic foreign bodies containing nickel and cobalt, *Cutis*, 19, 285–295, 1977.

Fisher, A.A., Nickel — the ubiquitous contact allergen, in *Contact Dermatitis*, Lea & Febiger, Philadelphia, 1986, pp. 745–761.

Fisher, A.A., Reactions of the mucous membrane to contactants, *Clin. Dermatol.*, 5, 123–136, 1987.

Fisher, J.R., Rosenblum, G.A., and Thomson, B.D., Asthma induced by nickel, *JAMA*, 248, 1065–1066, 1982.

Fisher, T., Occupational nickel dermatitis, in *Nickel and the Skin: Immunology and Toxicology*, Maibach, H.I. and Menné, T., Eds., CRC Press, Boca Raton, FL, 1989, pp. 117–132.

Fisher, T. and Rystedt, I., Influence of topical metal binding substances, vehicles, and corticosteroid creams on the allergic patch test reaction in metal-sensitive patients, *Dermatol. Clin.*, 8, 27–31, 1990.

Flessel, C.P., Furst, A., and Radding, S.B., A comparison of carcinogenic metals, in *Carcinogenicity and Metal Ions*, Sigel, H., Ed., Marcel Dekker, New York, 1980, pp. 23–53.

Forman, L. and Alexander, S., Nickel antibodies, *Br. J. Dermatol.*, 87, 320–326, 1972.

Francomano, M., Bertoni, L., and Seidenari, S., Sensitive skin as subclinical expression of contact allergy to nickel sulfate, *Contact Dermatitis*, 42, 169–170, 2000.

Frosch, P.J. et al., Evaluation of skin barrier creams. II. Ineffectiveness of a popular "skin protector" against various irritants in the repetitive irritation test of the guinea pig, *Contact Dermatitis*, 29, 74–77, 1993a.

Frosch, P.J., Kurte, A., and Pilz, B., Efficacy of skin barrier creams. III. The repetitive irritation test (RIT) in humans, *Contact Dermatitis*, 29, 113–118, 1993b.

Fullerton, A. et al., Permeation of nickel salts through human skin *in vitro*, *Contact Dermatitis*, 15, 173–177, 1986.

Fullerton, A., Andersen, J.R., and Hoelgaard, A., Permeation of nickel through human skin *in vitro* — effect of vehicles, *Br. J. Dermatol.*, 118, 509–516, 1988a.

Fullerton, A. and Hoelgaard, A., Binding of nickel to human epidermis *in vitro*, *Br. J. Dermatol.*, 119, 675–682, 1988b.

Fullerton, A. and Menné, T., In vitro and in vivo evaluation of the effect of barrier gels in nickel contact allergy, *Contact Dermatitis*, 32, 100–106, 1995.

Gaul, L., Development of allergic nickel dermatitis from earrings, *JAMA*, 200, 176–179, 1967.

Gawkrodger, D.J., Healy, J., and Howe, A.M., The prevention of nickel contact dermatitis: a review of the use of binding agents and barrier creams, *Contact Dermatitis*, 32, 257–265, 1995.

Gawkrodger, D.J., Nickel dermatitis: how much nickel is safe?, *Contact Dermatitis*, 35, 267–271, 1996.

Gilboa, R., Al-Tawil, N.G., and Marcusson, J.A., Metal allergy in cashiers, *Acta Derm. Venereol. (Stockh.)*, 68, 317–324, 1988.

Giménez-Arnau, A. et al., Metal-induced generalized pruriginous dermatitis and endovascular surgery, *Contact Dermatitis*, 43, 35–40, 2000.

Goh, C.L., An epidemiological comparison between occupational and non-occupational hand eczema, *Br. J. Dermatol.*, 120, 77–82, 1989.

Gollhausen, R. and Ring, J., Allergy to coined money: nickel contact dermatitis in cashiers, *J. Am. Acad. Dermatol.*, 25, 365–369, 1991.

Graham, J.A. et al., Influence of cadmium, nickel, and chromium on primary immunity in mice, *Environ. Res.*, 16, 77–87, 1978.

Grandjean, P., Human exposure to nickel, *IARC Sci. Publ.*, 53, 469–485, 1984.

Guéniche, A. et al., Effect of nickel on the expression of immune-associated antigens (1L-1 and 1CAM-1) by cultured normal human keratinocytes, *J. Invest. Dermatol.*, 100, 437, 1993.

Guerra, L. et al., Role of contact sensitizers in the "burning mouth syndrome," *Am. J. Contact Dermat.*, 4, 154–157, 1993.

Guimaraens, D., Gonzales, M.A., and Condé-Salazar, L., Systemic contact dermatitis from dental crowns, *Contact Dermatitis*, 30, 124–125, 1994.

Haley, P.J. et al., The immunotoxicity of three nickel compounds following 13-week inhalation exposure in the mouse, *Fund. Appl. Toxicol.*, 15, 476–487, 1990.

Hamann, C.P., Natural rubber latex protein sensitivity in review, *Am. J. Contact Dermat.*, 4, 4–21, 1993.

Hanson, C. and Ågrup, G., Stability of mercaptobenzothiazole compounds, *Contact Dermatitis*, 28, 29–34, 1993.

Harrison, P.V., A postal survey of patients with nickel and chromate dermatitis, *Contact Dermatitis*, 5, 29–232, 1979.

Harvell, J., Bason, M., and Maibach, H.I., Contact urticaria and its mechanisms, *Food Chem. Toxicol.*, 32, 103–112, 1994.

Haudrechy, P. et al, Nickel release from stainless steels, *Contact Dermatitis*, 37, 113–117, 1997.

Healy, J. et al., An *in vitro* study of the use of chelating agents in cleaning nickel-contaminated human skin: an alternative approach to preventing nickel allergic contact dermatitis, *Contact Dermatitis*, 39, 171–181, 1998.

Heese, A. et al., Allergic and irritant reactions to rubber gloves in medical health services, *J. Am. Acad. Dermatol.*, 25, 831–839, 1991.

Hensten-Pettersen, A., Nickel allergy and dental treatment procedures, in *Nickel and the Skin: Immunology and Toxicology*, Maibach, H.I. and Menné, T., Eds., CRC Press, Boca Raton, FL, 1989, pp. 195–205.

Hensten-Pettersen, A., Casting alloys: side-effects, *Adv. Dent. Res.*, 6, 38–43, 1992.

Hensten-Pettersen, A., Skin and mucosal reactions associated with dental materials, *Eur. J. Oral Sci.*, 106, 707–712, 1998.

Hildebrand, H.F., Veron, C., and Martin, P., Nickel, chromium, cobalt dental alloys and allergic reactions: an overview, *Biomater*, 10, 545–548, 1989a.

Hildebrand, H.F., Veron, C., and Martin, P., Non-precious dental alloys and allergy, *J. Biol. Buccale*, 17, 227–243, 1989b.

Hogan, D.J. et al., An international survey on the prognosis of occupational contact dermatitis of the hands, *Dermatosen*, 38, 143–147, 1990a.

Hogan, D.J., Dannaker, C.J., and Maibach, H.I., Contact dermatitis: prognosis, risk factors, and rehabilitation, *Semin. Dermatol.*, 9, 233–246, 1990b.

Hogan, D.J., Dannaker, C.J., and Maibach, H.I., The prognosis of contact dermatitis, *J. Am. Acad. Dermatol.*, 23, 300–307, 1990c.

Holti, G., Immediate and Arthus-type hypersensitivity to nickel, *Clinical Allergy*, 4, 437–438, 1974.

Hostýnek, J.J., Metals, in *Contact Urticaria Syndrome*, Amin, S., Lahti, A., and Maibach, H.I., Eds., CRC Press, Boca Raton, FL, 1997, pp. 189–211.

Hostýnek, J.J., Multiple allergic responses to metals, in *Metals and the Skin: Topical Effects and Systemic Absorption*, Marcel Dekker, New York, 1999, pp. 10–13.

Hostýnek, J.J. et al., Human stratum corneum adsorption of nickel salts: investigation of depth profiles by tape stripping in vivo, *Acta Derm. Venereol.*, Suppl. 212, 11–18, 2001a.

Hostýnek, J.J. et al., Human stratum corneum penetration by nickel: in vivo study of depth distribution after occlusive application of the metal as powder, *Acta Derm. Venereol.*, Suppl. 212, 5–10, 2001b.

Ingber, A., Klein, S., and David, M., The nickel released from jewelry in Israel and its clinical significance, *Contact Dermatitis*, 39, 195–197, 1997.

Ishii, N. et al., Nickel sulfate-specific suppressor T cells induced by nickel sulfate in drinking water, *J. Dermatol. Sci.*, 6, 159–164, 1993.

Ishikawaya, Y., Suzuki, H., and Kullavanija, P., Exposure of nickel in used and unused gold-plated earrings: a study using scanning electron microscopy and x-ray microanalysis, *Contact Dermatitis*, 36, 1–4, 1997.

Johansen, J. et al., Changes in the pattern of sensitization to common contact allergens in Denmark between 1985–86 and 1997–98, with a special view to the effect of preventive strategies, *Br. J. Dermatol.*, 142, 490–495, 2000.

Jones, T.K. et al., Dental implications of nickel hypersensitivity, *J. Prosth. Dent.*, 56, 507–509, 1986.

Kaaber, K. et al., Antabuse treatment of nickel dermatitis: chelation — a new principle in the treatment of nickel dermatitis, *Contact Dermatitis*, 5, 221–228, 1979.

Kaaber, K., Sjolin, K.E., and Menné, T., Elbow eruptions in nickel and chromate dermatitis, *Contact Dermatitis*, 9, 213–216, 1983.

Kaaber, K. et al., Some adverse effects of disulfiram in the treatment of nickel-allergic patients, *Dermatosen*, 35, 209–211, 1987.

Kalimo, K., Koulu, L., and Jansen, C.T., Effect of single UVB or PUVA exposure on immediate and delayed skin hypersensitivity reactions in humans, *Arch. Dermatol. Res.*, 275, 374–378, 1983.

Kalimo, K. et al., PUVA treatment of nickel contact dermatitis: effect on dermatitis, patch test sensitivity, and lymphocyte transformation reactivity, *Photodermatology*, 6, 16–19, 1989.

Kalimo, K. et al., Is it possible to improve the prognosis in nickel contact dermatitis, *Contact Dermatitis*, 37, 121–124, 1997.

Kanerva, L. et al., Occupational allergic contact dermatitis from mercury, *Contact Dermatitis*, 28, 26–28, 1993.

Kanerva, L., Estlander, T., and Jolanki, R., Occupational allergic contact dermatitis caused by thiourea compounds, *Contact Dermatitis*, 31, 242–248, 1994a.

Kanerva, L. et al., Nickel release from metals, and a case of allergic contact dermatitis from stainless steel, *Contact Dermatitis*, 31, 299–303, 1994b.

Kanerva, L., Estlander, T., and Jolanki, R., Bank clerk's occupational allergic nickel and cobalt contact dermatitis from coins, *Contact Dermatitis*, 38, 217–218, 1998.

Kanerva, L. et al., A multicenter study of patch test reactions with dental screening series, *Am. J. Contact Dermat.*, 12, 83–87, 2001.

Katchen, B.R. and Maibach, H.I., Immediate-type contact reaction: immunologic contact urticaria in *Exogenous Dermatoses: Environmental Dermatitis*, Menné, T. and Maibach, H.I., Eds., CRC Press, Boca Raton, FL, 1991, pp. 51–63.

Kerosuo, H. et al., Nickel allergy in adolescents in relation to orthodontic treatment and piercing of ears, *Am. J. Orthod. Dentofac. Orthop.*, 109, 148–154, 1996.

Kerosuo, H., Moe, G., and Hensten-Pettersen, A., Salivary nickel and chromium in subjects with different types of fixed orthodontic appliances, *Am. J. Orthod. Dentofac. Orthop.*, 111, 595–598, 1997.

Keskinen, H., Kalliomäki, P.-L., and Alanko, K., Occupational asthma due to stainless steel welding fumes, *Clin. Allergy*, 10, 151–159, 1980.

Kiec-Swierczynska, M., Occupational dermatoses and allergy to metals in Polish construction workers manufacturing prefabricated building units, *Contact Dermatitis*, 23, 27–32, 1990.

Kiec-Swierczynska, M., Occupational allergic contact dermatitis in Lodz: 1990–1994, *Occup. Med.*, 46, 205–208, 1996.

Kimber, I. and Dearman, R.J., Immune responses to contact and respiratory allergens, in *Immunotoxicology and Immunopharmacology*, Dean, J.H. et al., Eds., Raven Press, New York, 1994, pp. 663–679.

Kligman, A. M., The identification of contact allergens by human assay. 3. The maximization test: a procedure for screening and rating contact sensitizers, *J. Invest. Dermatol.*, 47, 393–409, 1966.

Kurtin, A. and Orentreich, N., Chelation deactivation of nickel ion in allergic eczematous sensitivity, *J. Invest. Dermatol.*, 22, 441–445, 1954.

Kusaka, Y., Occupational diseases caused by exposure to sensitizing metals, *Jpn. J. Ind. Health*, 35, 75–87, 1993.

Kwangsukstith, C.H. and Maibach, H.I., Contact urticaria from polyurethane-membrane hypoallergenic gloves, *Contact Dermatitis*, 33, 200–201, 1995.

Lachapelle, J.M., Principles of prevention and protection in contact dermatitis (with special reference to occupational dermatology), in *Textbook of Contact Dermatitis*, Rycroft, R.J.G., Menné, T., and Frosch, J.P., Eds., Springer, Berlin, 1995, pp. 695–702.

Lacroix, J., Morin, C.L., and Collin, P.-P., Nickel dermatitis from a foreign body in the stomach, *J. Pediat.*, 95, 428, 1979.

Lahti, A., Immediate contact reactions, in *Contact Dermatitis*, Rycroft, R.J.G. et al., Eds., Springer-Verlag, Heidelberg 1992, pp. 62–72.

Lahti, A. and Maibach, H.I., Contact urticaria syndrome, in *Dermatology*, Vol. 1, 3rd ed., Moschella, S.L. and Hurley, H.J., Eds., W.B. Saunders, Philadelphia, 1992, pp. 433–440.

Lahti, A. and Maibach, H.I., Immediate contact reactions, in *Allergy: Principles and Practice*, Middleton, E. et al., Eds., C.V. Mosby, St Louis, 1993, pp. 1641–1647.

Lammintausta, K. et al., Interrelationship of nickel and cobalt contact sensitization, *Contact Dermatitis*, 13, 148–152, 1985.

Laschi-Loquerie, A. et al., Influence of heavy metals on the resistance of mice towards infection, *Immunopharmacol. Immunotoxicol.*, 9, 235–241, 1987.

Levantine, A.V., Sensitivity to metal dental plate, *Proc. Royal. Soc. Med.*, 67, 1007, 1974.

Levin, C. and Maibach, H.I., An overview of the efficacy of topical corticosteroids in experimental human nickel contact dermatitis, *Contact Dermatitis*, 43, 317–321, 2000.

Lidén, C., Nickel in jewellery and associated products, *Contact Dermatitis*, 26, 73–75, 1992.

Lidén, C., Menné, T., and Burrows, D., Nickel-containing alloys and platings and their ability to cause dermatitis, *Br. J. Dermatol.*, 134, 193–198, 1996.

Lidén, C. et al., Nickel release from tools on the Swedish market, *Contact Dermatitis*, 39, 127–131, 1998.

Lim, J.T.E. et al., Changing trends in the epidemiology of contact dermatitis in Singapore, *Contact Dermatitis*, 26, 321–326, 1992.

Lisby, S. et al., Nickel-induced proliferation of both memory and naive T cells in patch test-negative individuals, *Clin. Exp. Immunol.*, 117, 217–222, 1999a.

Lisby, S. et al., Nickel-induced activation of T cells in individuals with negative patch test to nickel sulfate, *Arch. Dermatol. Res.*, 291, 247–252, 1999b.

Lundborg, M. and Camner, P., Lysozyme levels in rabbit lung after inhalation of nickel, cadmium, cobalt, and copper chlorides, *Environ. Res.*, 34, 335–342, 1984.

Maibach, H.I., Sensitive skin syndrome — what is it?, *Skin and Aging*, 60–65, 2000.

Malo, J.-L. et al., Occupational asthma caused by nickel sulfate, *J. Allergy Clin. Immunol.*, 69, 55–59, 1982.

Malo, J.-L. et al., Isolated late asthmatic reaction to nickel sulphate without antibodies to nickel, *Clinical Allergy*, 15, 95–99, 1985.

Malo, J.-.L. and Cartier, A., Occupational asthma due to fumes of galvanized metal, *Chest*, 92, 375–377, 1987.

Marks, J.G. et al., North American Contact Dermatitis Group patch test results for the detection of delayed-type hypersensitivity to topical allergens, *J. Am. Acad. Dermatol.*, 38, 911–918, 1998.

Marzulli, F.N. and Maibach, H.I., Contact allergy: predictive testing in man, *Contact Dermatitis*, 1–17, 1976.

Massone, L. et al., Positive patch test reactions to nickel, cobalt, and potasium dichromate in a series of 576 patients, *Cutis*, 47, 119–122, 1991.

Mattila, L. et al., Prevalence of nickel allergy among Finnish university students, *Contact Dermatitis*, 44, 218–223, 2001.

McConnell, L.H. et al., Asthma caused by nickel sensitivity, *Ann. Intern. Med.*, 78, 888–890, 1973.

McKenzie, A.W. and Aitken, C.V.E., Urticaria after insertion of Smith-Petersen Vitallium nail, *Br. Med. J.*, 4, 36, 1967.

Meding, B., Differences between the sexes with regard to work-related skin disease, *Contact Dermatitis*, 43, 65–71, 2000.

Memon, A.A., Molokhia, M.M., and Friedmann, P.S., The inhibitory effects of topical chelating agents and antioxidants on nickel-induced hypersensitivity reactions, *J. Am. Acad. Dermatol.*, 30, 560–565, 1994.

Meneghini, C. and Angelini, G., Intradermal test in contact allergy to metals, *Acta Derm. Venereol.*, 85 suppl., 123–124, 1979.

Menné, T. and Kaaber, K., Treatment of pompholyx due to nickel allergy with chelating agents, *Contact Dermatitis*, 4, 289–290, 1978.

Menné, T., Kaaber, K., and Tjell, J.C., Treatment of nickel dermatitis (the influence of tetraethylthiuramdisulfide, Antabuse) on nickel metabolism, *Ann. Clin. Lab. Sci.*, 10, 160–164, 1980.

Menné, T. and Maibach, H.I., Reactions to systemic exposure to contact allergens: systemic contact allergy reactions (SCAR), *Immunol. Allergy Practice*, 9, 373–385, 1987.

Menné, T. et al., Evaluation of the dimethylglyoxime stick test for the detection of nickel, *Dermatosen*, 35, 128–130, 1987.

Menné, T., Christophersen, J., and Green, A., Epidemiology of nickel dermatitis, in *Nickel and the Skin: Immunology and Toxicology*, Maibach, H.I. and Menné, T., Eds., CRC Press, Boca Raton, FL, 1989, pp. 109–115.

Menné, T. and Rasmussen, K., Regulation of nickel exposure in Denmark, *Contact Dermatitis*, 23, 57–58, 1990.

Menné, T. et al., Systemic contact dermatitis, *Am. J. Contact Dermat.*, 5, 1–12, 1994.

Mitchell, J.C., Type I without type II and type IV hypersensitivity reaction to nickel, *Contact Dermatitis*, 7, 270, 1981.

Mobacken, H. et al., Oral lichen planus: hypersensitivity to dental restoration material, *Contact Dermatitis*, 10, 11–15, 1984.

Möller, H., Attempts to induce contact allergy to nickel in the mouse, *Contact Dermatitis*, 10, 65–68, 1984.

Möller, H. and Svensson, A., Metal sensitivity: positive history but negative test indicates atopy, *Contact Dermatitis*, 14, 57–60, 1986.

Morris, D.L., Intradermal testing and sublingual desensitization for nickel, *Cutis*, 61, 129–132, 1998.

Mosmann, T.R. and Coffman, R.L., Heterogeneity of cytokine secretion patterns and functions of helper T cells, *Adv. Immunol.*, 46, 111–147, 1989.

Mosmann, T.R. et al., Diversity of cytokine synthesis and function of mouse CD4+ T cells, *Immunol. Rev.*, 123, 209–229, 1991.

Motolese, A., Truzzi, M., and Seidenari, S., Nickel sensitization and atopy, *Contact Dermatitis*, 26, 274–275, 1992.

Najem, N. and Hull, D., Langerhans cells in delayed skin reactions to inhalant allergens in atopic dermatitis — an electron microscopic study, *Clin. Exp. Dermatol.*, 14, 218–222, 1989.

Nethercott, J.R. and Holness, D.L., Cutaneous nickel sensitivity in Toronto, Canada, *J. Am. Acad. Dermatol.*, 22, 756–761, 1990.

Nieboer, E., Evans, S.L., and Dolovich, J., Occupational asthma from nickel sensitivity. II. Factors influencing the interaction of Ni2+, HSA, and serum antibodies with nickel related specificity, *Br. J. Ind. Med.*, 41, 56–63, 1984.

Nielsen, G.D. et al., Nickel-sensitive patients with vesicular hand eczema: oral challenge with a diet naturally high in nickel, *Br. J. Dermatol.*, 122, 299–308, 1990.

Nielsen, N.H. and Menné, T., Allergic contact sensitization in an unselected Danish population. The Glostrup Allergy Study, Denmark, *Acta Derm. Venereol.*, 72, 456–460, 1992.

Nielsen, N.H. et al., Effects of repeated skin exposure to low nickel concentrations: a model for allergic contact dermatitis to nickel on the hands, *Br. J. Dermatol.*, 141, 676–682, 1999.

NIOSH, Proposed National Strategies for the Prevention of Leading Work-Related Diseases and Injuries, Part 2, Association of Schools of Public Health/NIOSH, 1988.

NIOSH, National Occupational Research Agenda (NORA), U.S. Department of Health and Human Services, 1996, pp. 96–115.

Novey, H.S., Habib, M., and Wells, I.D., Asthma and IgE antibodies induced by chromium and nickel salts, *J. Allergy Clin. Immunol.*, 72, 407–412, 1983.

Orchard, S., Barrier creams, *Dermatol. Clin.*, 2, 619–629, 1984.

Osmundsen, P.E., Contact urticaria from nickel and plastic additives (butylhydroxytoluene, oleylamide), *Contact Dermatitis*, 6, 452–454, 1980.

Paliard, X. et al., Simultaneous production of IL-2, IL-4, and IFN-gamma by activated human CD4+ and CD8+ T cell clones, *J. Immunol.*, 141, 849–855, 1988.

Park, H.Y. and Shearer, T.R., In vitro release of nickel and chromium from simulated orthodontic appliances, *Am. J. Orthodont.*, 84, 156–159, 1983.

Peltonen, L., Nickel sensitivity in the general population, *Contact Dermatitis*, 5, 27–32, 1979.

Peters, M.S. et al., Pacemaker contact sensitivity, *Contact Dermatitis*, 11, 214–218, 1984.

Pigatto, P.D. et al., Are barrier creams of any use in contact dermatitis?, *Contact Dermatitis*, 26, 19, 1992.

Pirilä, V. and Kajanne, H., Sensitization to cobalt and nickel in cement eczema, *Acta Derm. Venereol.*, 45, 9–14, 1965.

Popa, V. et al., Bronchial asthma and asthmatic bronchitis determined by simple chemicals, *Dis. Chest*, 56, 395–404, 1969.

Räsänen, L. and Tuomi, M., Diagnostic value of the lymphocyte proliferation test in nickel contact allergy and provocation in occupational coin dermatitis, *Contact Dermatitis*, 27, 250–254, 1992.

Resl, V. and Sykora, J., In vitro testing of ointments designed to protect the skin from damage by chromium and nickel, *Dermatol. Wochenschr.*, 151, 1327–1340, 1965.

Ricciardi, L. et al., Nickel allergy, a model of food cellular hyersensitivity?, *Allergy*, 56, 109–112, 2001.

Richter, G., Dental materials — problem substances in allergologic diagnosis? II. Patch test diagnosis and relevance evaluation of selected dental material groups, *Hautarzt, Zeitschrift für Dermatologie, Venerologie und Verwandte Gebiete*, 47, 844–845, 1996.

Richter, G., Ergebnisse und Probleme mit Dentallegierungen im Epikutantest, *Occup. Environ. Dermatol.*, 49, 5–12, 2001.

Ring, J. and Thewes, M., The clinical expression of allergy in the skin, *Allergy*, 54, 192–197, 1999.

Roggeband, R. et al., Labelling of skin sensitizers: the new European Dangerous Preparations Directive, *Contact Dermatitis*, 44, 321–324, 2001.

Romaguera, C. and Grimalt, F., Pacemaker dermatitis, *Contact Dermatitis*, 7, 333, 1981.

Romaguera, C., Grimalt, F., and Vilaplana, J., Contact dermatitis from nickel: an investigation of its sources, *Contact Dermatitis*, 19, 52–57, 1988.

Romaguera, C., Vilaplana, J., and Grimalt, F., Contact stomatitis from a dental prosthesis, *Contact Dermatitis*, 21, 204, 1989.

Roshchin, A.V., Industrial aerosols of rare metals and their hygienic significance, in *Inhaled Particles III: Proceedings of an international symposium organized by the British Occupational Hygiene Society in London, 14–23 Sept., 1970*, Walton, W.H., Ed., Unwin Brothers, Old Woking, U.K., 1971, pp. 611–817.

Rostenberg, A. and Perkins, A.J., Nickel and cobalt dermatitis, *J. Allergy*, 22, 466–451, 1951.

Rougier, A., Lotte, C., and Dupuis, D., An original predictive method for in vivo percutaneous absorption studies, *J. Soc. Cosmetic Chemists*, 38, 397–403, 1987.

Samitz, M.H. and Pomerantz, H., Studies of the effects on the skin of nickel and chromium salts, *A.M.A. Arch. Ind. Health,* 18, 473–479, 1958.

Samitz, M.H. and Katz, S.A., Nickel–epidermal interactions: diffusion and binding, *Environ. Res.*, 11, 34–39, 1976.

Savolainen, H.,Biochemical and clinical aspects of nickel toxicity, *Rev. Environmental Health*, 11, 167–173, 1996.

Schubert, H.J., Nickel dermatitis in medical workers, *Dermatol. Clin.*, 8, 45–47, 1990.

Schurer, N.Y. and Elias, P.M., The biochemistry and function of stratum corneum lipids, *Adv. Lipid Res.*, 24, 27–56, 1991.

Seaton, A., Cherry, B., and Trunbull, J., Rubber glove asthma, *Br. Med. J.*, 296, 531–532, 1988.

Seidenari, S. et al., Comparison of 2 different methods for enhancing the reaction to nickel sulfate patch tests in negative reactors, *Contact Dermatitis*, 35, 308, 1996a.

Seidenari, S., Motolese, A., and Belletti, B., Pretreatment of nickel test areas with sodium lauryl sulfate detects nickel sensitivity in subjects reacting negatively to routinely performed patch tests, *Contact Dermatitis*, 34, 88–92, 1996b.

Sertoli, A. et al., Epidemiological survey of contact dermatitis in Italy (1984–1993) by GIRDCA, *Am. J. Contact Dermat.*, 10, 18–30, 1999.

Shah, M., Lewis, M., and Gawkrodger, D.J., Prognosis of occupational hand dermatitis in metalworkers, *Contact Dermatitis*, 34, 27–30, 1996.

Shah, M., Lewis, F.M., and Gawkrodger, D.J., Nickel as an occupational allergen, *Arch. Dermatol.*, 134, 1231–1236, 1998.

Shirakawa, T. et al., Positive bronchoprovocation with cobalt and nickel in hard metal asthma, *Am. Rev. Resp. Dis.*, 135, 233, 1987.

Shirakawa, T. et al., Hard metal asthma: cross immunological and respiratory reactivity between cobalt and nickel?, *Thorax*, 45, 267–271, 1990.

Shirakawa, T., Kusaka, Y., and Morimoto, K., Specific IgE antibodies to nickel in workers with known reactivity to cobalt, *Clin. Exp. Allergy*, 22, 213–218, 1992.

Sinigaglia, F., The molecular basis of metal recognition by T cells, *J. Invest. Dermatol.*, 102, 398–401, 1994.

Slaweta, G. and Kiec-Swierczynska, M., Contact allergy to nickel, *Medycyna Pracy,* 49, 305–308, 1998.

Sosroseno, W., A review of the mechanisms of oral tolerance and immunotherapy, *J. R. Soc. Med.*, 88, 14–17, 1995.

Spruit, D., Bongaarts, P.J.M., and De Jongh, G.J., Dithiocarbamate therapy for nickel dermatitis, *Contact Dermatitis*, 4, 350–358, 1978.

Stenman, E. and Bergman, M., Hypersensitivity reactions to dental materials in a referred group of patients, *Scand. J. Dent. Res.*, 97, 76–83, 1989.

Stoddard, J.D., Nickel sensitivity as a cause of infusion reactions, *Lancet*, 2, 741–742, 1960.

Sunderman, F.W., Jr. et al., Biological monitoring of nickel, *Toxicol. Ind. Health*, 2, 17–78, 1986.

Symanski, E., Kupper, L.L., and Rappaport, S.M., Comprehensive evaluation of long term trends in occupational exposure. I. Description of the database, *J. Sci. Occup. Environ. Health Safety*, 55, 300–309, 1998.

Symanski, E., Chang, C., and Chan, W., Long-term trends in exposure to nickel aerosols, *J. Sci. Occup. Environ. Health Safety*, 61, 324–333, 2000.

Symanski, E., Chan, W., and Chang, C., Mixed-effects models for the evaluation of long-term trends in exposure levels with an example from the nickel industry, *Ann. Occup. Hyg.*, 45, 71–81, 2001.

Tanojo, H. Hostýnek, J.J., Mountford, H.S., and Maibach, H.I., In vitro permeation of nickel salts through human stratum corneum, *Acta Derm. Venereol.*, Suppl. 212, 19–23, 2001.

Temesvári, E. and Racz, I., Nickel sensitivity from dental prosthesis, *Contact Dermatitis*, 18, 50–51, 1988.

Todd, D.J., Burrows, D., and Stanford, C.F., Atopy in subjects with a history of nickel allergy but negative patch tests, *Contact Dermatitis*, 21, 129–133, 1989.

Tosti, A. et al., Immediate hypersensitivity to nickel, *Contact Dermatitis*, 15, 95, 1986.

Trombelli, L. et al., Systemic contact dermatitis from an orthodontic appliance, *Contact Dermatitis*, 27, 259–260, 1992.

Uter, W. et al., Epidemiology of contact dermatitis, *Eur. J. Dermatol.*, 1, 36–40, 1998.

Valsecchi, R. and Cainelli, T., Contact urticaria from nickel, *Contact Dermatitis*, 17, 187, 1987.

van Hoogstraten, I.M.W. et al., Preliminary results of a multicenter study on the incidence of nickel allergy in relationship to previous oral and cutaneous contacts, in *Current Topics in Contact Dermatitis*, Frosch, P.J. et al., Eds., Springer-Verlag, Heidelberg, 1989, pp. 178–183.

van Hoogstraten, I.M.W. et al., Reduced frequency of nickel allergy upon oral nickel contact at an early age, *Clin. Exp. Immunol.*, 85, 441–445, 1991.

van Joost, T.H., van Ulsen, J., and van Loon, L.A., Contact allergy to denture materials in the burning mouth syndrome, *Contact Dermatitis*, 18, 97–99, 1988.

van Ketel, W.G. and Bruynzeel, D.P., The possible chelating effect of sodium diethylcarbamate of nickel allergic patients, *Dermatosen*, 30, 198–202, 1982.

van Loon, L.A.J. et al., Contact stomatitis and dermatitis to nickel and palladium, *Contact Dermatitis*, 11, 294–297, 1984.

van Loveren, H., Meade, R., and Askenase, P.W., An early component of delayed-type hypersensitivity mediated by T-cells and mast cells, *J. Exp. Med.*, 157, 1604–1617, 1983.

Varigos, G.A. and Dunt, D.R., Occupational dermatitis — an epidemiological study in the rubber and cement industries, *Contact Dermatitis*, 7, 105–110, 1981.

Veien, N.K. et al., Antibodies against nickel-albumin in rabbits and man, *Contact Dermatitis*, 5, 378–382, 1979.

Veien, N.K., Systemically induced eczema in adults, *Acta Derm. Venereol.*, 147 (Supp.), 12–55, 1989.

Veien, N.K. and Menné, T., Nickel contact allergy and nickel restricted diet, *Semin. Dermatol.*, 9, 197–205, 1990.

Veien, N.K. et al., New trends in the use of metals in jewelry, *Contact Dermatitis*, 25, 145–148, 1991.

Veien, N.K. et al., Stomatitis or systemically-induced contact dermatitis from metal wire in orthodontic materials, *Contact Dermatitis*, 30, 210–213, 1994.

Vilaplana, J., Romaguera, C., and Cornellana, F., Contact dermatitis and adverse oral mucous membrane reactions related to the use of dental prostheses, *Contact Dermatitis*, 30, 80–84, 1994.

Volden, G., Molin, L., and Thomsen, K., PUVA-induced suppression of contact sensitivity to mustine hydrochloride in mycosis fungoides, *Br. Med. J.*, 2, 865–866, 1978.

von der Burg, C.K.H. et al., Hand eczema in hairdressers and nurses: a prospective study, *Contact Dermatitis*, 14, 275–279, 1986.

von Krogh, G. and Maibach, H.I., The contact urticaria syndrome, *Semin. Dermatol.*, 1, 59–66, 1982.

Wahlberg, J.E. and Skog, E., Nickel allergy and atopy. Threshold of nickel sensitivity and immunoglobulin E determinations, *Br. J. Derm.*, 85, 97–104, 1971.

Wahlberg, J.E., Nickel: animal sensitization assays, in *Nickel and the Skin: Immunology and Toxicology*, Maibach, H.I. and Menné, T., Eds., CRC Press, Boca Raton, FL, 1989, pp. 65–73.

Wall, L.M., Nickel penetration through rubber gloves, *Contact Dermatitis*, 6, 461–463, 1980.

Warin, R.P. and Smith, R.J., Chronic urticaria: investigations with patch and challenge test, *Contact Dermatitis*, 8, 117–121, 1982.

Wataha, J.C., Biocompatibility of dental casting alloys: a review, *J. Prosth. Dentistry*, 83, 223–234, 2000.

Waters, M.D. et al., Metal toxicity for rabbit alveolar macrophages *in vitro*, *Environ. Res.*, 9, 32–47, 1975.

Watt, T.L. and Baumann, R.R., Nickel earlobe dermatitis, *Arch. Dermatol.*, 98, 155–158, 1968.

Weerheim, A. and Ponec, M., Determination of stratum corneum lipid profile by tape stripping in combination with high-performance thin-layer chromatography, *Arch. Dermatol. Res.*, 293, 191–199, 2001.

Weismann, K. and Menné, T., Nickel allergy and drug intraction, in *Nickel and the Skin: Immunology and Toxicology*, Maibach, H.I. and Menné, T., Eds., CRC Press, Boca Raton, FL, 1989, pp. 179–186.

Wertz, P.W., Epidermal lipids, *Semin. Dermatol.*, 11, 106–113, 1992.

Weston, W.L. and Weston, J.A., Allergic contact dermatitis in children, *Am. J. Dis. Child.*, 138, 932–936, 1984.

Wilkinson, J.D., Nickel allergy and orthodontic prostheses, in *Nickel and the Skin: Immunology and Toxicology*, Maibach, H.I. and Menné, T., Eds., CRC Press, Boca Raton, FL, 1989, pp. 187–193.

Wilson, A.G. and Gould, D.J., Nickel dermatitis from a dental prosthesis without buccal involvement, *Contact Dermatitis*, 21, 53, 1989.

Wöhrl, S. et al., A cream containing the chelator DTPA (diethylenetriaminepenta-acetic acid) can prevent contact allergic reactions to metals, *Contact Dermatitis*, 44, 224–228, 2001.

Wrangsjö, K. and Meding, B., Occupational allergy to rubber chemicals: a follow-up study, *Dermatosen*, 42, 184–189, 1994.

Young, E., van Weelden, H., and van Osch, L., Age and sex distribution of the incidence of contact sensitivity to standard allergens, *Contact Dermatitis*, 19, 307–308, 1988.

Zachariae, C.O.C., Agner, T., and Menné, T., Chromium allergy in consecutive patients in a country where ferrous sulfate has been added to cement since 1981, *Contact Dermatitis*, 35, 83–85, 1996.

Zhai, H. and Maibach, H.I., Dermatopharmacokinetics in evaluating barrier creams, in *Prevention of Contact Dermatitis*, Elsner, P. et al., Eds., S. Karger, Basel, 1996, pp. 193–205.

2 Nickel Allergic Hypersensitivity: Prevalence and Incidence by Country, Gender, Age, and Occupation

Jurij J. Hostýnek, Katherine E. Reagan, and Howard I. Maibach

CONTENTS

Abstract 40
2.1   Introduction 40
2.2   Clarification of Terms 41
    2.2.1   Patch Testing 41
    2.2.2   Standard Series of Allergens...55
    2.2.3   Incidence 56
    2.2.4   Prevalence..56
    2.2.5   Repeat Open Application Test (ROAT) 56
    2.2.6   Thin Layer Rapid Use Epicutaneous Test (T.R.U.E.® TEST) 56
    2.2.7   MOAHL Index 57
    2.2.8   Finn Chambers 57
    2.2.9   Heredity 57
    2.2.10 Atopy..57
2.3   Study Highlights 58
    2.3.1   Nickel Allergic Hypersensitivity According to Gender
         and Geographic Location...58
    2.3.2   Population Studies of Nickel Allergy...63
    2.3.3   Prevalence and Incidence of Nickel Allergy According to Age 65
    2.3.4   Prevalence/Incidence of Nickel Allergy According
         to Occupation 68
2.4   Summary and Conclusions 72
2.5   Confounders and Data Gaps..75
2.6   Suggested Further Studies 76
2.7   Acknowledgment..76

0-8493-1072-5/02/$0.00+$1.50
© 2002 by CRC Press LLC

2.8   Appendix: Variables Determining NAH and Test Results 76
References..77

ABSTRACT

Consistently, nickel ranks as the most common cause of allergic contact dermatitis
(ACD) in the countries where statistics on occurrence of sensitization are recorded,
and population as well as patient studies indicate that the prevalence of nickel
hypersensitivity may be on a slow but steady increase. For that reason the literature
has been scoured for epidemiological studies run over the past century, in order to
create an overview of trends and differences in particular populations, ages, occupations, and genders.

The female population is particularly affected due to its frequent use of jewelry
and accessories. Although not always of overt clinical relevance, the incidence of
nickel allergic hypersensitivity (NAH) in patch-tested women rose from 12% in
1967 to 21% in 1976, and in men from 1 to 4% over the same time interval. At
present it is seen to reach 22% of the female and 4.7% of the male dermatology
patients in the U.S. and Europe. In both female and male cohorts nickel often ranks
as the number one contact allergen.

Such prevalence of NAH in both women and men is attributed mainly to the
use of costume jewelry, often involving perforation of the skin on various parts of
the body, and to the prolonged and intimate contact with buttons, rivets, and other
types of metallic fasteners on clothes.

2.1   INTRODUCTION

The objective of the review is to document new aspects and trends in the immune
response to nickel as revealed by patch testing and clinical manifestation of allergy
over the past 30 years, by country, age group, and type of exposure, and to evaluate
them against the background of earlier data. Since nickel became the most common
of all causes of human skin sensitization and epidemiological studies began track-
ing the occurrence of NAH in the population, frequency of allergy was deduced
mainly from the number of positive patch tests obtained from surveys of dermatology clinic patients. Initial studies indicated a prevalence of 10% for women
and 1% for men, approximately consistent throughout the industrialized world.
Such surveys were considered a relevant indicator until it became evident that,
since a significant part of the general population was sensitized to nickel without
overt symptoms of allergy, NAH was not part of clinical rosters or statistics, and
thus eluded epidemiological survey. An additional element of uncertainty in population studies stems from the inadequately explained observation that negative
nickel patch tests can even result in patients with a classical history suggestive of
nickel allergy. Also the question whether atopics are less likely to develop hypersensitivity to nickel or are simply less reactive to patch test challenge remains *sub
judice* (Möller and Svensson, 1986; Todd et al., 1989). Certainly part of the
increase in frequency of NAH data registered in more recent time now reflects

increased awareness of NAH risk and wider testing for nickel sensitivity. The general population cohorts studied to that end involve specific segments, however, focusing on those recognized to be at higher risk of NAH, e.g., children and adolescents given to personal embellishment with metal objects (body piercing). Conversely, also cohorts developing tolerance to elicitation of NAH through early exposure to orthodontic appliances have become subjects of statistical evaluation. Such in-depth investigations focusing on particular causative (or preventive) factors (selection bias) result in a cluster effect, potentially leading to skewed data that can be difficult to interpret and cannot be used for generalizations, applicable to the entire population. The majority of studies published are based on patient populations from dermatology clinics and may not present a realistic picture of the occurrence of NAH in the general population. Conclusions from those numbers may serve as an indication of disease trends, or serve for risk-factor analysis, with due consideration given to the specific intent by investigators and the potential bias introduced in the studies reported. Risk evaluation will become more meaningful and revealing when it becomes based on unselected populations.

Atopy as an endogenous factor in susceptibility to systemic nickel sensitization and to contact dermatitis is still considered an unsettled issue, particularly in context with NAH prevalence studies, as clinical investigations report conflicting results and conclusions on the subject. (See Section 2.2.10.)

For overview and quick reference, the literature is organized in tables grouped by categories, presenting prevalence and incidence data generated in national or regional dermatology clinics (Table 2.1), from the general population (Table 2.2), specific age groups (Table 2.3), and occupation (Table 2.4). Particular aspects of certain studies and relevant information not amenable to tabulation are excerpted in respective Highlights, listed by category in chronological order. When studies summarized as Highlights address more than one such category, the data are presented in more than one table, but only once in the narrative. The many variables that determine induction of NAH and the outcome of test results are listed in Section 2.8.

2.2 CLARIFICATION OF TERMS

2.2.1 PATCH TESTING

The widely accepted test establishing ACD is the skin patch test. In most instances reviewed, the patch procedures are similar, but there may be variations to accommodate special situations or the practitioners' skills. The most important factor in successful patch testing is the knowledge and experience of the interpreting physican. Furthermore, optimum outcome of the test depends on appropriate dose (concentration and volume), technique of application (vehicle and type of occlusion), and occlusion time. The test is an occluded patch system commonly using Finn Chambers®, which contain the suspected causative allergen standardized for concentration and vehicle, most often petrolatum. (See Section 2.2.2.) In cases where a new allergen is under consideration, the highest concentration that does not irritate the patient's skin (highest nonirritating dose) is determined experimentally. Upper back or forearm is the most appropriate site of patch application.

TABLE 2.1
Nickel Allergic Hypersensitivity Seen in Patch Test Clinics According to Gender and Geographical Location

Reference (specifics)	Year	Location	Cohort Tested			Prevalence		
			M	F	Total	M (%)	F (%)	Total (%)
Rudner et al., 1973 (NACDG)	1971–72	U.S.	509	691	1,200	28 (2.3)	103 (19)	131 (11)
Menné, 1978		Denmark		213			20 (9.4)	
Dooms-Goossens et al., 1980	1975–77	Belgium	396	604	1,000	8 (2)	62 (10.2)	70 (7.0)
Lynde, 1982	1972–73	Canada	80	119	199	(6.3)	(13.4)	(11.6)
	1973–74		162	309	471	(3.7)	(15.2)	(11.3)
	1974–75		149	256	405	(12.8)	(10.9)	(11.6)
	1975–76		170	281	351	(13.0)	(22.1)	(18.6)
	1976–77		192	288	480	(5.7)	(22.0)	(15.6)
	1977–78		152	289	441	(7.2)	(18)	(14.3)
	1978–79		164	311	475	(5.0)	(29.3)	(22.0)
	1979–80		156	370	526	(1.3)	(18.0)	(13.1)
	1980–81		267	475	742	(5.5)	(22.7)	(16.4)
Total 1972–81 (23 Allergens)			1,492	2,698	4,190	(6.7)		
Schubert et al., 1987		Eastern Europe	913	1,487	2,400	19 (2.1)	157 (10.5)	176 (7.3)
Lunder, 1988		Slovenia						
	1972–76				1,945	41	89	130 (6.7)
	1977–81				2,082	28	104	132 (6.3)
	1982–86				2,373	21	195	216 (9.1)
Total 1972–86					6,400	90	388	478 (7.5)
Gollhausen et al., 1988	1977–83	Germany	4,785	7,177	11,962	311 (2.6)	1,639 (13.7)	(9.2)
	1977							(6.2)

Reference	Year	Country						
van Hoogstraten et al., 1989	1983	Western						(12.7)
	1988	Europe						
(Age ≤31)								
(Pierced)			41	568	609	8 (19.5)	225 (39.6)	233 (38)
(Not pierced)			149	48	197	4 (2.7)	3 (6.3)	7 (4)
(Brace only)					200			7 (3.5)
(Brace and pierced)					431			168 (39)
(Brace before pierced)					86			24 (30)
Todd, 1989		Ulster						
(Pierced)			6	241	247	2 (33)	75 (31)	77 (31)
(Not pierced)			20	27	47	2 (10)	1 (4)	3 (6)
(Brace)					6			1 (17)
(No brace; not pierced)					185			55 (30)
(Brace before pierced)					36			9 (25)
(Brace after pierced)					26			13 (36)
Enders et al., 1989	1987	Germany	684	1,161	1,845	31 (4.5)	277 (23.9)	308 (16.7)
	1977–83		4,785	7,177	11,962	311 (2.6)	1,639 (13.7)	1,950 (9.2)
Storrs et al., 1989 (NACDG)	1984–85	U.S.			1,123			109 (9.7)
Stransky and Krasteva, 1989	1975	Bulgaria			220			(5)
	1978				232			(5)
	1981				270			(9)
	1984				275			(10)
	1987				240			(9)
	Total 1975–87				1,237			
Christophersen, 1989	1985–86	Denmark	696	1,470	2,166	35 (5.1)	303 (20.7)	338 (15.6)

(continued)

TABLE 2.1 (CONTINUED)
Nickel Allergic Hypersensitivity Seen in Patch Test Clinics According to Gender and Geographical Location

Reference (specifics)	Year	Location	Cohort Tested			Prevalence		
			M	F	Total	M (%)	F (%)	Total (%)
Lipozencic et al., 1989		Croatia			1,412			(11.4)
	1984							28 (17.6)
	1985							62 (27.6)
	1986							69 (23.1)
	1987							63 (23.2)
Sertoli, 1989 (GIRDCA)	1984	Italy			4,850			1,121 (23.1)
	1985				4,469			982 (21.9)
	1986				4,952			1,705 (34.4)
	1987				4,226			1,493 (35.3)
	Total				18,497			5,301 (28.7)
Widström, 1989	1982–89	Sweden	216			3		3 (1.4)
(Male recruits; pierced)			48			2		2 (4.2)
(Not pierced)			168			1		1 (0.6)
Freeman, 1990		Australia			3,300			226 (6.9)
Nethercott and Holness, 1990 (2.5%)	1981–87	Canada	246	201	447	(7.7)	(16.9)	(11.9)
(5%)			335	294	629	(5.1)	(16.7)	(10.5)
Shehade et al., 1991		U.K.			4,719			873 (18.5)
Nethercott et al., 1991 (2.5%) (NACDG)	1985–89	U.S.-Canada	2,170	2,876	5,046			530 (10.5)
Lim, 1992	1984–85	Singapore			2,471			343 (13.9)
	1986–90		2,634	2,923	5,557			986 (17.7)
Marks, 1998 (NACDG)	1994–96	U.S.			3,108			444 (14.3)

Reference / Group								
Dawn, 2000	Scotland	1992–94	307	493	3,508	18 (7)	111 (22)	(14.3)
		1985–89	191	669	3,969	13 (7)	174 (26)	(10.5)
		1982			800			129 (16)
		1997			860			187 (22)
Johansen, 2000	Denmark	1985–86 (Total patients)	397	835	1,232	(4.2)	(18.3)	(13.8)
		(Children 0–18 years)			145			36 (24.8)
		(Atopic children, Ni sens.)						(11.5)
		(Nonatopic children, Ni sens.)						(32.2)
		1997–98 (Total patients)	423	884	1,267	(4.9)	(20.0)	(15)
		Children 0–18 years)			120			11 (9.2)
		(Atopic children, Ni sens.)						(10.5)
		(Nonatopic children, Ni sens.)						(7.9)
Veien et al., 2001	Denmark	1986–89						
		(Age <20)	303	702	1,005	9 (3)	155 (22.1)	164 (16.3)
		(Age >20)	832	2,322	3,154	26 (3.1)	474 (20.4)	500 (15.8)
		1996–99						
		(Age <20)	133	324	457	7 (5.3)	54 (16.7)	61 (13.3)
		(Age >20)	971	1,869	2,840	41 (4.2)	370 (19.8)	411 (14.5)

TABLE 2.2
Population Studies of NAH

Reference (specifics)	Year	Location	Cohort Tested			Prevalence		
			M	F	Total	M (%)	F (%)	Total (%)
Kieffer, 1979 (students)		Denmark	247	168	415	7 (2.8)	6 (9.5)	23 (5.5)
Peltonen and Terho, 1989	1987–88							
(Age 7, pierced and not pierced)			108	31/57	196	3	3/1	6
(Age 11, pierced and not pierced)			121	110/38	269	3	11/2	14
(Age 14, pierced and not pierced)			104	103/18	225	1	22/0	23
(Age 17, pierced and not pierced)			73	132/10	215	1	39/0	40
(Overall)			406	499	905	8 (2)	78 (16)	86 (9.5)
Dotterud and Falk, 1994 (age 7–12)	1992–93	Norway						
(Pierced)			11	78	89	1 (9.1)	24 (30.8)	25 (28)
(Not pierced)			212	123	335	18 (8.5)	20 (16.3)	38 (11)
(Overall)			223	201	424	19 (9.5)	44 (21.9)	63 (15)
Meijer et al., 1995 (military)		Sweden	520					
(Pierced)			152			7 (4.6)		
(Not pierced)			368			3 (0.8)		

Kerosuo et al., 1996	1992–93	Finland						
(Age group 14–18)								
(Ear pierced before orthodontics)			283			3 (9)	123 (32)	126 (31)
(Not pierced)			96			6 (2)	0	6 (2)
(Overall)						9 (3)	123 (30)	132 (19)
Mattila et al., 2001	1995	Finland						
(Female, pierced)				417			(42)	
(Female, not pierced)				188			(14)	
(Overall)							(39)	
(Male, pierced)					700	(3)		
(Male, not pierced)					284	(7)		
(Overall)						(3)		

TABLE 2.3
NAH by Age

Reference (specifics)		Year	Location	Cohort Investigated			Prevalence		
				M	F	Total	M (%)	F (%)	Total (%)
Prystowsky, 1979			California						
Age group	<24			182	243	425	0 (0)	26 (11)	26 (6.1)
	25–34			96	219	415	3 (1.5)	20 (9.1)	23 (5.5)
	>35			82	236	318	1 (2.4)	17 (7.2)	18 (5.7)
	Total			460	698	1,158	4 (0.9)	63 (9.0)	67 (5.8)
Peltonen, 1979		1976–77	Finland						
Age group	10–19			84	95	179	1	2	3
	20–29			164	146	310	1	12	13
	30–39			111	89	200	2	6	8
	40–49			66	69	135		7	7
	50–59			26	62	88		9	9
	>60			27	41	68		4	4
	Total			478	502	980	4 (0.8)	40 (8)	44 (4.5)
Menné, 1982		1978	Denmark						
Female, age group	16–19					139		16 (11)	16 (11)
	20–29					351		65 (19)	65 (19)
	30–39					383		66 (17)	66 (17)
	40–49					289		55 (19)	55 (19)
	50–59					308		34 (11)	34 (11)
	60–69					239		29 (12)	29 (12)
	70–79					188		18 (9.6)	18 (9.6)
	Total				1,976	1,976		286 (14.5)	286 (14.5)

Study, year	Period	Country	Age group	No. tested		No. positive (%)	
Menné, 1983							
Female, twins, age			50–59	315		40 (12.7)	
			60–69	598		83 (13.9)	
			70–75	185		14 (7.6)	
			Total	1,098		137 (12.5)	
General population, age 50–59			50–59	308		34 (11)	
			60–69	239		29 (12.1)	
			70–75	188		18 (9.6)	
			Total	735		81 (11)	
Larsson-Stymne, 1985	1982–83	Sweden					
Age group			8	285		22 (8)	22 (8)
			11	304		26 (9)	26 (9)
			15	371		43 (12)	43 (12)
			Total	960		91 (9)	91 (9)
Gawkrodger, 1986	1982–85	Scotland					
Age group			10–19			18	
			20–29			38	
			30–39		2	19	
			40–49		3	20	
			50–59		6	14	
			60–69		3	8	
			70–79		1	1	
			Total	501	15	119	
Schubert, 1987	1982	Central/Eastern Europe					
Female, age group			<16			(30)	
			16–19			(25.8)	
			20–24			(27.1)	
			25–29			(17.2)	134 (27)

(continued)

TABLE 2.3 (CONTINUED)
NAH by Age

Reference (specifics)	Year	Location	Cohort Investigated			Prevalence		
			M	F	Total	M (%)	F (%)	Total (%)
30–34							(7.2)	
35–39							(5.4)	
40–44							(1.3)	
45–49							(4.9)	
50–54							(1.3)	
55–59							(5.3)	
≥60							(3.8)	
Young, 1987 (2.5% patch)	1974	Holland	115	135	250	(3.3)	(13.3)	22 (8.8)
(5% patch)	1984		198	416	614	(5.6)	(19.7)	93 (15.1)
Age groups 1984: <30					250			57 (22.7)
30–50					256			29 (11.3)
>50					108			7 (6.5)
van Hoogstraten, 1991	1987–88	Western Europe	641	1,535	2,176			
Female; pierced; age<35				755				(37.9)
>35				400				(20.5)
n/pierced <35				84				(4.8)
>35				281				(10.0)
Male; pierced			67					(21.6)
n/pierced			563					(2.7)
McDonagh, 1992		U.K.						
Age group <30			59	143	202	4 (7)	65 (45)	69 (34)
30–59			143	168	311	5 (3.5)	46 (27)	51 (16)
>60			46	53	99	2 (4.3)	8 (15)	10 (10)

				248	364	612	11 (4.4)	119 (32.7)	130 (21)
Nielsen, 1993	Denmark		Total	248	364	612	11 (4.4)	119 (32.7)	130 (21)
Age			15–34	85	112	197	(2.4)	(19.6)	(12.2)
			35–49	95	101	196	(1.1)	(7.9)	(4.6)
			50–69	99	75	174	(3.0)	(2.7)	(2.9)
			Total	279	288	567	(2.2)	(11.1)	(6.7)
Mangelsdorf, 1996	U.S.								
Age asymptomatic		68–87				82			5(6)
Brasch, 1997	Germany								
Age group			6–15	142	241	383	(5.6)	(22.0)	(15.9)
			6–13	89	109	198	(4.5)	(18.3)	(12.1)
			14–15	53	132	185	(7.5)	(25)	(20)
			Total	284	482	766			
Schnuch, 1997	Germany/Austria	1990–95				36,720	(4.8)	(18.3)	(15.7)
Age group		20–29						(36.2)	

TABLE 2.4
NAH by Occupation

Reference (specifics)	Year	Location	Cohort Tested			Prevalence		
			M	F	Total	M (%)	F (%)	Total (%)
Wahlberg, 1975 hairdressers	1970–71	Sweden			35			(17)
Lynde, 1982	1973–81	Canada			66			18 (27)
Boss, 1982 female hairdressers		Denmark		43			11 (25.6)	
Gawkrodger, 1986	1982–85	Scotland						
office						3	37	
cleaning							37	
catering							15	
nursing							7	
engineering						4	7	
hairdressing							6	
clothing							6	
building						3		
other						5		
Total					501	15	119	134
van der Burg, 1986	1982–83	Holland						
nursing			29	188	217	0 (0)	25 (13)	25 (12)
hairdressing			12	74	86	2 (17)	20 (27)	22 (26)
Schubert, 1987		Central and East Europe	913	1,487	2,400	19 (2.1)	157 (10.5)	176 (7.3)
electroplater						2	7	
metal worker							10	
hairdresser							7	
nurse							7	
tailor							5	

Study	Period	Country					
cook						4	
cleaning						2	
typists					7	2	
other						7	
Matsunaga, 1988	1982–86	Japan	12			1 (8)	
beauticians							
Schubert, 1989	1980–83	Germany		1,585			150 (9.5)
concrete fabrication				726			12 (1.6)
Schubert, 1990	1986–87	Germany	180			17 (9.4)	
medical workers	1981–88		130			34 (26.2)	
Holness (1990)		Canada		53			(17)
hairdresser							
Kiec-Swierczynska, 1990	1972–87	Poland	230	1,782			19 (1.1)
building industry			1,552				
Seidenari, 1990		Italy					
ceramic workers		Italy		139	2	6	8 (6)
Gola, 1992 (GIRDCA)	1984			4,850			1,115 (23)(181/934)[a]
	1985			4,469			910 (20)(88/822)[a]
	1986			4,952			1,568 (32)(195/1373)[a]
	1987			4,226			1,351 (32)(137/1214)[a]
	1988			5,044			1,670 (33)(218/1452)[a]
total	1984–88			23,541			6,614 (28.1)(819/5,795)[a]
Kanerva, 1994 misc. occup.;	1991	Finland	165	412	2 (1)	36 (15)	38 (9)
1314 allergy cases/412 ACD			247				
Kiec-Swierczynska, 1996	1990–94	Poland		1,619	30 (1.8)	72 (4.4)	102 (6.3)
misc. occupations							
Kanerva, 1997		Finland	48	103	2 (4.2)	8 (15)	10 (9.7)
electroplaters			55				

[a] Occupational/nonoccupational.

Reaction to the patch is evaluated after 48, 72, or 96 h, or 1 week later since some reactions may be delayed, like those to gold thiosulfate, where reaction at first remains negative but in isolated cases may turn positive ten days after test application (Bruze et al., 1995).

Reading of reactions can assign them into four categories: irritant, doubtful, positive, and negative reactions. Scoring of the response follows degree of reaction based on certain morphologic features, starting from erythematous infiltration or erythematous infiltration with coalescing vesicles. Erythema without infiltration makes the reaction doubtful, borderline between irritant and marginally allergic, unlikely to be clinically relevant. In that case further testing is appropriate, either at a higher concentration or in a different vehicle. Severity increases going from erythema to formation of papules, oedema or vescicles, to spreading bullous or ulcerative reactions.

False-positive and false-negative reactions are problems that render correct interpretation of patch test results difficult, distorting the outcome in epidemiological studies. False positives are defined as positive reactions in absence of ACD, and may be irritant reactions instead. This potentially happens in tests with nickel salts that are intrinsically irritating. Irritant reactions have the same morphology as ACD and are indistinguishable from allergic reactions except by histological examination of the tissue involved or through appropriate dose-response studies. False positives can result from excessive dose or an irritant vehicle, or are attributable to "angry back syndrome." Inadequate dispersion of the test substance in the vehicle can result in foci of excessive (thus irritating) concentration, as may happen with nickel sulfate crystals in petrolatum. "Excited skin" and angry back syndrome are terms coined to describe a hyperirritable skin condition potentially occurring when multiple, concomitant skin reactions occur. Such a state may also lead to false-positive patch test results (van Hoogstraten et al., 1991).

False-negative reactions may result in patients who are idiosyncratic "late reactants," when the allergen is applied at too low a concentration or the duration of contact is too brief. False negative can also be a test outcome resulting from inadequate diffusion of the test material through the stratum corneum (SC) barrier, thus failing to reach the epidermis at the minimum sensitizing dose; this may happen in patch tests with nickel sulfate routinely applied to the back, a site where diffusion of that xenobiotic appears to be less than optimal (Hostýnek et al., 2001). The choice of the sulfate salt as patch test standard represents a compromise; although the chloride is the more sensitive agent and would be the better penetrant (Wahlberg, 1990; Hostýnek et al., 2001; Räsänen et al., 1999), it also proves to be more irritating.

Adding to the uncertain significance of patch test outcome is a large inter- and intra-individual variation in nickel patch test reactivity noted by Hindsén when retesting a cohort of females over several months. The outcome was different for each of four iterations. Thus, when a patient with a history of nickel allergy tests negative, retesting appears indicated to ascertain the significance of the test result (Hindsén et al., 1997; Hindsén, 1999).

Patch tests with nickel sulfate in petrolatum in particular appear associated with the occurrence of negative test results in patients who have a well-defined history of allergy due to contact with metal jewelry, supposedly the prime correlate in NAH etiology (Burrows, 1989; Kieffer, 1979; Mattila et al., 2001). Faulty execution of the skin patch procedure can be excluded when repeat tests with nickel chloride, a better SC penetrant than the sulfate (Hostýnek et al., 2001), does not substantially alter the test outcome (Möller and Svensson, 1986). Suggested is an association with atopy in those cases, where the observed reaction to nickel is one of irritation, rather than hypersensitivity (Gilboa et al., 1988; Möller and Svensson, 1986).

Appropriate application of the patch onto the test site is but one of the factors critical for the correct test outcome and its interpretation in ACD diagnosis. Several criteria have been defined in an algorithm that appear important in demonstrating clinical relevance of ACD (Ale and Maibach, 1995): personal history of exposure to a particular chemical or compound needs to be established in dialogue with the patient; the site of dermatitis must correspond with the site of contact with the putative allergen, established through careful clinical examination; and test material concentration used must be nonirritating, to be determined through preliminary application of a dilution series of the agent, yielding a dose-response relation. If occurrence of Excited Skin Syndrome (ESS) is suspected, the patch test is to be repeated on an alternate site; the (occluded) patch test is to be complemented with a use test or open patch. (See Section 2.2.5.)

It is likely that quality (reproducibility) and homogeneity of patch tests has benefited thanks to improved patch test materials since the Fischer publication (Fischer and Maibach, 1984).

2.2.2 STANDARD SERIES OF ALLERGENS

Of some 3700 allergens known (de Groot, 1994), various series are established based on experience gathered at dermatology clinics and based on population allergy incidence reports. The typical 20 to 25 test substances making up such series consist of chemically defined synthetic compounds and mixes of natural allergens. They change over time as they are reviewed regularly by national and international contact dermatitis groups, composed of dermatology specialists who review test methods, standardize techniques, and monitor information relating to the allergic sensitization potential of products and chemicals in their respective geographical areas (Andersen et al., 1992; Bruynzeel et al., 1995; Lachapelle et al., 1997). Thus several national (GIRDCA, Italy; JSDA, Japan; DKG, Germany) and supranational standard series are in use: the International Contact Dermatitis Research Group (NCDRG), the North American Contact Dermatitis Group (NACDG) (Storrs et al., 1989), and the European Environmental and Contact Dermatitis Research Group (EECDRG) (Fullerton et al., 1988). Various sublists address special occupational or population exposures, such as the test series for dental materials, metal compounds, photographic chemicals, and so on (Axéll et al., 1983).

Nickel is one of the test materials of the Standard Series, as it is the most common allergen in the population of industrialized countries (Marks et al., 1998; Marks et al., 2000; Storrs et al., 1989). The standardized nickel patch test concentrations in petrolatum used are either 2.5% (U.S., Japan), or 5% (Europe) (Nakada et al., 1998).

2.2.3 INCIDENCE

Incidence describes the number of specified new illnesses, such as persons developing NAH, as recorded in a specified population over a specified period of time. The finding of increased incidence of NAH over a number of years, for example, indicates that more people have developed that condition year after year.

2.2.4 PREVALENCE

Prevalence refers to the number of people with NAH in a given population at a specific time period. Period prevalence includes cases with long-lasting NAH, diagnosed in prior years and up to the present, and often is based on (potentially unreliable) patient recall. Point prevalence represents cases only at a particular moment and includes only subjects with actual NAH. The incidence of X cases of NAH in a given year with a prevalence of Y, for example, indicates that X new cases are diagnosed in the year and that Y number of people live with that condition.

2.2.5 REPEAT OPEN APPLICATION TEST (ROAT)

The ROAT or PUT (Provocative Use Test) is used to confirm the relevance of a positive or negative patch test reaction (Nakada et al., 2000). They are use tests more approximating the real-life condition of exposure to a suspected allergen. The substance is applied once or twice a day for 7 to 14 days on the flexor forearm or other relevant anatomic site (Chang et al., 1997). A positive reaction is usually seen within 4 days, less frequently between 5 and 7 days. In approximately half of the positive patch tests the (open) use test is negative, an indication that the individual threshold of response may not have been reached. A test with higher concentrations is then indicated. Should the open test be positive, then a repeat test using samples with and without allergen will clarify whether the reaction may be irritant in nature (both sites reacting).

2.2.6 THIN LAYER RAPID USE EPICUTANEOUS TEST (T.R.U.E.® TEST)

The T.R.U.E. TEST is a ready-to-use system, developed to overcome some of the inaccuracies inherent in conventional skin patch testing. It is a commercially available, ready-to-use system comprising the standard panel of test materials by the NACDG, except for formaldehyde. The test allergens are prepared in advance and incorporated into a hydrophilic, multilayered, moisture-sensitive patch, and the practitioner has only to remove the covering material before applying it on the patient's skin. Taped onto the skin, the patch releases the test substance as perspiration hydrates the protactive film, transforming it into a permeable gel (Fisher, 1989; Lachapelle et al., 1988).

Although it lacks the flexibility of conventional patch testing and represents only a limited choice of allergens, advantages of the T.R.U.E. system are exact standardized dosage; stability of the test material, which is warranted by airtight and light-proof packaging; and ease of application and reproducibility of test results

(Lachapelle et al., 1988). It is a screening tool for the dermatologist who does not specialize in contact dermatitis.

2.2.7 MOAHL INDEX

Comparison of the frequencies of skin disease in different populations (e.g., comparison between different dermatology centers), is meaningful only if the results are standardized, accounting for such factors as age, sex, atopy, diseased skin, or occupational exposure. For more adequate analysis of patch test results these characteristics have been combined in the MOAHL index, introduced by Wilkinson. It specifically accounts for the *m*ale-to-female ratio, *o*ccupational dermatitis, *a*topy, *h*and dermatitis, and *l*eg ulcers or stasis dermatitis, and serves to show the variance occurring between subpopulations (Andersen and Veien, 1985; Burrows, 1989; Christophersen et al., 1989a; Veien, 1989; Wilkinson et al., 1980).

2.2.8 FINN CHAMBERS

Available commercially as ready-to-use screening trays, Finn Chambers are shallow aluminum cups, mounted on nonsensitizing and low-irritant acrylate adhesive tape, that contain preformulated standard series compounds (Andersen et al., 1992).

2.2.9 HEREDITY

Addressing the question of heredity, Fleming et al. examined familial disposition to NAH among 258 patients, based on questionnaire and interview. Having determined a risk ratio of 2.83 for first-degree relatives of a NAH patient (parents, siblings, and offspring), the authors concluded that relatives of patients with NAH are at increased risk of developing the condition (Fleming et al., 1999).

2.2.10 ATOPY

Atopy (Greek for uncommonness) describes conditions that manifest Type I hypersensitivity, including asthma, hay fever, and eczema, believed to be due to genetic predisposition. Definition of atopy, however, is not uniform. Some include family and personal history, while others distinguish between subjects with atopic eczema and those with respiratory allergy. Others again only consider prick-test positives as atopics. History of atopy is recognized as having a bearing on irritant contact dermatitis, but not on ACD, as the latter does not seem to be more prevalent among atopics (Klas et al., 1996; Rystedt, 1985). Between 10 and 20% of the population appear to belong to that group. Those sensitized by environmental antigens such as pollen, dust, plants, or fungi can exhibit typical anaphylactic symptoms when in contact with antigen.

Several studies have been conducted with the intent to clarify the importance and the effect of atopy as a contributing factor to the occurrence and course of NAH in normal subjects also. In a study investigating atopy as a factor in NAH susceptibility among hairdressers, Wahlberg (1975) noted a divergent trend between atopy and nickel allergy. Hindsén et al. (1994) indicated that in atopics a potential difference may exist in gastrointestinal nickel absorption, through urine analysis after controlled oral dosing. Increased levels of nickel seen in urine from atopics after oral challenge were significant when compared to controls. Atopics have deficient T-lymphocyte function, which could result in diminished susceptibility to allergens (Hanifin, 1983; Hanifin and Rajka, 1980).

Clinical studies addressing both occurrence of irritant and allergic contact dermatitis in atopics are not consistent, however. Elevated transepidermal water loss on exposure to irritants in individuals with active atopic hand eczema was taken as an indication of impaired skin barrier function (Nassif et al., 1994). This can lead to enhanced susceptibility to irritant reactions, an explanation for the frequent recording of false-positive skin patch reactions to nickel sulfate. This was observed to occur in some atopics, but not consistently in all (Gehring et al., 1998).

Thus, the divergent characteristics and thus potentially confounding factors noted in atopics were:

- Increased permeability of the skin barrier
- Lessened immune reactivity due to reduced T-lymphocyte function
- Heightened GI nickel absorption

They contribute to the uncertainty in attempts to assess the role that such state may have on the susceptibility for systemic or skin-contact-induced NAH in atopic individuals. They help explain the less than consistent outcome of epidemiological studies.

2.3 STUDY HIGHLIGHTS

2.3.1 Nickel Allergic Hypersensitivity According to Gender and Geographic Location

2.3.1.1 Rudner et al., 1973 (Table 2.1)

In 10 North American dermatology clinics, 1200 patients patch tested with nickel sulfate and 15 other allergens showed an overall incidence of NAH of 11%. Such high incidence was attributed to the large number of female patients sensitized to nickel contained in jewelry (103 out of 691). Several among the centers involved in the survey did not include cases of obvious earlobe nickel dermatitis in their tests. The reactivity of 11% seen in the North American Contact Dermatitis Group (NACDG) test program was found to be comparable to the 6.7% reactivity in a corresponding International Contact Dermatitis Research Group (ICDRG) study.

2.3.1.2 Menné, 1978 (Table 2.1)

In a Danish hospital 213 female patients were queried for NAH by anamneses. Twenty (9.4%) had a history pointing to nickel allergy, with a mean age of eczema onset of 25 years. Most frequent causes for sensitization were earrings and suspenders.

2.3.1.3   Dooms-Goossens et al., 1980 (Table 2.1)

One thousand dermatitis patients in Belgium were patch tested for NAH, and as follow-up, those found positive were screened for ongoing allergy by questionnaire 3 to 30 months later. In 62 women found allergic to nickel, 54 reactions (87%) were considered relevant to their dermatitis. Of the 45 NAH patients who answered the questionnaire, 34 (75%) continued to suffer from contact eczema after therapeutic measures were taken and instruction given to avoid contact with nickel-releasing materials. In the view of the authors, prognosis for hand eczema is very poor.

2.3.1.4   Edman and Möller, 1982 (Not Tabulated)

Data from 12 years of standardized patch testing conducted in a dermatology clinic were analyzed statistically to determine incidence and trends in contact allergy in the city of Malmö, Sweden. The steepest increase was noted for NAH in females, attributed to metal in earrings and clothing accessories. While the prevalence seen in the general population was on the order of 10%, the prevalence in the hospital cohort reached 21.2% in 1980 (data presented in the report are not amenable to tabulation).

2.3.1.5   Lynde, Warshawski, and Mitchell, 1982 (Table 2.1)

Changes in sensitization patterns in 4190 eczema patients in Vancouver, Canada were recorded over 10 years, from 1972 to 1981. Changing incidence of reactions to a standard screen of patch test chemicals was noted over that period among men: annual positive patch test results to nickel sulfate (2.5% in petrolatum) ranging between 1.3 and 12.8%, 6.7% of the total 1388 tested. Among women, however, nickel was the most frequently recorded allergen throughout, with 19.1% NAH cases registered among the 2534 women tested.

2.3.1.6   Schubert et al., 1987 (Tables 2.1, 2.3, 2.4)

Epidemiology of NAH in 8 clinics in 5 Eastern European countries, based on 300 patients tested in each city, revealed an incidence ranging from 5.0% in Sofia to 12.7% in Erfurt. Of those testing positive for nickel out of a total 2400 patients, 19 were male (2.1%) and 157 female (10.5%).

2.3.1.7   Lunder, 1988 (Table 2.1)

For a group of 6400 patients patch tested over a period of 15 years in Slovenia (1972–86), overall rate of NAH positivity rose from 6.7 to 9.1%. Striking was the shift in the female-to-male ratio: from 2:1 for 1972–76, doubling to 4:1 for 1977–81, and doubling again to 9:1 for 1982–86. Over the 15-year period, incidence declined in males while it steadily increased in females. There also nickel-releasing jewelry was seen as the main risk factor. Average annual prevalence over the three periods studied was steadily increasing among the youngest set (11 to 20 years of age): 2.3, 3, and 10.8%, respectively. Consistently the greatest prevalence of NAH was noted in the 21- to 30-year age group over the 15 years of the survey: 9, 10.2, and 19.1%.

2.3.1.8   Gollhausen et al., 1988 (Table 2.1)

Results from patch testing of 11,962 dermatology patients in West Germany showed that overall NAH seen in that population more than doubled in the 6 years from 1977 to 1983: from 6.2 to 12.7%, with a mean frequency of 2.6% among males and 13.7% among females.

2.3.1.9   van Hoogstraten et al., 1989 (Table 2.1)

In Western European clinics, 1252 females and 485 males were patch tested and interviewed by questionnaire, with a specific focus on the potential relationship between wearing of orthodontic devices and piercing of ears. The study shows that NAH is promoted by ear piercing, but also that, if orthodontic treatment precedes ear piercing at an early age, the frequency of NAH can be significantly reduced. In a group of 568 females and 41 males with pierced ears, the frequency of NAH was 39.6 and 19.5%, respectively. In contrast, NAH was observed in only 6.3% of 48 unpierced female and in 2.7% of 149 unpierced male patients. Of patients with pierced earlobes the frequency of NAH was markedly reduced (from 39 to 27.9%) when orthodontic treatment had preceded ear piercing. This supports the view that oral contact with allergen may induce immunological tolerance.

2.3.1.10   Todd and Burrows, 1989 (Table 2.1)

Relationships between development of NAH and previous ear piercing or orthodontic treatment with nickel-containing appliances were studied in 294 patients. Seventy-seven (31.2%) of patients with pierced ears were allergic to nickel compared with only 3 (6.4%) of patients without pierced ears, representing a significant difference. When orthodontic treatment followed ear piercing the frequency of NAH was 36%, compared with 25% when orthodontic treatment preceded ear piercing. These results confirmed the correlation between ear piercing and the frequency of NAH, although statistically significant in female patients only. This also supported the view that oral exposure to low and steady levels of nickel at an early age, such as occurs through leaching of the metal ions from dental metal prostheses, may induce a state of immunological tolerance to nickel.

2.3.1.11   Enders et al., 1989 (Table 2.1)

A review of patch test results from 11,962 patients from 1977 to 1983 and 18,456 patients in 1987 in a West German clinic showed a frequency in NAH that virtually doubled in both males and females, to 4.5 and 23.9%, respectively.

2.3.1.12   Storrs et al., 1989 (Table 2.1)

Ten investigating centers in North America participated in studying prevalence and relevance of allergic reactions to nickel among the NACDG Standard Series. Of 1123 patients patch tested, 109 (9.7%) were found to be allergic. Gender in that cohort was not indicated.

2.3.1.13   Stransky and Krasteva, 1989 (Table 2.1)

In 3-year intervals, 1237 patients from a dermatology clinic in Bulgaria were patch tested from 1975 to 1987. The increasing importance of nickel as allergen in Bulgaria over a 12-year period is noted, the incidence having risen from 5% in 1975 to 9% in 1987. Still, in contrast to its first rank in industrialized countries, in 1987 nickel as allergen ranked fourth in importance, following chromium, IPPD, and PPD.

2.3.1.14   Christophersen et al., 1989 (Table 2.1)

Of 2166 patients tested for contact allergies in seven different Danish medical centers, 35 men (5.1%) and 303 women (20.7%) gave positive skin patch test reactions to nickel sulfate tested at 5%, making it the most common sensitizer in that cohort (15.6% of all patients). The relative risk for sensitization was seen in women of the age group under 30 years.

2.3.1.15   Lipozencic, Kansky, Peris et al., 1989 (Table 2.1)

In five dermatology centers in Croatia, 1412 patients were examined for contact dermatitis by skin patch testing over 5 years from 1980 to 1986, 953 resulting in positives. The greatest percentage of patients were sensitive to chromium (321; 13.44%), followed by nickel (273; 11.43%). The high chromium sensitization is attributed to materials exposure in the construction industry (cement dermatitis).

2.3.1.16   Sertoli et al., 1989 (Table 2.1)

NAH epidemiology based upon review of 18,497 patients patch tested in Italy showed a steady rise in prevalence from 23.1% in 1984 to 35.3% by 1987. Those numbers combined occupational and nonoccupational patch test positives. While nickel still ranked first as nonoccupational allergen, it was in second place in an industrial environment, following chromium.

2.3.1.17   Widström and Erikssohn, 1989 (Table 2.1)

A patch test study of NAH among military recruits showed that men with pierced ears (22% of cohort) had a prevalence of 4.2%, lower than that generally observed among women (8% among girls of age 8; 12% of age 15; almost 20% in women of age 20 to 30).

2.3.1.18   Freeman, 1990 (Table 2.1)

In 3300 eczema patients tested over 7.5 years from 1982 to 1989 in Sydney, Australia, the most common allergen seen was nickel, with 6.85%. A previously unsuspected allergy was confirmed by using the ROAT.

2.3.1.19   Nethercott and Holness, 1990 (Table 2.1)

Two cohorts of a total of 1074 patients in a contact dermatitis clinic in Toronto were patch tested separately with two concentrations of nickel sulfate: 2.5 (447 patients) and 5% (629 patients). 10% responded at the 5% level, 12% at 2.5%. The difference in response between the two eliciting concentrations was significant and directionally counterintuitive, possibly due to a number of confounding factors in the execution of the patch test. Sensitization in both cohorts was attributed to domestic rather than occupational exposure to the allergen.

2.3.1.20   Shehade, Beck, and Hillier, 1991 (Table 2.1)

Out of a total of 4719 patients tested in a patch test clinic in Manchester, 873 (18.5%) had a positive reaction to nickel sulfate. Response on day two versus day four post application of test patches was analyzed for occurrence of late-onset reactions. A significant difference was observed in reactions to nickel sulfate patches between the two readings, leading to the conclusion that day-two reading only of patch test reactions is insufficient.

2.3.1.21   Nethercott et al., 1991 (Table 2.1)

Between 1985 and 1989, 5046 patients in 14 North American clinics were examined for NAH by skin patch test. 10.5% were found positive to 2.5% nickel sulfate, an increase from 9.7% seen in the previous study done in 1984–85.

2.3.1.22   Lim et al., 1992 (Table 2.1)

Of the 17.7% found sensitized to nickel in the multiracial cohort of 5557 dermatology patients in Singapore, in the majority (15.8%) the cause was attributed to nonoccupational exposure. The incidence had increased from the 13.9% recorded in the previous study, conducted there in 1994–95.

2.3.1.23   Marks et al., 1998 (Table 2.1)

Of 3120 patients patch tested by the North American Contact Dermatitis Group from 1994 to 1996, 66.5% had positive reactions, and 57% were assessed as clinically relevant. Of the 3108 individuals tested with nickel sulfate, the most frequent contact allergen was nickel sulfate, with 444 (14.3%) reactants, the same percentage as in the previous survey (1992–94), but up from 10.5% in 1985–89.

2.3.1.24   Dawn, Gupta, and Forsyth, 2000 (Table 2.1)

The aim of a study conducted in Scotland was to assess the change in trend of NAH by analyzing data collected for 1-year periods set 15 years apart. Data analysis covered patch test results from 800 (307 male, 493 female) and 860 patients (191 male, 669 female), in 1982 and 1997, respectively, also reviewing each patient's clinical presentation, demographics, symptoms, and affected sites, toward establishing a MOAHL index. A total of 129 (16% overall; 7% male, 22% female) patients in 1982, and 187 (22% overall; 7% male, 26% female) patients in 1997 developed relevant positive patch test reactions to nickel sulfate. The female preponderance increased from 1982 (female/male = 6:1) to 1997 (female/male = 13:1), and the rate of atopy in patients with NAH grew from 23% in 1982 to 33% in 1997. In both years, the vast majority of patients developed eruptions below the age of 30, with the most found in the 11 to 20 year age group in 1982 (40%), and in those aged 21 to 30 (35%) in 1997.

2.3.1.25 Johansen et al., 2000 (Table 2.1)

Prevalence of NAH was studied in a Danish patient population by skin patch testing with nickel sulfate (5% in petrolatum) over the periods 1985–86 and 1997–98. While a small increase was noted among both males and females (4.2 to 4.9% and 18.3 to 20.0%, respectively, among children age 0 to 18) NAH decreased significantly, from 24.8 to 9.2%. Analysis of the numbers for that young cohort along lines of atopic status revealed that the decrease was mainly due to the decrease of nickel allergy among nonatopic children. While the decrease among atopic children remained virtually unchanged (11.5 to 10.5%), among nonatopics NAH went from 32.2% in 1986–87 to 7.9% in 1997–98.

2.3.1.26 Veien, Hattel, and Laurberg, 2001 (Table 2.1)

In a retrospective study of patients with NAH seen in dermatological practice in Denmark, the comparison was made between the number of cases before and after implementation in 1991 of limits that regulate nickel exposure in that country. A marked decrease of cases was seen in the female age group under 20, which from 22.1% in the earlier period went to 16.7% ($p < 0.05$) in the postregulatory time span.

2.3.2 POPULATION STUDIES OF NICKEL ALLERGY

2.3.2.1 Kieffer, 1979 (Table 2.2)

The possible correlation between patch test results with a history of dermatitis was documented in a survey of unselected male and female veterinary students. The number of false-positive (13 of 28) and false-negative (8 of 23) predictions obtained from history or interview when compared with patch test outcome led the view that a number of variables were involved that preclude definite conclusions from being reached on NAH status of an individual, short of actual patch testing.

2.3.2.2 Peltonen, 1989 (Table 2.2)

In a patch test study of NAH among schoolchildren in Finland, occurrence was compared between boys (n = 406) and girls (n = 499) with pierced and unpierced ears. Notable was the fact that besides the (expected) low incidence of nickel allergy among boys overall (2%), none of the boys with pierced ears (3%) was sensitized.

2.3.2.3 Dotterud and Falk, 1994 (Table 2.3)

The study by patch testing and questionnaire involving 424 school children showed NAH among girls twice as high for those with pierced ears (30.8%) than the nonpierced (16.3%), while no such difference was noted among boys (9.1

versus 8.5%). Even among girls without pierced ears, the rate of positive reactions was relatively high (16.3%). Also a high incidence of NAH among boys without pierced ears resulted from that study (8.5%) When atopic status was noted, atopic girls had twice the positive patch test reactions (30.8%) to nickel when compared to nonatopics (17%). No such difference resulted from the survey of boys (12.4 versus 9.3%).

2.3.2.4 Meijer et al., 1995 (Table 2.2)

Questionnaires and patch tests of 520 Swedish (male) military conscripts age 20 to 24 revealed a significantly higher incidence in positive reactions among 152 with pierced earlobes (4.6%), as compared to the cohort without pierced earlobes (368, 0.8%). This was taken as an indication that the practice of piercing the skin can be considered a major factor in the etiology of increasing NAH also seen among women. No correlation resulted from this study between the occurrence of hand eczema and ear piercing or NAH.

2.3.2.5 Kerosuo, 1996 (Table 2.2)

Prevalence of NAH was investigated in adolescents in relation to sex, onset, duration and type of orthodontic treatment, and the age at which ears were pierced. The subjects were 700 Finnish adolescents, from 14 to 18 years of age, of which 476 (68%) had a history of orthodontic treatment with metallic appliances. The study consisted of patch testing for nickel allergy and a patient history obtained by a questionnaire and from patient records. The frequency of nickel sensitization in the entire group was 19%, significantly higher in girls (30%) than in boys (3%), and in subjects with pierced ears (31%) than in those with no piercing of ears (2%). None of the girls who were treated with fixed orthodontic appliances before ear piercing showed hypersensitivity to nickel, whereas 35% of the girls who had experienced ear piercing before the onset of orthodontic treatment were sensitized to nickel. The results suggest that orthodontic treatment per se does not seem to increase the risk for nickel hypersensitivity. Rather, the data suggests that treatment with nickel-containing metallic orthodontic appliances before ear piercing may have reduced the prevalence of NAH.

2.3.2.6 Mattila et al., 2001 (Table 2.2)

In Finland, 284 university students were tested for delayed- and immediate-type sensitivity to nickel, by questionnaire, patch testing, prick testing, and serum-specific IgE levels. Overall, NAH was determined in 39% of the female students, in 42% of those with pierced skin, and in 14% without pierced skin. In the male cohort the corresponding numbers were 3, 7, and 3%, respectively. At the time of individual examination, dermatologists noted that 82% among females and 74% of males had skin contact with metal items. No association was noted between immediate-type reaction to allergens and nickel allergy. The authors note that from 1986 to 1995 the prevalence of NAH in females has increased from 13 to 39%, while among males it stayed at 3%.

2.3.3 PREVALENCE AND INCIDENCE OF NICKEL ALLERGY ACCORDING TO AGE

2.3.3.1 Prystowsky, 1979 (Table 2.3)

A cohort of 1158 adult volunteers chosen from the general population in the San Francisco Bay Area was patch tested for nickel sensitivity and the numbers categorized by age group. Highest incidence was seen in those under age 24 (6.1% of total). 9% of 698 women reacted positively, compared to 0.9% of the 460 men. There was a strong correlation of NAH with a history of pierced ears, earlobe rash, and jewelry rash. Of 127 dermatology clinic patients presenting with contact dermatitis, 11% yielded positive tests to nickel.

2.3.3.2 Peltonen, 1979 (Table 2.3)

Prevalence of NAH in the Finnish general population was studied through epicutaneous tests on 980 individuals, subdivided by groups in function of age in 10-year segments, and correlated with incidence of eczema. A tenfold overall preponderance of hypersensitive female over male subjects is recorded (8% versus 0.8%), a ratio also observed in other study groups of that time. The most positive female reactors (14.5% of total females) were seen in the 50 to 59-year age group, with the highest percentage of reactors seen among the female staff of a newspaper and printing plants (10.3%). Overall, NAH was observed in 44 cases (4.5%), 42 of which had a history of dermatitis from metal contact. At the time of testing, 16 (34%) of the NAH subjects also presented with eczema, 1.6% of the total population tested (2.8% females and 0.4% males).

2.3.3.3 Menné, Borgan, and Green, 1982 (Table 2.3)

Based on a retrospective cohort study conducted by interview among a stratified sample of the Danish female population, incidence density of NAH was found to have doubled in all age groups from 1948 to 1973. Out of a total population sample of 1976, 286 recalled a history of allergy to suspenders, metal buttons, fasteners, or costume jewelry (14.2%). This was taken as an indication of the sources of nickel allergy in this study. Based on recall, the highest incidence in the onset of nickel allergy appeared to occur in the age bracket of 10 to 19 years (114; 40%); the highest prevalence of nickel allergy appeared to occur in the age brackets of 20 to 29 and 40 to 49 years at 19%.

2.3.3.4 Menné and Holm, 1983 (Table 2.3)

In Denmark, 1546 female twins were screened by questionnaire and some by patch testing for NAH with the intent to establish possible genetic predisposition of nickel allergy. The pairwise concordance rate based on a history of nickel allergy showed a statistically significant difference of 0.32 for the monozygotic and 0.14 for the dizygotic twins. Concerning the patch tests, the difference in pairwise concordance rate between the two classes was not statistically significant but did show the same trend as the results from the personal interviews. In a different study of genetic predesposition for NAH, Fleming et al. (1999) also came to the conclusion that first-degree relatives of parents with NAH were at increased risk of developing the condition, with a risk ratio of 2.83.

When in the Menné and Holm study the prevalence rate in the history of nickel allergy among twins was compared with questionnaire results from a female cohort of the general population, no significant difference between the two became evident.

2.3.3.5   Larsson-Stymne and Widström, 1985 (Table 2.3)

In Sweden, 960 schoolgirls between the ages of 8 and 15 years, of whom 72% had pierced ears, were patch tested for NAH prevalence. Overall, hypersensitivity was noted in 9%; among those with pierced ears it reached 13%, and only 1% in those without. Thereby a clear correlation was noted between ear piercing and the prevalence of NAH.

2.3.3.6   Gawkrodger et al., 1986 (Tables 2.3, 2.4)

Data analysis of 134 patch test nickel-positive allergy clinic patients ages 15 to 78 identified women in the age group 20 to 29 and men in the 50 to 59 bracket as the most frequently presenting with NAH. In descending order, the areas most frequently involved were the hand, wrist, face, arm, and neck. The majority of affected women had had their ears pierced; in two thirds NAH followed ear piercing, and in one third it occurred before piercing. Remarkable is the delay between ear piercing and the onset of dermatitis, the mean figure being 13.5 years for women. The investigators concluded that the following factors influence the incidence for developing NAH: female gender, fashion jewelry, and wet work. Classified by occupation, the highest incidence (with equal number of cases) was seen among women office workers and building maintenance (37 cases; 7.4% of cohort tested).

2.3.3.7   Schubert et al., 1987 (Table 2.3)

A survey of 2400 dermatology patients in 5 Central and Eastern European countries identified 176 cases (7.3%) of NAH, of which 19 were male (0.8%) and 157 (6.5%) female. Classification of cases by age showed that nickel dermatitis was highest in prevalence for schoolgirls and young women, the highest rate seen in the group younger than 25 years (60.6% of all female cases). Most cases were ascribed to contact with costume jewelry, watches, and clothing accessories. Citing data from Kuwait and Nigeria, the authors detect patterns according to which NAH is a sex-indifferent occurrence in certain countries, especially in third-world countries, as a result of such exposure (Kanan, 1969; Olumide, 1985). Data from Sweden point to a similar trend (Meijer et al., 1995). Positive patch test reactions to nickel sulfate without a dermatitis history were found in only nine cases (5%).

2.3.3.8 Young and Houwing, 1987 (Table 2.3)

Based on patch test results from dermatitis patients, the change in NAH incidence in Holland is compared over a 10-year interval (1974–84), and stratified by age groups in the survey. By 1984, prevalence among the group younger than 30 years old was 22.7%. A significant increase in prevalence of NAH was observed for females: from 13.3% in 1974 to 19.7% in 1984, but not in males (from 3.3 to 5.6%, respectively). Although testing was performed with 2.5% $NiSO_4$ in 1974 and 5% in 1984, based on similar studies the number of responses should not be radically affected by that difference in challenge concentration.

2.3.3.9 Van Hoogstraten et al., 1991 (Table 2.3)

In Western European clinics, 1,535 females and 641 males were patch tested and interviewed by questionnaire, with a specific focus on the potential relationship between wearing of orthodontic devices and piercing of ears. The study showed that NAH is promoted by ear piercing, but also that, if orthodontic treatment preceded ear piercing at an early age, the frequency of NAH could be significantly reduced. In a group of 568 females and 41 males with pierced ears the frequency of NAH was 39.6 and 19.5%, respectively. In contrast, NAH was observed in only 6.3% of 48 unpierced female and in 2.7% of 149 unpierced male patients. Of patients with pierced earlobes the frequency of NAH was markedly reduced (from 39 to 27.9%) when orthodontic treatment had preceded ear piercing. This supported the view that oral contact with allergen may induce immunological tolerance (van Hoogstraten et al., 1991).

2.3.3.10 McDonagh et al., 1992 (Table 2.3)

In a contact dermatitis clinic in Sheffield, 612 patients were patch tested with the European standard series of contact allergens. A definite female preponderance in NAH over men with 32.7 versus 4.4% is noted. No evidence of altered susceptibility to nickel sensitization in atopic individuals was observed, and occurrence of hand dermatitis did not differ significantly between the two groups. A correlation between pierced ears and NAH was evident.

2.3.3.11 Nielsen and Menné, 1993 (Table 2.3)

The distribution of ACD was assessed in an unselected population living in Western Copenhagen, Denmark, by patch testing with 23 haptens and mixtures of haptens by means of the T.R.U.E. TEST. Among 567 participants, overall sensitization was less frequent in men than in women (11.5 versus 18.8%, $p < 0.03$). For the 23 chemicals tested, positive reactions to nickel were most frequent with 6.7%. Nickel sensitivity in particular was less frequent in men than in women (2.2 versus 11.1%, $p < 0.0001$). A clear association between NAH and ear piercing resulted from that study, with 14.8% sensitized among those with pierced ears versus 1.8% among the nonpierced. In the youngest age group, all women with NAH also had pierced ears. A history of metal-contact eczema was researched by questionnaire. Fewer men than women reported such effects (21% versus 48%).

2.3.3.12 Mangelsdorf, Fleischer, and Sherertz, 1996 (Table 2.3)

Patch test reactivity and its prevalence and relevance were investigated in the aging population of the U.S. Of 82 healthy individuals ranging in age from 68 to 87 years, 5 (6%) reacted to nickel, revealing the presence of positive reactions without a history of dermatitis. This was taken to signify a retained ability to develop contact allergy following a lifetime of exposure.

2.3.3.13 Brasch and Geier, 1997 (Table 2.3)

Children were tested by gender and age group for contact allergy to 16 allergens in 22 centers in Germany from 1990 to 1995. Nickel sulfate elicited the highest number of positive reactions, ascribed to the wearing of costume jewelry, with 25% of 132 girls tested of age 14 to 15. The least number of reactions was seen among boys age 6 to 13: 4.5% positives of the 89 tested. Contact allergy in children appeared to be related to sex as well as age.

2.3.3.14 Schnuch et al., 1997 (Table 2.3)

Sensitization rates to test allergens were studied in data for 40,004 patients from 24 dermatology centers in Germany and Austria from 1990 to 1995. Reactions to nickel sulfate in the 36,720 patients tested for that allergen showed the highest number overall, with 12.9% when standardized by sex and age. Standardized by age and gender, overall NAH was 12.9%, and among women age 20 to 29 the rate was 36.2%. Standardized by age and gender and applying the MOAHL index, the authors concluded that atopic dermatitis did not impact sensitization rates for a majority of allergens in the ICDRG standard series.

2.3.4 PREVALENCE/INCIDENCE OF NICKEL ALLERGY ACCORDING TO OCCUPATION

2.3.4.1 Wahlberg, 1975 (Table 2.4)

Of 35 Swedish hairdressers examined for NAH, 40% gave positive skin patch test reactions. Investigation of atopy as a contributing factor (by IgE determination) indicated that prevalence of personal atopy was higher in those negative to the nickel patch.

2.3.4.2 Lynde and Mitchell, 1982 (Table 2.4)

In a program screening for allergic reactions, 66 dermatology patients (ages 16 to 65) in Vancouver working as hairdressers were skin patch tested from 1973–81, using the NACDG screening tray. Nickel sulfate patch testing produced 18 (27%) positive reactions, second after paraphenylenediamine (45%).

2.3.4.3 Boss and Menné, 1982 (Table 2.4)

NAH prevalence was evaluated in Denmark among young females attending a school for hairdressers who had had their ears pierced. One part of the survey was conducted exclusively by questionnaire, which included the question of subsequent lack of reactivity to costume jewelry earrings. The second group included patch testing with nickel sulfate. Of 53 individuals, 32 (60%) reported having had some reaction to costume jewelry; of 43 patch tested in the study, 11 reacted to nickel, indicating a sensitization rate of a minimum of 20%. The use test showed a higher degree of intolerance, pointing to a certain incidence of false negatives on patch testing.

2.3.4.4 van der Burg et al., 1986 (Table 2.4)

In a prospective study of 303 hairdressers and nurses in Amsterdam, an effect contrary to sensitization was noted for the first time if exposure to nickel occurred in the form of orthodontic treatment at an early time in life, mainly prior to ear piercing. The incidence of nickel allergy among hairdressers was 26%, more than twice that seen among nurses (12%). Questioning of the cohorts' ear piercing history revealed that 13% of the nurses who had their ears pierced were sensitive to nickel, while none were sensitive among those without pierced ears; 16 of the 61 hairdressers with pierced ears were sensitive to nickel (28%).

2.3.4.5 Schubert et al., 1987 (Tables 2.3, 2.4)

In the study of 2400 dermatology patients in Central and Eastern Europe, also listed above (see Section 2.3.1.6) by age, job-dependent NAH was mostly seen associated with wet work. In decreasing order of incidence, among men jobs at risk are electroplaters, engine fitters, and turners; among women, they were metal workers, electroplaters, hairdressers, nurses, tailors, cooks, and waitresses.

2.3.4.6 Matsunaga et al., 1988 (Table 2.4)

Skin patch testing of 13 Japanese beauticians with hand dermatitis identified one of 12 as sensitized to nickel (8%), while 12 of 13 reacted to para-phenylenediamine (92%). Exposure to hair dyes thereby appears to be the highest risk factor for acquiring ACD in that profession.

2.3.4.7 Schubert, Lück, and Auermann, 1989 (Table 2.4)

Analysis of NAH etiology in 12 construction workers among 1585 consecutive dermatology patients in Berlin failed to identify cement (known to contain up to 900 ppm nickel) as a causative factor; rather, nonoccupational sensitization due to common articles of everyday use was identified as the cause. Background investigation of exposure of a different cohort of 726 construction workers (12 sensitized) led to the same conclusion, explained by the low solubility of nickel compounds in those matrices.

2.3.4.8   Schubert, 1990   (Table 2.4)

Prevalence and incidence of nickel dermatitis among female medical workers observed in Erfurt, Germany (26.2%) is not significantly different from that seen in the general female population (27.4%). It was acquired in 70.6% of all cases before exposure to nickel ion in occupational activities. Secondary NAH was attributed to fashion jewelry, watch bands, and clothing fasteners, but the main source of primary sensitization is seen to be piercing of the ears.

2.3.4.9   Holness and Nethercott, 1990 (Table 2.4)

Assessment of NAH in hairdressers by epicutaneous testing leads the authors to the conclusion that allergy to nickel (seen in 17% of 53 subjects) due to potential on-the-job exposure to nickel-releasing utensils was not more frequent in that profession. They also see no convincing evidence from their own or earlier, similar studies that atopics were at greater risk of developing NAH on the job or that they should be discouraged from pursuing their profession as hairdressers.

2.3.4.10   Kiec-Swierczynska, 1990 (Table 2.4)

In a total of 1782 male and female workers engaged in the manufacture of building components and exposed to cement, waste fly ash, and asbestos cement, NAH was seen in 2.7% of the cohort and confirmed in 1.1% by definitely positive patch tests. Such low incidence was attributed to the low solubility of nickel compounds present in those materials.

2.3.4.11   Seidenari et al., 1990 (Table 2.4)

While 37 (27%) of 139 workers examined in 3 ceramics factories in Italy by skin patch test were diagnosed as sensitized to one or more substances from the standard and occupational patch test series, only in 18 subjects did sensitization express as dermatitis. In the 52 cases of dermatitis, 37% were diagnosed as ACD, while the other 63% were attributed to irritation.

   Six women and two men (6% of total; three of the atopics) were positive to nickel sulfate. It was the most frequent sensitizing agent in the cohort, but the incidence was similar to that seen among the general population.

   In that study 26 subjects were classified as atopics: 22 cases determined by positive prick tests, and 4 based on history of asthma or allergic rhinitis. This may put in doubt the immunologic nature of the 37% level of dermatitis afflicting the workforce, as atopy is associated with heightened skin susceptibility to irritant xenobiotics. The overall level of sensitization at 21% of the workforce was higher than that in the control group (11%), leading to the conclusion that work in that industry carries a risk of sensitization.

2.3.4.12   Gola et al., 1992 (Table 2.4)

The Italian multicenter study of 23,541 dermatology patients showed a continuing increase in NAH, both occupationally and nonoccupationally, to 38.7% overall in

1988, with 4.3 and 28.8%, respectively. This compared with the 1987 data of 35.3% overall and 3.2 and 28.7%, respectively. The most frequent cause of occupational sensitization, accounting for 70% of cases, was activity in housework, construction, metallurgy and mechanical, hairdressing, and health care.

2.3.4.13   Kanerva, Jolanki, and Toikkanen, 1994 (Table 2.4)

Frequencies of occupational allergic diseases and gender differences were studied in Finland for 1991. Of a total of 1314 cases of occupational allergic diseases reported, comprising 14.2% of all registered occupational diseases, 412 cases were allergic contact dermatitis. Women were overrepresented in that category (247 women versus 165 men), taken as an indication of women's predisposition to delayed-type allergy as was also noted in other studies (Jordan and King, 1977; Leyden and Kligman, 1977; Rees et al., 1989) or women's greater occupational exposure to contact allergens. Prevalence of NAH among women tested was significantly higher than that noted in men: 36 of 247 (15%) versus 2 of 165 (1%). While NAH is also generally ten times more common in women than in men (Christensen, 1990), the number noted in that study may be due to changes in Finnish law that are reflected in census numbers; according to such law, preexisting conditions that have been aggravated by work are also considered occupational.

2.3.4.14   Kiec-Swierczynska, 1996 (Table 2.4)

Consistent with surveys conducted in other socialist countries in Eastern Europe, nickel as occupational allergen in Poland is listed in third place only, following chromates and cobalt. A cohort of 1619 industry workers was included in a dermatological survey. The cases identified as NAH in Table 2.4 (102 out of a total of 332 diagnosed with occupational contact dermatitis; 30.7%) are expressed as percent of the total diagnosed with occupational allergic contact dermatitis due specifically to nickel (30/173 = 17.3% males; 72/159 = 45.3% females). Compared to a previous rate of NAH seen in 9.5% of subjects tested in 1987, in the most recent 5-year period studied (1990–94) occupational NAH in that country had risen to 30.7% of all occupational contact allergy cases, also confirmed by positive patch test results. In decreasing frequency by occupation, NAH was seen in fitters, seamstresses, lab assistants, masons, turners, and nurses.

2.3.4.15   Kanerva et al., 1997 (Table 2.4)

A study of nickel allergy by patch testing and questionnaire among 163 electroplaters (94 men, 69 women) in Finland led to the conclusion that, although history (recall) of hand eczema among men and women was a common occurrence (30 and 35%, respectively) and significantly higher than patch test positivity (4 and 15%), workers did not necessarily have to change jobs because of allergy, presumably due to good industrial hygiene practices.

2.4 SUMMARY AND CONCLUSIONS

As results from a review of the literature, a constant effort is expended to gain insight into factors that determine induction and elicitation of nickel allergy or a silent immune response to that allergen. The quality of the data found in the literature is not necessarily equivalent to the quantity of data reported. Knowledge of the relationship of patch test response and clinical disease is based on questionnaires and patch test data. Both approaches may give false-positive and false-negative readings. Over time, patch test results can vary, because they have been generated using an entire spectrum of changing test materials, from crude patches to Al-test® to Finn Chamber. (See also Section 2.8.) With patch testing utilizing standard commercial allergens, some patients have a history strongly suggestive of nickel allergy but a negative patch test, whereas others are patch-test positive but do not have a clinical history of NAH due to contact with nickel releasing objects (Kieffer, 1979). In earlier years, such an apparent paradox could be due to departures from the label concentration of commercial test materials (Fischer and Maibach, 1984), a problem that now appears to have come under control (Nakada et al., 1998). Only a closely supervised prospective study utilizing defined chemical and historical criteria and physical examination by trained observers, combined with serial dilution patch testing, will likely lead to the next level of quantitative insight. This type of analysis may not be of the highest priority at present, but will eventually be required to provide a gold standard for ascertaining the relationship between patch test positivity and clinical disease.

While several epidemiological studies of NAH have been performed, most are cross sectional, providing an assessment of prevalence. Incidence data are hard to come by because the condition is associated with relatively low rates of hospitalization and mortality. It thus is not considered serious enough to warrant prospective follow-up studies among the general population, and data from different dermatological clinics provide a base that is inadequate for estimating the prevalence rate (Rutstein et al., 1983). On the other hand, NAH may be underreported because individuals with a history of metal allergy have given false-negative patch test results. At least in part this may be attributed to the slow diffusion through the SC by $NiSO_4$ used in epidermal patch testing, which could be circumvented by intradermal testing. This confirms nickel sensitivity in nickel patch test positive individuals. However, 48 h occluded patch testing was recommended until more controlled studies can be conducted (Christensen and Wall, 1987).

The opposite observation has also been recorded, because incidence of false-positive patch test reactions to nickel were seen in patients who never experienced skin reactions from metal contact (Kieffer, 1979). It is possible that some of these were misread irritant reactions (Fisher, 1985; Podmore et al., 1984).

While in the first part of the twentieth century NAH was an occupational hazard, the emphasis now has shifted to the side of the consumer. Clothing accessories first were the main cause of sensitization, followed by metal buttons, and finally by the habit of ear piercing. Nickel now continues as the most common cause of allergic sensitization in Western industrialized countries. Prevalence reports indicate that nickel sensitization has been on a steady increase since World War II, and a doubling in NAH numbers over a period of 10 years is not unusual (Diepgen and Coenraads, 1999; Enders et al., 1989; Gollhausen et al., 1988; Johansen et al., 2000; Kanerva et al., 2001; Kiec-Swierczynska, 1996; Massone et al., 1991; Mattila et al., 2001; Menné et al., 1982; Romaguera et al., 1988). In the early 1990s, population patch test data from Denmark showed a prevalence of 20% among women and 2 to 4% among men (Nielsen and Menné, 1992). Although such an increase continues especially among some cohorts of younger women (Brasch and Geier, 1997; Brasch et al., 1998; Dickel et al., 1998; Massone et al., 1991; Young et al., 1988), the gender difference in NAH seems to become less pronounced, as is seen several studies (Dotterud and Falk, 1994; Goh, 1988; Meijer et al., 1995; Nethercott and Holness, 1990; Widström and Erikssohn, 1989). Most recent data shows that a decrease in the prevalence among the young population and a leveling out of prevalence for the older population is now occurring, particularly in Denmark, where since 1991 regulation has limited nickel exposure (Johansen et al., 2000; Veien et al., 2001).

The high female-to-male ratio still persists when comparing nonoccupational exposure, mainly due to the predilection for ear piercing by women. Prevalence of NAH in the work environment, still prevalent in the former socialist countries of Eastern Europe, on the other hand, seems to be leveling out (Table 2.4). Prevalence statistics by country thus roughly fall into two groups, distinguishable by social and economic patterns. While the steady rise in NAH among women appears to be concordant with lifestyle and affluence prevailing in the Western industrial environment, in countries where occupational activities are less segregated by gender this trend is less pronounced. Where tradition along lines of occupation is not a determinant, and industrial hygiene is not a preeminent issue, the differences between the sexes due to ear piercing appear less pronounced, and nickel still ranks third or fourth, after chromates and cobalt.

Reports of ear piercing as a causative factor for NAH among males are inconsistent: while Widström and Erikssohn (1989), Todd and Burrows (1989), van Hoogstraten et al. (1989), and Meijer et al. (1995) found that the frequency of NAH in men with pierced ears was significantly elevated over that of nonpierced, Dotterud and Falk (1994) noted no such difference among school-age boys. Finally, an earlier study conducted by Olumide (1985) in Nigeria had registered equally high NAH rates for both men and women, explained by similar traditions between the genders in wearing jewelry. The increase in NAH frequency in women with pierced ears compared with unpierced ears is highly significant, and the growing prevalence recorded at the end of the 1980s continues its ascent into the 1990s, particularly among the young (Table 2.3). With time, however, this trend is also becoming more pronounced among the young male population, which apparently is increasingly adopting the fashion of permanent adornment with metal objects through intradermal traumatization of the integument (van Hoogstraten, 1989; Christophersen, 1989; Nethercott, 1990; Dawn, 2000; Dotterud, 1994; Brasch, 1997). Such concordance between fashion and prevalence can be explained as the consequence of the insertion of metal objects immediately following scarring of dermal tissues. Intimate contact between nickel-containing metal and living tissue results in corrosion (oxidation) and solubilization of nickel, and the cellular response to the foreign agent in the dermis constitutes systemic exposure, distinct from epicutaneous contact with allergen resulting from simple wearing of jewelry. Occurrence of distal eczema some-times observed in challenged patients can be seen as a reaction pointing to such systemic sensitization.

In summary on the gender issue, the difference in susceptibility to NAH remains controversial. While the earlier 10:1 ratio seems to be closing due to changing lifestyle in the Western industrialized world, conflicting data from the few and relatively heterogeneous prevalence studies still make it difficult to arrive at clear and unambiguous conclusions due to the many confounding factors seemingly crit-ical in this issue. Studies conducted in Europe show higher NAH prevalence levels than those from America, a difference that can be explained by the selection of cohorts examined in a number of European studies. The lesser focus on gender and occupation, particularly in the youngest sector among women in studies conducted in America precludes drawing corresponding conclusions on NAH prevalence that can claim general validity.

The function of gender as factor in susceptibility to hypersensitivity has been raised by some investigators for allergens in general (Christensen, 1990; Jordan and King, 1977; Leyden and Kligman, 1977; Polak et al., 1968) and for nickel, specif-ically concerning the female population: based on interviews of 1546 Danish female twins, the difference in pairwise concordance rate for predisposition to NAH between monozygotic and dizygotic twins was statistically significant (60%), but not when it was based on patch testing with nickel sulfate (Menné and Holm, 1983). This led the authors to the conclusion that a genetic predisposition is of possible importance in the development of nickel allergy. While some individuals may be sensitized more easily by nickel than others due to genetic background, the total number sensitized in the population will depend on the degree of exposure.

Atopy as a condition impacting on the development of NAH has been investi-gated, with differing results. Certain studies characterize atopics as exhibiting an increased frequency of NAH (Diepgen et al., 1989). Others see a correlation between atopy and occurrence of dermatitis, but not necessarily of the immunologic type (Seidenari et al., 1990). Thus the predisposition of atopics for irritant hand dermatitis is considered by Möller to be a confounding factor in the interpretation of diagnostic skin patch testing for NAH (Möller and Svenson, 1986).

Todd et al. (1989) specifically investigated the phenomenon of patients with a history of nickel allergy but negative patch test results by closely analyzing reactants and nonreactants for markers of atopy. The authors concluded that indi-viduals with a nickel-positive history but negative patch test results do not show a higher than normal incidence of atopy. A separate study of school children, on the other hand, observed that atopic girls were twice as likely to develop metal sensitization than nonatopics (Dotterud and Falk, 1994). In a cohort of hairdresser professionals, a group at high risk for eczema and NAH, atopy correlated with eczema, but a diverging trend was noted between individuals with NAH and atopics (Wahlberg, 1975).

In a series of studies, Hindsén (1999) correlated atopic state with intestinal nickel absorption and skin reactivity to oral nickel provocation. Significantly more urinary nickel was present in atopics than in controls, taken as an indication of increased intestinal nickel absorption, which also correlated with stronger clinical reactions seen in atopics. A significant positive correlation between urinary nickel and total iron-binding capacity in female atopics may also indicate that the iron status of atopic females may have significance for nickel absorption.

2.5 CONFOUNDERS AND DATA GAPS

A number of experimental variables can be discerned that may alter the outcome of future prevalence studies. (See Section 2.8.) Investigations should become more comparable when these factors are considered:

- Most publications are of uncorrected patch test data; they do not account for false negatives or false positives. It is likely that approximately one third of the positives are false positives, due to the ESS. Some studies (Andersen et al., 1993; Menné, 1983) have been performed with a limited number of patches applied at the same time in a "normal" population free of dermatitis. These studies avoid ESS and they presumably have few false-positive responses.
- It is standard procedure to test with 2.5% nickel sulfate in North America, with 5% in Europe, and with both concentrations in Japan. Depending on the idiosyncrasy of the SC and the microenvironment of the skin, 2.5% may be too low for elicitation, and conversely, 5% may cause nonspecific irritation.
- Few of the studies on record are dose–response in nature. Important exceptions are those of Andersen et al. (1993). That experiment defines the patch test dose response and dramatically demonstrates the tenfold variation of positivity (end-point dilutions) in the test population (N = 72). A larger population would be expected to demonstrate an even greater range of end-point sensitivity. Today we realize that allergy is not "all-or-none," but a graded level of sensitivity in the general population.
- This review was mainly a computer, key-reference, and key-textbook search. Performing a hand search and contacting key government, industry, and academic centers might provide additional information.

To summarize, from a synopsis of earlier and more recent investigations, a number of risk factors for NAH emerge that are reasonably secure:

- Young age
- Female gender
- Wearing of (nickel-releasing) costume jewelry
- Hand eczema
- Systemic exposure to nickel ion by piercing of the skin

However, the historical gender gap is closing as skin piercing becomes a common denominator.

2.6 SUGGESTED FURTHER STUDIES

In spite of the considerable efforts expended to date in the epidemiology of nickel allergic contact dermatitis, numerous gaps require filling:

- Consistent dosing with equivalent and accurate challenge concentrations.
- Measurement of percutaneous penetration to explain individual reactivity. The method of SC stripping could lead to actual assessment of exposure.
- Strict dose-response NAH studies.
- Studies simulating actual use could be conducted with application of disks of known nickel content to verify the dose from contact with metal objects, such as tools and coins, to quantify nickel released from metal objects under use conditions.

2.7 ACKNOWLEDGMENT

We gratefully acknowledge the financial support by the Nickel Producers Environmental Research Association (NiPERA) toward this review project.

2.8 APPENDIX: VARIABLES DETERMINING NAH AND TEST RESULTS

- Reproducibility of nickel patch testing, i.e., "left-right" comparison
- Reproducibility of nickel release from petrolatum (Fischer and Maibach, 1984)
- Purity of nickel, free from cobalt and other metals
- Solubility and penetration ability of various salts
- Use of petrolatum in Finn Chamber technique versus T.R.U.E. TEST
- Patch utilized: Finn Chamber, Al-test, T.R.U.E. TEST
- 24 h versus 48 h patching
- 48 h versus 72 h versus 96 h test reading
- Difference between European standard (5%) versus NACDG standard (2.5%), expressed as nickel concentration
- Eliciting dose–response curve (Andersen et al., 1993)
- "Normals" versus dermatitis patients tested
- Earlier diagnosis, increasing frequency of patch testing
- Correlations with Provocative Use Test (Repeat Open Application Test)
- Correction of data for ESS and the MOAHL index (Ale and Maibach, 1995)
  - (M = male versus female)
  - (O = occupational versus non-occupational)
  - (H = hand)
  - (L = leg ulcers versus none)
- Ear and body piercing method
- Changing personal habits over time (multiple piercing, etc.)

- Age of surveyed population, high prevalence of subclinical dermatitis in the aged (Mangelsdorf et al. 1996)
- Altered percutaneous absorption in the aged

REFERENCES

Ale, S.I. and Maibach, H.I., Clinical relevance in allergic contact dermatitis, *Dermatosen in Beruf und Umwelt,* 43, 119–121, 1995.

Andersen, K., Burrows, D., and White, I.R., Allergens from the standard series, in *Textbook of Contact Dermatitis,* Rycroft, R.J.G. et al., Eds., Springer-Verlag, Heidelberg, 1992, pp. 416–456.

Andersen, K.E. et al., Dose-response testing with nickel sulphate using TRUE test in nickel-sensitive individuals, *Br. J. Dermatol.,* 129, 50–56, 1993.

Axéll, T. et al., Standard patch test series for screening of contact allergy to dental materials, *Contact Dermatitis,* 9, 82–84, 1983.

Boss, A. and Menné, T., Nickel sensitization from ear piercing, *Contact Dermatitis,* 8, 211–213, 1982.

Brasch, J. and Geier, J., Patch test results in schoolchildren: results from the Information Network of Departments (IVDK) and the German Contact Dermatitis Research group (DKG), *Contact Dermatitis,* 37, 286–293, 1997.

Brasch, J., Geier, J., and Schnuch, A., Differentiated contact allergy lists serve in quality improvement, *Hautarzt, Zeitschrift fur Dermatologie, Venerologie und Verwandte Gebiete,* 49, 184–191, 1998.

Bruynzeel, D.P. et al., The European standard series, *Contact Dermatitis,* 33, 145–148, 1995.

Bruze, M. et al., The development and course of test reactions to gold sodium thiosulfate, *Contact Dermatitis,* 33, 386–391, 1995.

Burrows, D., Prosser White oration, mischievous metals — chromate, cobalt, nickel and mercury, *Clin. Exp. Dermatol.,* 14, 266–272, 1989.

Chang, Y., Clarke, G., and Maibach, H.I., The provocative use test (PUT) and repeat open application test (ROAT) in topical corticosteroid allergic contact dermatitis, *Contact Dermatitis,* 37, 309–311, 1997.

Christensen, O.B. and Wall, L.M., Open, closed and intradermal testing in nickel allergy, *Contact Dermatitis,* 16, 21–26, 1987.

Christensen, O.B., Nickel dermatitis — an update, *Dermatologic Clinics,* 8, 37–40, 1990.

Christophersen, J. et al., Clinical patch test data evaluated by multivariate analysis, *Contact Dermatitis,* 21, 291–299, 1989a.

Christophersen, J. et al., Impact of individual factors on clinical patch test results with special reference to age, *Semin. Dermatol.,* 8, 127–129, 1989b.

Dawn, G., Gupta, G., and Forsyth, A., The trend of nickel allergy from a Scottish tertiary referral centre, *Contact Dermatitis,* 43, 27–30, 2000.

de Groot, A.C., *Patch Testing. Test Concentrations and Vehicles for 3700 Allergens,* Elsevier, Amsterdam, 1994.

Dickel, H. et al., Patch testing with a standard series, *Dermatosen,* 46, 234–243, 1998.

Diepgen, T.L., Fartasch, M., and Hornstein, O.P., Evaluation and relevance of atopic basic and minor features in patients with atopic dermatitis and in the general population, *Acta Derm. Venereol. Suppl. (Stockh.),* 144, 50–54, 1989.

Diepgen, T.L. and Coenraads, P.J., The epidemiology of occupational contact dermatitis, *Int. Arch. Occup. Environ. Health,* 72, 496–506, 1999.

Dooms-Goossens A. et al., Follow-up study of patients with contact dermatitis caused by chromates, nickel and cobalt, *Dermatologica*, 160, 249–260, 1980.

Dotterud, L.K. and Falk, E.S., Metal allergy in north Norwegian schoolchildren and its relationship with ear piercing and atopy, *Contact Dermatitis*, 31, 308–313, 1994.

Edman, B. and Möller, H., Trends and forecasts for standard allergens in a 12-year patch test material, *Contact Dermatitis*, 8, 95–104, 1982.

Enders, F. et al., Patch test results in 1987 compared to trends from the period 1977–1983, *Contact Dermatitis*, 20, 230–232, 1989.

Fischer, T. and Maibach, H.I., Amount of nickel applied with a standard patch test, *Contact Dermatitis*, 11, 285–287, 1984.

Fisher, A.A., Allergic stomatitis from dental impression compounds, *Cutis*, 36, 295–296, 1985.

Fisher, T., Occupational nickel dermatitis, in *Nickel and the Skin: Immunology and Toxicology*, Maibach, H.I. and Menné, T., Eds., CRC Press, Boca Raton, FL, 1989, pp. 117–132.

Fleming, C.J., Burden, A.D., and Forsyth, A., The genetics of allergic contact hypersensitivity to nickel, *Contact Dermatitis*, 41, 251–253, 1999.

Freeman, S., Fragrance and nickel: old allergens in new guises, *Am. J. Contact Dermat.*, 1, 47–52, 1990.

Fullerton, A., Andersen, J.R., and Hoelgaard, A., Permeation of nickel through human skin in vitro — effect of vehicles, *Br. J. Dermatol.*, 118, 509–516, 1988.

Gawkrodger, D.J. et al., Contact clinic survey of nickel-sensitive subjects, *Contact Dermat.*, 14, 165–169, 1986.

Gehring, W., Gloor, M., and Kleesz, P., Predictive washing test for evaluation of individual eczema risk, *Contact Dermatitis*, 39, 8–13, 1998.

Gilboa, R., Al-Tawil, N.G., and Marcusson J.A., Metal allergy in cashiers: an in vitro and in vivo study for the presence of metal allergy, *Acta Derm. Venereol. (Stockh.)*, 68, 317–324, 1988.

Goh, C.L., Epidemiology of contact allergy in Singapore, *Int. J. Derm.*, 27, 308–311, 1988.

Gola, M. et al., GIRDCA Data Bank for Occupational and Environmental Contact Dermatitis (1984 to 1988), *Am. J. Contact Dermat.*, 3, 179–188, 1992.

Gollhausen, R. et al., Trends in allergic contact sensitization, *Contact Dermatitis*, 18, 147–154, 1988.

Hanifin, J.M. and Rajka, G., Diagnostic features of atopic dermatitis, *Acta Derm. Venereol.*, 92, 44–47, 1980.

Hanifin, J.M., Atopic dermatitis: Special clinical complications, *Postgraduate Medicine*, 74, 188–193, 1983.

Hindsén, M., Christensen, O.B., and Möller, H., Nickel levels in serum and urine in five different groups of eczema patients following oral ingestion of nickel, *Acta Derm. Venereol. (Stockh.)*, 74, 176–178, 1994.

Hindsén, M., Bruze, M., and Christensen, O.B., The significance of previous allergic contact dermatitis for elicitation of delayed hypersensitivity to nickel, *Contact Dermatitis*, 37, 101–106, 1997.

Hindsén, M., Clinical and experimental studies in nickel allergy, *Acta Derm. Venereol. (Suppl.)*, 204, 1–22, 1999.

Holness, D.L. and Nethercott, J.R., Dermatitis in hairdressers, *Dermatol. Clin.*, 8, 119–126, 1990.

Hostýnek, J.J. et al., Human stratum corneum adsorption of nickel salts: investigation of depth profiles by tape stripping in vivo, *Acta Derm. Venereol. (Suppl.)*, 212, 5–10, 2001.

Johansen, J. et al., Changes in the pattern of sensitization to common contact allergens in Denmark between 1985–86 and 1997–98, with a special view to the effect of preventive strategies, *Br. J. Dermatol.*, 142, 490–495, 2000.

Jordan, W. and King, S., Delayed hypersensitivity in females: sex differences, *Contact Dermatitis*, 3, 19–26, 1977.

Kanan, M.W., Contact dermatitis in Kuwait, *J. Kuwait Med. Assoc.*, 3, 129–137, 1969.

Kanerva, L., Jolanki, R., and Toikkanen, J., Frequencies of occupational allergic diseases and gender differences in Finland, *Int. Arch. Occup. Environ. Health*, 66, 111–116, 1994.

Kanerva, L. et al., Hand dermatitis and allergic patch test reactions caused by nickel in electroplaters, *Contact Dermatitis*, 36, 137–140, 1997.

Kanerva, L. et al., A multicenter study of patch test reactions with dental screening series, *Am. J. Contact Dermat.*, 12, 83–87, 2001.

Kerosuo, H. et al., Nickel allergy in adolescents in relation to orthodontic treatment and piercing of ears, *Am. J. Orthodont. Dentofacial Orthoped.*, 109, 148–154, 1996.

Kiec-Swierczynska, M., Occupational dermatoses and allergy to metals in Polish construction workers manufacturing prefabricated building units, *Contact Dermatitis*, 23, 27–32, 1990.

Kiec-Swierczynska, M., Occupational allergic contact dermatitis in Lodz: 1990–1994, *Occup. Med.*, 46, 205–208, 1996.

Kieffer, M., Nickel sensitivity: relationship between history and patch test reaction, *Contact Dermatitis*, 5, 398–401, 1979.

Klas, P.A. et al., Allergic and irritant patch test reactions and atopic disease, *Contact Dermatitis*, 34, 121–124, 1996.

Lachapelle, J.-M. et al., European multicenter study of the TRUE test, *Contact Dermatitis*, 19, 91–97, 1988.

Lachapelle, J.-M. et al., Proposal for a revised international standard series of patch tests, *Contact Dermatitis*, 36, 121–123, 1997.

Larsson-Stymne, B. and Widström, L., Ear-piercing — a cause of nickel allergy in schoolgirls?, *Contact Dermatitis*, 13, 289–293, 1985.

Leyden, J. and Kligman, A., Allergic contact dermatitis: sex differences, *Contact Dermatitis*, 3, 333–338, 1977.

Lim, J. et al., Changing trends in the epidemiology of contact dermatitis in Singapore, *Contact Dermatitis*, 26, 321–326, 1992.

Lipozencic, A. et al., Epidemiology of contact allergic dermatitis in Croatia, in *Current Topics in Contact Dermatitis*, Frosch, P.J. et al., Eds, Springer-Verlag, Heidelberg, 1989, pp. 57–80.

Lunder, M., Variable incidence of nickel dermatitis, *Contact Dermatitis*, 18, 287–289, 1988.

Lynde, C.W. and Mitchell, J.C., Patch test results in 66 hairdressers 1973–1981, *Contact Dermatitis*, 8, 302–307, 1982.

Lynde, C.W., Warshawski, L., and Mitchell, J.C., Screening patch tests in 4190 eczema patients 1972–81, *Contact Dermatitis*, 8, 417–421, 1982.

Mangelsdorf, H.C., Fleischer, A.B., and Sherertz, E.F., Patch testing in an aged population without dermatitis: high relevance of patch test positivity, *Am. J. Contact Dermat.*, 7, 155–157, 1996.

Marks, J. et al., North American Contact Dermatitis Group patch test results for the detection of delayed-type hypersensitivity to topical allergens, *J. Am. Acad. Dermatol.*, 38, 911–918, 1998.

Marks, J. et al., North American Contact Dermatitis Group Patch-Test Results, *Arch. Dermatol.*, 136, 272–273, 2000.

Massone, L. et al., Positive patch test reactions to nickel, cobalt, and potassium dichromate in a series of 576 patients, *Cutis*, 47, 119–122, 1991.

Matsunaga, K. et al., Occupational allergic contact dermatitis in beauticians, *Contact Dermaitis*, 18, 94–96, 1988.

Mattila, L. et al., Prevalence of nickel allergy among Finnish university students, *Contact Dermatitis*, 44, 218–223, 2001.

McDonagh, A.J.G. et al., Nickel sensitivity: the influence of ear piercing and atopy, *Br. J. Dermatol.*, 126, 16–18, 1992.

Meijer, C. et al., Ear piercing, and nickel and cobalt sensitization, in 520 young Swedish men doing compulsory military service, *Contact Dermatitis*, 32, 147–149, 1995.

Menné, T., The prevalence of nickel allergy among women, *Dermatosen*, 26, 123–125, 1978.

Menné, T., Borgan, O., and Green, A., Nickel allergy and hand dermatitis in a stratified sample of the Danish female population: an epidemiological study including a statistic appendix, *Acta Derm. Venereol. (Stockh.)*, 62, 35–41, 1982.

Menné, T. and Holm, N.V., Nickel allergy in a female twin population, *Int. J. Derm.*, 22, 22–28, 1983.

Menné, T., Reactions to systemic exposure to contact allergens, in *Dermatotoxicology*, Marzulli, F.N. and Maibach, H.I.., Eds., Hemisphere, Washington, 1983, pp. 483–499.

Möller, H. and Svensson, A., Metal sensitivity: positive history but negative test indicates atopy, *Contact Dermatitis*, 14, 57–60, 1986.

Nakada, T., Hostýnek, J.J., and Maibach, H.I., Nickel content of standard patch test materials, *Contact Dermatitis*, 39, 68–70, 1998.

Nakada, T., Hostýnek, J.J., and Maibach, H.I., Use tests: ROAT (repeated open application test)/PUT (provocative use test): an overview, *Contact Dermatitis*, 43, 1–3, 2000.

Nassif, A. et al., Abnormal skin irritancy and atopic dermatitis and in atopy without dermatitis, *Arch. Dermatol.*, 130, 1402–1407, 1994.

Nethercott, J.R. and Holness, D.L., Cutaneous nickel sensitivity in Toronto, Canada, *J. Am. Acad. Dermatol.*, 22, 756–761, 1990.

Nethercott, J. et al., Patch testing with a routine screening tray in North America, 1985 through 1989. I. Frequency of response, *Am. J. Contact Dermat.*, 2, 122–129, 1991.

Nielsen, N.H. and Menné, T., Allergic contact sensitization in an unselected Danish population, The Glostrup Allergy Study, Denmark, *Acta Derm. Venereol.*, 72, 456–460, 1992.

Nielsen, N.H. and Menné, T., Nickel sensitization and ear piercing in an unselected Danish population, *Contact Dermatitis*, 29, 16–21, 1993.

Olumide, Y.M., Contact dermatitis in Nigeria, *Contact Dermatitis*, 12, 241–246, 1985.

Peltonen, L., Nickel sensitivity in the general population, *Contact Dermatitis*, 5, 27–32, 1979.

Peltonen, L. and Terho, P., Nickel sensitivity in schoolchildren in Finland, in *Current Topics in Contact Dermatitis*, Frosch, P.J. et al., Eds., Springer-Verlag, Heidelberg, 1989, pp. 184–187.

Podmore, P., Burrows, D., and Bingham, E.A., Prediction of patch tets results, *Contact Dermatitis*, 11, 283–284, 1984.

Polak, L., Barnes, J.M.,,and Turk, J.L., The genetic control of contact sensitization to inorganic metal compounds in guinea-pigs, *Immunology*, 14, 707–711, 1968.

Prystowsky, S.D. et al., Allergic contact hypersensitivity to nickel, neomycin, ethylenediamine, and benzocaine, *Arch. Dermatol.*, 115, 959–962, 1979.

Räsänen, L., Mattila, U., and Kalimo, K., Patch testing with nickel sulfate versus nickel chloride, *Contact Dermatitis*, 40, 287–288, 1999.

Rees, J.L., Friedmann, P.S., and Matthews, J.N., Sex differences in susceptibility to development of contact hypersensitivity to dinitrochlorobenzene (DNCB), *Br. J. Dermatol.*, 120, 371–374, 1989.

Romaguera, C., Grimalt, F., and Vilaplana, J., Contact dermatitis from nickel: an investigation of its sources, *Contact Dermatitis*, 19, 52–57, 1988.

Rudner, E.J. et al., Epidemiology of contact dermatitis in North America, *Arch. Dermatol.*, 108, 537–540, 1973.

Rutstein, D.D. et al., Sentinel health events (occupational): a basis for physician recognition and public health surveillance, *Am. J. Publ. Health*, 73, 1054–1062, 1983.

Rystedt, I., Hand eczema and long-term prognosis in atopic dermatitis, *Acta Derm. Venereol.*, 117, 1–59, 1985.

Schnuch, A. et al., National rates and regional differences in sensitization to allergens of the standard series, Population-adjusted frequencies of sensitization (PAFS) in 40,000 patients from a multicenter study (IVDK), *Contact Dermatitis*, 37, 200–209, 1997.

Schubert, H. et al., Epidemiology of nickel allergy, *Contact Dermatitis*, 16, 122–128, 1987.

Schubert, H.J., Lück, H., and Auermann, E., Nickel dermatitis in construction workers, in *Current Topics in Contact Dermatitis*, Frosch, P.J. et al., Eds., Springer-Verlag, Heidelberg, 1989, pp. 191–194.

Schubert, H.J., Nickel dermatitis in medical workers, *Dermatol. Clin.*, 8, 45–47, 1990.

Seidenari, S. et al., Contact sensitization among ceramic workers, *Contact Dermatitis*, 22, 45–49, 1990.

Sertoli, A. et al., Epidemiology of Contact Dermatitis, *Semin. Dermatol.*, 8, 120–126, 1989.

Shehade, S.A., Beck, M.H., and Hillier, V.F., Epidemiological survey of standard series patch test results and observations on day 2 and day 4 readings, *Contact Dermatitis*, 24, 119–122, 1991.

Storrs, F.J. et al., Prevalence and relevance of allergic reactions in patients patch tested in North America — 1984–1985, *J. Am. Acad. Dermatol.*, 20, 1038–1045, 1989.

Stransky, L. and Krasteva, M., Dynamics of the pattern of contact dermatitis, *Contact Dermatitis*, 20, 224, 1989.

Todd, D.J. and Burrows D., Nickel allergy in relationship to previous oral and cutaneous nickel contact, *Ulster Med. J.*, 58, 168–171, 1989.

Todd, D.J., Burrows, D., and Stanford, C.F., Atopy in subjects with a history of nickel allergy but negative patch tests, *Contact Dermatitis*, 21, 129–133, 1989.

van der Burg, C.K.H. et al., Hand eczema in hairdressers and nurses: a prospective study, *Contact Dermatitis*, 14, 275–279, 1986.

van Hoogstraten, I.M. et al., Preliminary results of a multicenter study on the incidence of nickel allergy in relationship to previous oral and cutaneous contacts, in *Current Topics in Contact Dermatitis*, Frosch, P.J. et al., Eds., Springer-Verlag, Heidelberg, 1989, pp. 178–183.

van Hoogstraten, I.M.W. et al., Reduced fequency of nickel allergy upon oral nickel contact at an early age, *Clin. Exp. Immunol.*, 85, 441–445, 1991.

Veien, N.K., Systemically induced eczema in adults, *Acta Derm. Venereol. (Stockh.)*, 147 (Suppl.), 12–55, 1989.

Veien, N.K., Hattel, T., and Laurberg, G., Reduced nickel sensitivity in young Danish women following regulation of nickel exposure, *Contact Dermatitis*, 45,104–106, 2001.

Wahlberg, J.E., Nickel allergy and atopy in hairdressers, *Contact Dermatitis*, 1, 161–165, 1975.

Wahlberg, J.E., Nickel chloride or nickel sulfate? Irritation from patch-test preparations as assessed by laser doppler flowmetry, *Dermatol. Clin.*, 8, 41–44, 1990.

Widström, L. and Erikssohn, I., Nickel allergy and ear piercing in young men, in *Current Topics in Contact Dermatitis*, Frosch, P.J. et al., Eds., Springer-Verlag, Heidelberg, 1989, pp. 188–190.

Wilkinson, J.D., Hambly, E.M., and Wilkinson, D.S., Comparison of patch test results in two adjacent areas of England, *Acta Derm. Venereol.*, 60, 245–249, 1980.

Young, E. and Houwing, R.H., Patch test results with standard allergens over a decade, *Contact Dermatitis*, 17, 104–107, 1987.

Young, E., van Weelden, H., and van Osch, L., Age and sex distribution of the incidence of contact sensitivity to standard allergens, *Contact Dermatitis*, 19, 307–308, 1988.

3 Oxidative Properties of the Skin: A Determinant for Nickel Diffusion

Jurij J. Hostýnek, Katherine E. Reagan, and Howard I. Maibach

CONTENTS

Abstract 83
3.1   Introduction 84
3.2   Characterization of Human Sweat 85
    3.2.1   Collection Methods 86
    3.2.2   The Major Sweat Components 87
        3.2.2.1   Macro-Electrolytes 87
        3.2.2.2   Amino Acids 89
        3.2.2.3   Proteins 89
        3.2.2.4   Lactate and Pyruvate 90
        3.2.2.5   Trace Metals 90
3.3   The Acid Mantle of the Skin (Sebum) 91
3.4   Diffusion of Nickel in Contact with the Skin 92
3.5   Release of Nickel in Synthetic Sweat 92
3.6   Conclusions 93
3.7   Acknowledgment 94
References 94

ABSTRACT

Skin exudates can corrode (oxidize, dissolve) metal surfaces they contact. Their composition varies as a function of physical, pharmacological and environmental conditions, gender, age, sweat rate, body site, and methods of collection, also in a healthy organism. This overview includes sweat composition and discusses components that constitute the skin's acid mantle: low molecular weight acids in sweat, and fatty acids in sebum, with a particular potential to solubilize nickel-containing metal objects contacting skin. They can form nickel salts whose molecular characteristics will determine the preferred route of penetration: either appendageal diffusion, or through the intercellular lipid domains, besides the commonly assumed transcellular path. Considering the ease with which elicitation reactions set in when highly sensitized individuals come into prolonged contact with nickel-containing metal objects, these two alternatives appear to represent pathways that are more likely routes than is conventional transcellular diffusion. Occlusive application of micronized nickel powder on human skin *in vivo* in fact leads to a time-dependent concentration gradient of the metal in the stratum corneum, as was demonstrated in our laboratory using inductively coupled plasma mass spectroscopy to analyze the spatial nickel distribution within the superficial layer of the skin.

3.1 INTRODUCTION

To understand the phenomenon of skin penetration by metals, it is important to account for the role played in that process by the chemical microenvironment prevailing on the skin surface. By the action of salts and acids present in sweat and sebum, metals in their elemental state can be converted to the hydrophilic or lipophilic salt form, respectively. Only then do they become diffusible via the transcellular, intercellular, and transappendageal routes. This overview describes in detail the microenvironment of the skin as a factor in the corrosion of metallic surfaces containing nickel. Exposure to potentially allergenic corrosion products resulting from intimate and prolonged skin contact with articles of daily use can lead to elicitation of nickel allergic hypersensitivity (NAH). This overview is part of the discussion of nickel released from metal alloys in various media and its effects.

Using the brick-and-mortar model to describe it, the stratum corneum (SC) consists of proteinaceous corneocytes (bricks) imbedded in an intercellular matrix of lipids (mortar), rendering the skin poorly permeable to water and other polar compounds (Elias, 1983). Interspersed in this envelope are appendageal orifices comprised of hair follicles and sweat ducts. An overall envelope covering that outer layer of the epidermis is a thin film that complements its barrier function; it consists of two main components of endogenous origin: sweat and sebum, secreted by the respective glands. An abundance of eccrine sweat glands occurs widely distributed over all exposed skin areas; its function is to dissipate body heat through evaporation. Sebaceous glands, closely asociated with hair follicles, produce an oily secretion, sebum (Sens et al., 1985). Combined, these secretions form a chemical environment that fluctuates in function of endogenous processes and environmental factors, and that can corrode metal. Organometallic compounds, such as derivatives of lead (Rasetti et al., 1961), mercury (Toribara et al., 1997), or tin (Stoner, 1966), have been characterized as relatively good skin penetrants. Nickel reacting with fatty acids may thus also form lipophilic salts that are equally diffusible. The pathways that nickel oxidation products can follow in the process of diffusion through the skin will depend on the polarity of the salts formed with exudates, and can be anticipated in light of those earlier investigations on skin penetration by xenobiotics.

Overall, depending on the polarity of the ion pair formed, three routes of entry appear available for skin penetration by nickel:

- Shunts may serve for rapid passage of hydrophilic salts as an early-stage event.
- This can be followed by slower but continuous, potentially more important intercellular diffusion. It appears reasonable to postulate that nickel ion pairs formed with fatty acids on the skin surface will preferably partition into the lipophilic environment. The intercellular lipid domains in the SC may present a ready pathway for diffusion of lipophilic compounds, since transcellular penetration does not explain such phenomena as provocation of allergic reactions due to simple handling of metallic nickel. It is not likely that nickel, solubilized by palmar sweat, for instance, will penetrate callus on the palms (of the order of 0.8 mm thickness) in amounts sufficient to elicit an allergic reaction. Even urushiol, one of the most potent allergens, rarely causes dermatitis of the palms.
- The route of transcellular diffusion would appear to be of marginal immunological importance; it would be limited to adsorption in the outermost layers of the SC, and possibly the epithelium of appendages. Such adsorption may well be terminal, resulting in the depot formation repeatedly described (Fullerton and Hoelgaard, 1988; Samitz and Katz, 1976).

These three modes of diffusion available to xenobiotics thus puts in evidence the characteristics of the skin, which can function as a barrier, a reservoir, and a filter, depending on the polarity and chemical reactivity of the solute.

The components of skin exudates will determine the diffusible form of nickel responsible for the easy onset of allergic reactions, and help explain the observations of nickel allergic reaction on prolonged skin contact. Highly sensitized individuals may react to contact with coinage, or nickel-containing tools, jewelry, or articles of daily use (Gollhausen and Ring, 1991; Preininger, 1934; Rothman, 1930; Samitz and Pomerantz, 1958). Also, the occurrence of "nickel rash" observed in the metalworking industry (Buckley and Lewis, 1960; Bulmer and Mackenzie, 1926) might be explained by the ready formation of skin-diffusible, lipophilic salts by nickel on contact with the skin. Such transformation may also account for significant increased risk of the more general adverse health effects observed among nickel refinery workers (Chashschin et al., 1994).

3.2 CHARACTERIZATION OF HUMAN SWEAT

Sweat is the most copious bodily secretion after urine and feces; it can also be an important pathway in metabolism, maintaining the balance of minerals and other substances critical for normal physiology, as well as providing a detoxification route. This latter role has been investigated for metals, using different methods of sweat collection. However, for purposes of diagnosing disease, indicating body burden for a specific metal, or assessing the nutritional status of the organism, the interpretation of data is associated with problems due to a variety of factors discussed in the following. Analytical samples must originate only from the eccrine sweat gland and not include glandular and skin-derived components. In elemental analysis, allowance must be made for the different levels of desquamated cells present, versus data

---

TABLE 3.1
Mean Levels of Eccrine Sweat Components*

Sodium	Men	51.9 meq/l
	Women	36.5 meq/l
Potassium	Men	7.5 meq/l
	Women	10.0 meq/l
Chloride		29.7 meq/l
Urea		260–1220 mg/l
Lactic acid		360–3600 mg/l
Amino acids		270–2590 mg/l
Ammonia		60–110 mg/l

* Excerpted from *Geigy Scientific Tables,* 7th ed., 1975.

---

obtained from cell-free sweat. As an example, "cell-rich" sweat averaged 1.15 µg/ml iron, compared to 0.34 µg/ml iron for the cell-free sweat (Morris, 1987). The rate of elimination follows element- and individual-specific patterns, such as acclimatization or, in the case of essential elements, reabsorption governed by homeostasis (Cage and Dobson, 1965).

With respect to detoxification, the levels of lead found in human sweat, for instance, were equal to those in urine; for nickel, on the other hand, sweat levels exceeded those found in urine, underscoring the importance of sweat glands as an excretory organ (Cohn and Emmett, 1978; Suzuki, 1976).

Values for the main components of sweat have repeatedly been investigated over time, yielding increasingly accurate data reflecting improvements in analytical techniques. The main categories of solutes are discussed here. Table 3.1 lists the prevalent ranges; they are approximations, because values are unavoidably subject to variation even in normal subjects due to the type of stress applied for sweat stimulation, environmental and individual temperature, environmental humidity, diet and nutritional status, age, gender, sweat rate, skin area of collection, local skin temperature, and muscular activity.

3.2.1 COLLECTION METHODS

Sweat composition varies with collection method — gauze pad, filter-paper disks, arm bag, or total wash-down technique — as well as the site of collection: arm, back, chest, abdomen, forehead, or total body. The mean total concentration of components routinely measured including sodium, potassium, chloride, nitrogen, calcium, and magnesium was lowest in total body sweat (Costa et al., 1969), and thus the total body washdown method appears to be most representative when measuring total solute eliminated from the skin surface. The collection of sweat limited to discrete body sites and under occlusion, such as the most frequently used arm-bag sweat-collection method, yields variable results, and the values thus obtained cannot be extrapolated to predict body losses accurately (Cohn and Emmett, 1978).

3.2.2 The Major Sweat Components

3.2.2.1 Macro-Electrolytes

Elevated levels of sodium and chloride concentrations in sweat are a hallmark of environmental deprivation (malnutrition) as well as of cystic fibrosis (CF) of the pancreas and other disorders (Beck et al., 1986). This appears as a criterion that may lead to erroneous diagnosis (Christoffel et al., 1985; Davis et al., 1983; Sekelj et al., 1973). Due to this, data on those two elements are the most common values found in the literature. The validity of these electrolyte levels in adults are often questioned, however, due to their particular susceptibility to methods of analysis and sweat stimulation (physiological, physical, or pharmacological).

Literature values define levels of less than 50 mmol/l of sodium in sweat as normal, 50 to 70 mmol/l as equivocal, and greater than 70 mmol/l as abnormal.

Values comparing electrode readings in normal subjects without local stimulation and data from pilocarpine electrophoresis of palmar sweat were equivalent. The upper limit for both sodium and chloride falls below 50 meq/l in 99% of subjects tested and lower than 65 meq/l in all 649 volunteers (Sekelj et al., 1973). Another study of sweat induced by pilocarpine iontophoresis in 187 healthy subjects contained chloride concentrations below 70 meq/l in 99% of those tested, and less than 60 meq/l in 96% (Davis et al., 1983).

Using direct-reading ion-selective electrodes on normal volunteers, mean sodium concentration in forearm transudate was 1.7 meq/l $\pm$ 0.7, and chloride concentration 2.8 meq/l $\pm$ 3.5 (n = 6). In normally nourished, healthy patients sweat chloride values ranged from 50 to 60 mmol/l. Malnourished children had chloride values greater than 60 mmol/l (Grice et al., 1975). The range of ionic forearm sweat composition in meq/l was measured as: Na = 10 to 146; K = 2.7 to 10; Ca = 0.41 to 12.4; Mg = 0.03 to 0.58; and Cl = 16 to 100 (Verde et al., 1982).

The range of chloride ion concentration in thermally induced sweat measured from 5 to 148 meq/l (Robinson and Robinson, 1954). Sodium content in thermally induced sweat of normal women, collected on filter paper, is of isotonic concentration, and is the same as that seen in men (Brown and Dobson, 1967). Mean body sweat induced through exercise contained 24.2 $\pm$ 2.2 meq/l chloride ion in men, and 26.0 $\pm$ 4.6 in women (Yousef and Dill, 1974). Sodium and potassium content of pharmacologically stimulated sweat in men (pilocarpine, methylcholine, and acetylcholine) was seen to be higher than that measured in thermal sweat: mean values (in meq/l) are 8.3 $\pm$ 0.66 and 4.9 $\pm$ 0.17, respectively (Sato et al., 1970).

Elevated concentrations of sodium in sweat are considered diagnostic for CF, a pulmonary obstructive disease due to a genetic defect. While differences in electrolyte concentration are significant between healthy and CF patients at an early age, the standard diagnostic marker for that condition becomes blurry with advancing age. Kirk and Westwood arrived at a definition of less than 50 mmol/l as normal, 50 to 70 mmol/l as equivocal, and greater than 70 mmol/l as abnormal. They determined values in prepubertal children to verify the relevance of such data: sodium levels induced by pilocarpine iontophoresis in children without cystic fibrosis (n = 595) rose from mean values of 23.0 mmol/l in babies below 4 months in age, to 41.3 in children aged 6 to 11 years (Kirk and Westwood, 1989). Environmental (nutritional) deprivation in children (n = 5; age 1 to 6) leads to elevated electrolyte levels (Na, K, and Cl) in sweat. They rapidly return to normal levels upon return to a normal diet; this may also serve as a caveat in diagnosing CF in infants (Christoffel et al., 1985). Further, for diagnostic purposes it must be ascertained that sweat collected is indeed from eccrine sweat glands. Sebaceous sweat glands outnumber eccrine glands on the forehead; at other sites such as the forearm the inverse ratio holds true. Experimental method for obtaining so-called pure (or eccrine) sweat has been described (Sens et al., 1985).

Sweat osmolality values in normal adults were seen to increase with increasing age. Range/mean (SD) values for men are 49 to 151/117 mmol/kg (33.4) and for women 66 to 187/134 mmol/kg (38.6). An increase in osmolality was observed to increase in tandem with the (normal) increase in sodium concentration in sweat on aging (Willing and Gamlen, 1987).

The main cause for corrosion of metal surfaces from skin contact in individuals referred to as "rusters" is not due to elevated electrolyte concentration, as generally assumed, but rather seems to coincide with palmar hyperhydrosis. When the sodium concentration measured in normal subjects was compared to that of "rusters," no significant difference could be observed (mean values of 49.6 versus 49.1 meq/l, respectively) (Jensen and Nielsen, 1979).

Mean ion concentrations in sweat collected from normal subjects (n = 10) upon iontophoretic stimulation with pilocarpine were compared with values from patients (n = 22) with chronic renal failure (Table 3.2) (Prompt et al., 1978). Predialysis concentrations of Ca, Mg, and phosphate from patients were significantly elevated when compared with controls (p = 0.05), while concentrations of Na, K, and Cl were equal to normal values.

Differences in sweat composition between sweat induced by thermal stress and physical exercise were determined in seven healthy male volunteers (Fukumoto, et al., 1988).

TABLE 3.2
Ion Concentrations in Sweat (Normal vs. Renal Failure)

	Controls	Predialysis
Na	46.1 ± 24.5 mM	34.2 ± 17.1 mM
K	11.5 ± 4.7 mM	14.9 ± 6.6 mM
Cl	45.6 ± 24.5 mM	33.9 ± 17.2 mM
Mg	0.10 ± 0.09 mM	0.31 ± 0.11 mM
Ca	0.45 ± 0.08 mM	0.90 ± 0.39 mM
PO_4, × 10^{-2}	5.7 ± 3.3 mM	8.0 ± 3.0 mM
Urea	13.9 ± 6.0 mM	66 ± 31.1 mM

3.2.2.2 Amino Acids

Proteins and amino acids (AAs) are normal components of mammalian sweat. Quantitative analysis for AAs has become facile thanks to ion-exchange chromatography. The data documented for man differ significantly, however, probably due to differences in the stimulation methods applied, to regional differences in anatomical site, or to the sampling methods used. Substantial variations were observed in relative concentrations of AAs in sweat collected from various body parts. AAs excreted in sweat are independent of dietary intake (Hier et al., 1946), although their concentrations increase markedly in blood and urine on oral protein intake. No differences in AA patterns are seen between young and middle-aged adults, or between men and women (Coltman et al., 1966). In contrast to essential elements, AAs are neither selectively excreted nor reabsorbed (Gitlitz et al., 1974).

In skin washings from forehead and both arms of three males and two females, the acids occurred in the free state in significantly greater amounts than do proteins, at 97 versus 3%. At rest, the presence of virtually all essential AAs has been determined there, detected in an approximate total amount of 72 mg/m²/h at 40°C thermal stimulation (McEwan Jenkinson et al., 1974). Large individual differences occur in AA composition between eccrine forearm sweat from men under controlled exercise conditions. Comparison of AA excretions analyzed in sweat and urine by ion exchange chromatography shows comparable losses in those two media. As a rule, AA concentrations are considerably higher in the exercise sweat of trained men than in the sweat of untrained men determined by thermal and physiological stimulation. Total average AA values collected from 20 untrained men and 20 trained men) were 12,797 and 24,855 μmol/l, respectively. Highest values were seen for serine (3954/7782), glycine (2239/4392), alanine (1559/3029), and threonine (1057/1856) (Liappis et al., 1979).

3.2.2.3 Proteins

It has become possible to analyze sweat for qualitative and quantitative protein content on a sub-picogram level by several techniques: agarose-gel isotachaphoresis (McEwan Jenkinson et al., 1974; Uyttendaele et al., 1977), two-dimensional polyacrylamide gel electrophoresis, or isoelectric focusing (Rubin and Penneys, 1983; Sens et al., 1985). Thus the occurrence of over 400 polypeptide components in the molecular weight range of 10,000 to 70,000 has been revealed in eccrine sweat (Marshall, 1984). Departure from the norm and variations in peptide patterns thus detectable are a valuable assist in the diagnosis of pathological conditions such as CF, renal failure, and diabetes. The main protein components of sweat have been tentatively identified as serum albumin and alpha-1-antitrypsin, present in roughly equal amounts (Rubin and Penneys, 1983). While isolation and quantitative analysis in absolute terms are not possible, the identity and relative abundance of macromolecules in sweat are determined by analogy based on molecular weight, isoelectric point, and multiple-charge characteristics. Protein material in human skin washings accounts for about 3% of amino acids, and the mean output from forehead and arms at rest was determined at 1.44 mg/m²/h at 15°C and 2.28 mg/m²/h at 40°C (McEwan Jenkinson et al., 1974).

TABLE 3.3
Sweat Composition under Thermal and Exercise Stress

	Thermal	Exercise
Na (meq/l)	84 ± 31	123 ± 33
K (meq/l)	14 ± 4	11 ± 3
Cl (meq/l)	67 ± 31	104 ± 31

By pattern recognition in proteinograms it was demonstrated that proteins in sweat are sex-specific. Thus isoelectric focusing demonstrated that the proteins present in sweat samples from adult males are absent in sweat from females or prepubertal males, and that samples from different healthy females have identical sweat protein composition regardless of age and sexual maturity (Sens et al., 1985).

Total nitrogen content of sweat varies with variations in nitrogen content in the diet (Ashworth and Harrower, 1967).

3.2.2.4 Lactate and Pyruvate

Lactate is the major organic compound secreted in sweat. At rest and low sweating rates, lactate concentrations are 30 to 40 mmol/l; at higher sweat levels they are 10 to 15 mmol/l. During passive heat tests and also during exercise, lactate concentration decreases with increasing sweating rate, while it remains constant in blood. Differences in the excretion of lactate were also observed in function of physical fitness of three male volunteers: Mean value for the sedentary individual was 21.71 ± 0.85 mM, for the fit individual 16.75 ± 0.99, and for the very fit individual 12.75 ± 0.50 mM (Fellmann et al., 1983).

In contrast, pyruvic acid (pyruvate) concentrations in sweat are very low, found to vary between 0.1 and 1.2 µmol/l. The ratio of the two metabolites, lactate and pyruvate, increases even further with rising heart rate (Pilardeau et al., 1988).

3.2.2.5 Trace Metals

Human studies conducted at sustained elevated temperatures (thermal stimulation) underscore the significance of sweat secretion to essential trace element balance, as extreme losses of Na, K, Mg, and Fe can result (Consolazio et al., 1963). The average sodium content is 60 mM and that of potassium 8 mM, but these values fluctuate significantly as a function of sweat rate, hormonal control, diet (Dobson and Sato, 1972), and, particularly in the case of sodium, their reabsorption (Cage and Dobson, 1965). Also for zinc and copper, sweat can be a critical excretory pathway, possibly resulting in significant depletion leading to adverse acute or even chronic manifestations such as heat stroke and iron deficiency anemia, respectively. Whole body sweat collected during a 90-min exercise period from six male and three female volunteers by the whole body washdown technique was analyzed for trace metal concentration by atomic absorption spectroscopy (Cohn and Emmett, 1978). The mean values by gender are in Table 3.4.

TABLE 3.4
Gender Difference in Exercise Sweats

Element	Males (n = 6)	Females (n = 3)
Zn (μg/l)	960	507
Cu (μg/l)	1427	1533
Fe (μg/l)	630	163
Ni (μg/l)	57	57
Pb (μg/l)	62	53
Mn (μg/l)	23	17
Na (meq/l)	11.5	21.8
Cl (meq/l)	7.6	19.2

For nickel the concentration in sweat was higher than that in urine; for lead it was approximately equivalent.

3.3 THE ACID MANTLE OF THE SKIN (SEBUM)

Human skin features an acid mantle of pH 4 to 6 at the surface of the SC, which increases with depth to pH 7 at the juncture with live tissue (Öhman and Vahlquist, 1998). Determinants of this pH are protons, which gradually reach the surface of the skin, originating in the epidermis or as products of sebaceous gland activity. They stem from three classes of compounds:

- Amino acids, e.g., urocanic acid, pyrrolidone carboxylic acid
- Alpha-hydroxy acids, e.g., lactic and butyric acid, also present in sweat
- Acidic lipids, e.g., cholesteryl sulfate and free fatty acids, primarily oleic and linoleic (Elias, 1983; Lampe et al., 1983; Schurer and Elias, 1991).

At its point of origin, in the viable epidermis, sebum as secreted by the sebaceous glands is a complex mixture of lipids consisting of glycerides but no free fatty acids.

The occurrence of free acids in the SC and on the skin surface is the result of hydrolysis of phospholipids and glycerides by lipolytic enzymes occurring in the sebaceous ducts and on the skin surface, and of bacterial decomposition. On the skin surface, lipids of epidermal origin contain up to 20% free fatty acids; lipids originating in the pilosebaceous glands contain 16% (Schurer and Elias, 1991). They consist for the greater part of C16 and C18 acids, but their full range reaches from C5 to C22, with an average length of C16. Such an acid milieu plays a regulating role for SC homeostasis with relevance to the integrity of the barrier function and regeneration of the SC barrier (Feingold, 1991). It is widely believed that the acid environment on the skin surface both controls moisture loss from the epidermis and protects the skin from fungal and bacterial infection.

These acid components making up the sebum play an important role in solubilizing ("corroding") metal surfaces in amounts apparently sufficient to elicit an allergic reaction when nickel-containing alloys contact the skin of sensitive individuals (Roth-man, 1930; Preininger, 1934; Menné and Maibach, 1987; Menné and Solgaard, 1979).

3.4   DIFFUSION OF NICKEL IN CONTACT WITH THE SKIN

The tape-stripping assay is used to detect xenobiotics present on the skin or diffusing into the skin (Pinkus, 1951; Rougier et al., 1986). Such sequential tape stripping was implemented on healthy volunteers to investigate the diffusion of nickel through human SC *in vivo* following occlusive application of the metal as finely divided powder on the volar forearm.

Exposure sites were stripped 20 times at intervals from 5 min to 96 h post-dosing and the strips analyzed for metal content by inductively coupled plasma mass spectroscopy.

The gradients of nickel distribution profiles increase proportionally with occlu-sion time, but level off with increasing depth after the tenth strip, to continue at constant levels to the twentieth strip.

Total nickel removed with 20 SC strips to the level of the glistening layer after maximum occlusion of 96 h was 41.6 $\mu g/cm^2$ (average, n = 3). In order to normalize the nickel depth distribution profiles obtained, SC removed by stripping of untreated skin after occlusion was determined by weighing. Following application of nickel dust over 24 h, analysis of the twentieth strip still indicates nickel present at 1.42 $\mu g/cm^2$ (± 0.68; average, n = 3). This serves to demonstrate that, in contact with skin, nickel metal is oxidized to form lipophilic, SC-diffusible compounds that penetrate via the intracellular route. This appears to be a contributing factor in the elicitation of allergic reactions (Hostýnek et al., 2001).

3.5   RELEASE OF NICKEL IN SYNTHETIC SWEAT

Leaching or release of nickel ion from metal objects in contact with sweat is a continuous variable that defeats prediction. Aside from immediate environmental factors, the microenvironment within the particular alloy in contact with a conducting medium is a principal determinant, due to the action of electromotive forces gener-ated by the presence of a multitude of possible accompanying metals (Cavelier et al., 1985). Review of published data on corrosion rates by Lidén et al. (1998) shows that release rates do not correlate with nickel content. That study also concluded that the wear and corrosion test adopted as directive in the European Union is suited for articles of personal adornment (jewelry, clothing fasteners, etc.), but may not be adequate for hand-held nickel-containing tools.

Other metals in immediate proximity with nickel form a galvanic element (or pile), whereby an electron current flows from the more electro-negative to the more electro-positive one, resulting in oxidation or solution ("corrosion") of the more electro-negative metal.

The most frequently used synthetic sweat formulations used experimentally are given in Table 3.5.

TABLE 3.5
Synthetic Sweat Formulations

Author	Formula
Bang Pedersen et al., 1974	0.5% NaCl
	0.1% lactic acid
	0.1% urea
	pH 6.5 (NH$_4$OH)
Hemingway and Molokhia, 1987	0.3% NaCl
	0.1% NaSO$_4$
	0.2% urea
	0.2% lactic acid
	0.19% glycerol trioleate
	0.01% Na oleate
	0.019% glycerol tristearate
	0.01% Na stearate

The amount of nickel liberated from metal objects immersed in synthetic sweat has been determined in several model experiments (Table 3.6).

Analysis of new and used articles of personal adornment in particular showed that they all released nickel to some degree upon a 1-week storage in synthetic sweat, and neither gold nor silver plating prevented this. Release ranged between 0.005 and 442 µg nickel (Fischer et al., 1984).

3.6 CONCLUSIONS

Definition, and thereby reconstitution of human sweat in absolute terms is not feasible because of variability in its composition and pH. Gender differences are marked, and even in normal and healthy subjects fluctuations occur due to environmental as well as subjective, endocrine factors.

TABLE 3.6
Nickel Release from Metal Objects in Synthetic Sweat

Reference	Object	Nickel Released
Bang Pedersen et al., 1974	Coins	96–137 µg
Emmett et al., 1988	Earrings	1.6–103 µg/cm^2
Fischer et al., 1984	White gold	0.09–0.82 µg
Haudrechy et al., 1994	Ni metal/steel	0.03–100 µg
Hemingway and Molokhia, 1987	Wire	2×10^{-6}–10^{-4} mg/cm^2/min
Kanerva et al., 1994	Jewelry	<0.5–435 µg/cm^2/wk
Menné and Solgaard, 1979	Buttons	<0.5–7µg
	Coins	409–691 µg
Santucci et al., 1989	Clips	49–103 µg

Most striking are changes in sweat composition due to the rate of sweat secretion. Sodium and chloride content, one decisive factor in the corrosivity of sweat, is as low as 5 meq/l under quiescent conditions, due to the reabsorption (conservation) mechanism. As sweating rate increases, that control mechanism is overwhelmed and the sodium concentration can rise to approximate that occurring in plasma.

Conversely, other significant components of sweat — urea, lactic acid, and potassium ions — increase at high rates of secretion, and their concentrations can reach the levels of plasma.

Most publications reflect state-of-the-art analytical science and cutaneous biology at the time written. Repetition with current analytical technology detecting ppb levels, larger cohorts, special populations (race, age, gender, etc.) and current biology should provide refinement. This validation can and should be pursued.

Possible future studies could include:

- Analytical chemistry; as noted above, current methods would refine the data, at the ppb level
- Comparison of artificial and "natural" sweat in leaching properties
- Inadequate validation exists to document that artificial sweat will mimic the more complex natural sweat in leaching and other studies
- Dose of nickel on and through skin

The interest in sweat in nickel toxicology relates to sweat's ability to solubilize nickel from alloys and permit entry of the ion into the stratum corneum. This field was largely theoretical because of the lack in technology to relate this directly to flux. There is now analytical and tape strip technology to define surface dose at the ppb level. This information should be merged with previous studies.

Recently evolved technology combined with improvements in quantitative chemistry of nickel will permit fundamental refinement and possibly provide new insights into the role of eccrine sweat in human percutaneous penetration.

3.7 ACKNOWLEDGMENT

We gratefully acknowledge the financial support by the Nickel Producers Environmental Research Association (NiPERA) toward this review project.

REFERENCES

Ashworth, A. and Harrower, A.D.B., Protein requirements in tropical countries: nitrogen losses in sweat and their relation to nitrogen balance, *Br. J. Nutr.*, 21, 833–839, 1967.

Bang Pedersen et al., Release of nickel from silver coins, *Acta Derm.Venereol. (Stockh.)*, 54, 231–234, 1974.

Beck, R. et al., Malnutrition: a cause of elevated sweat chloride concentration, *Acta Paed. Scand.*, 75, 639–644, 1986.

Brown, G. and Dobson, R.L., Sweat sodium excretion in normal women, *J. Appl. Physiol.*, 23, 97–99, 1967.

Buckley, W.R. and Lewis, C.E., The "ruster" in industry, *J. Occup. Med.*, 2, 23–31, 1960.

Bulmer, F.M.R. and Mackenzie, E.A., Studies in the control and treatment of nickel rash, *J. Ind. Hyg.*, 8, 517–527, 1926.

Cage, G.W. and Dobson, R.L., Sodium secretion and reabsorption in the human eccrine sweat gland, *J. Clin. Invest.*, 44, 1270–1276, 1965.

Cavelier, C., Foussereau, J., and Massin, M., Nickel allergy: analysis of metal clothing objects and patch testing to metal samples, *Contact Dermatitis,* 12, 65–75, 1985.

Chashschin, V.P., Artunina, G.P., and Norseth, T., Congenital defects, abortion and other health effects in nickel refinery workers, *Sci. Tot. Environ.*, 148, 287–291, 1994.

Christoffel, K.S. et al., Environmental deprivation and transient elevation of sweat electrolytes, *J. Pediatr.*, 107, 231–234, 1985.

Cohn, J.R. and Emmett, E.A., The excretion of trace metals in human sweat, *Ann. Clin. Lab. Sci.*, 8, 270–275, 1978.

Coltman, C.A., Rowe, N.J., and Atwell, R.J., The amino acid content of sweat in normal adults, *J. Clin. Nutr.*, 18, 373, 1966.

Consolazio, C.F. et al., Excretion of sodium, potassium, magnesium and iron in human sweat and the relation of each to balance and requirements, *J. Nutr.*, 79, 407–415, 1963.

Costa, F., Howes Calloway, D., and Margen, S., Regional and total body sweat composition of men fed controlled diets, *Am. J. Clin. Nutr.*, 22, 52–58, 1969.

Davis, P.A. et al., Sweat chloride concentration in adults with pulmonary diseases, *Am. Rev. Resp. Dis.*, 128, 34–37, 1983.

Dobson, R.L. and Sato, K., The secretion of salt and water by the eccrine sweat gland, *Arch. Dermatol.*, 105, 366–370, 1972.

Elias, P., Epidermal lipids, barrier function, and desquamation, *J. Invest. Dermatol.*, 80, 44s–49s, 1983.

Emmett, E.A. et al., Allergic contact dermatitis to nickel: bioavailability from consumer products and provocation threshold, *J. Am. Acad. Dermatol.*, 19, 314–322, 1988.

Feingold, K.R., The regulation of epidermal lipid synthesis by permeability barrier requirements, *Crit. Rev. Ther. Drug Carrier Syst.*, 8, 193–210, 1991.

Fellmann, N., Grizard, G., and Coudert, J., Human frontal sweat rate and lactate concentration during heat exposure and exercise, *J. Appl. Physiol.*, 54, 355–360, 1983.

Fischer, T. et al., Nickel release from ear piercing kits and earrings, *Contact Dermatitis*, 10, 39–42, 1984.

Fukumoto, T. et al., Differences in composition of sweat induced by thermal exposure and by running exercise, *Clin. Cardiol.*, 11, 707–709, 1988.

Fullerton, A. and Hoelgaard, A., Binding of nickel to human epidermis in vitro, *Br. J. Dermatol.*, 119, 675–682, 1988.

Gitlitz, P.H., Sunderman, F.W., and Hohnadel, D.C., Ion-exchange chromatography of amino acids in sweat collected from healthy subjects during sauna bathing, *Clin. Chem.*, 20, 1305–1312, 1974.

Gollhausen, R. and Ring, J., Allergy to coined money: nickel contact dermatitis in cashiers, *J. Am. Acad. Dermatol.*, 25, 365–369, 1991.

Grice, K. et al., An evaluation of Na, Cl and pH ion-specific electrodes in the study of the electrolyte contents of epidermal transudate and sweat, *Br. J. Dermatol.*, 92, 511–518, 1975.

Haudrechy, P. et al., Nickel release from nickel-plated metals and stainless steel, *Contact Dermatitis*, 31, 249–255, 1994.

Hemingway, J. D. and Molokhia, M.M., The dissolution of metallic nickel in artificial sweat, *Contact Dermatitis*, 16, 99–105, 1987.

Hier, S.W., Cornbleet, T., and Bergheim, O., The amino acids of human sweat, *J. Biol. Chem.*, 166, 327, 1946.

Jensen, O. and Nielsen, E., "Rusters" The corrosive action of palmar sweat: 2 physical and chemical factors in palmar hyperhidrosis, *Acta Derm. Venereol.*, 59, 139, 1979.

Kanerva, L. et al., Nickel release from metals, and a case of allergic contact dermatitis from stainless steel, *Contact Dermatitis*, 31, 299–303, 1994.

Kirk, J. M. and Westwood, A., Interpretation of sweat sodium results — the effect of patient age, *Ann. Clin. Biochem.*, 26, 38–43, 1989.

Lampe, M.A. et al., Human stratum corneum lipids: characterization and regional variations, *J. Lipid Res.*, 24, 120–130, 1983.

Liappis, N. et al., Quantitative study of free amino acids in human eccrine sweat excreted from the forearms of healthy trained and untried men during exercise, *Eur. J. Appl. Physiol.*, 42, 227–234, 1979.

Lidén, C. et al., Nickel release from tools on the Swedish market, *Contact Dermatitis*, 39, 127–131, 1998.

Marshall, T., Analysis of human sweat proteins by two-dimensional electrophoresis and ultrasensitive silver staining., *Anal. Biochem.*, 139, 506–509, 1984.

McEwan Jenkinson, D., Mabon, R.M., and Manson, W., Sweat proteins, *Br. J. Dermatol.*, 90, 175–181, 1974.

Menné, T. and Solgaard, P., Temperature-dependent nickel release from nickel alloys, *Contact Dermatitis*, 5, 82–84, 1979.

Menné, T. and Maibach, H.I., Reactions to systemic exposure to contact allergens: systemic contact allergy reactions (SCAR), *Immunol. Allergy Pract.*, 9, 373–385, 1987.

Morris, E.R., Iron. II. Iron metabolism, in *Trace Elements in Human and Animal Nutrition*, Vol. 1, Mertz, W., Ed., Academic Press, New York, 1987, pp. 91–108.

Öhman, H. and Vahlquist, A., The pH gradient over the stratum corneum differs in X-linked recessive and autosomal dominant ichthyosis: a clue to the molecular origin of the "Acid Skin Mantle," *J. Invest. Dermatol.*, 111, 674–677, 1998.

Pilardeau, P.A. et al., Effect of different work-loads on sweat production and composition in man, *J. Sports Med. Phys. Fitness*, 28, 247–252, 1988.

Pinkus, H., Examination of the epidermis by the strip method of removing horny layers. I. Observation on thickness of the horny layer, and on mitotic activity after stripping, *J. Invest. Dermatol.*, 383–386, 1951.

Preininger, T., Überempfindlichkeit gegen Nickelgeld, *Dermatol. Wochenschr.*, 99, 1082–1084, 1934.

Prompt, C.A., Quinton, P.M., and Kleeman, C.R., High concentrations of sweat calcium, magnesium and phosphate in chronic renal failure, *Nephron*, 20, 4–9, 1978.

Rasetti, L., Cappellaro, F., and Gaido, P., Contribution to the study of saturnism by inhibited oils, *Rass. Med. Ind. Igiene Lavoro*, 30, 71–75, 1961.

Robinson, S. and Robinson, A.H., Chemical composition of sweat, *Physiol. Rev.*, 34, 202–209, 1954.

Rothman, S., Überempfindlichkeit gegen Hartgeld, *Dermatol. Wochenschr.*, 90, 98–99, 1930.

Rougier, A. et al., Regional variation in percutaneous absorption in man: measurement by the stripping method, *Arch. Dermatol. Res.*, 278, 465–469, 1986.

Rubin, R.W. and Penneys, N.S., Subpicogram analysis of sweat proteins using two-dimensional polyacrylamide gel electrophoresis, *Anal. Biochem.*, 131, 520–524, 1983.

Samitz, M.H. and Pomerantz, H., Studies of the effects on the skin of nickel and chromium salts, *AMA Arch. Ind. Health*, 18, 473–479, 1958.

Samitz, M.H. and Katz, S.A., Nickel–epidermal interactions: diffusion and binding, *Environ. Res.*, 11, 34–39, 1976.

Santucci, B. et al., Nickel dermatitis from cheap earrings, *Contact Dermatitis*, 21, 245–248, 1989.

Sato, K., Feibleman, C., and Dobson, R.L., The electrolyte composition of pharmacologically and thermally stimulated sweat: a comparative study, *J. Inv. Dermatol.*, 55, 433–438, 1970.

Schurer, N.Y. and Elias, P.M., The biochemistry and function of stratum corneum lipids, *Adv. Lipid Res.*, 24, 27–56, 1991.

Sekelj, P. et al., Survey of electrolytes of unstimulated sweat from the hand in normal and diseased adults, *Am. Rev. Resp. Disease*, 108, 603–609, 1973.

Sens, D.A., Simmons, M.A., and Spicer, S.S., The analysis of human sweat proteins by isoelectric focusing. I. Sweat collection utilizing the Macroduct® system demonstrates the presence of previously unrecognized sex-related proteins, *Pediatr. Res.*, 19, 873–878, 1985.

Stoner, H.B., Toxicity of triphenyltin, *Br. J. Ind. Med.*, 23, 222–229, 1966.

Suzuki, T., Study on dermal excretion of metallic elements (Na, K, Ca, Mg, Fe, Mn, Zn, Cu, Cd, Pb), in *Proceedings of the Tenth International Congress of Nutrition, August 3–9, 1975, Kyoto, Japan*, Kyoto: International Congress of Nutrition, 1976, pp. 568–.

Toribara, T.Y., Clarkson, T.W., and Nierenberg, D.W., Chemical safety: more on working with dimethylmercury, *C. and E. News*, 75, 6, 1997.

Uyttendaele, K. et al., Analysis of the proteins in sweat and urine by agarose-gel isotachophoresis, *J. Chromatogr.*, 132, 261–266, 1977.

Verde, T. et al., Sweat composition in exercise and in heat, *J. Appl. Physiol.*, 53, 1540–1545, 1982.

Willing, S.K. and Gamlen, T.R., Sweat osmolality values in normal adults, *Clin. Chem.*, 33, 612–613, 1987.

Yousef, M.K. and Dill, D.B., Sweat rate and concentration of chloride in hand and body sweat in desert walks: male and female, *J. Appl. Physiol.*, 36, 82–85, 1974.

4 Release of Nickel Ion from the Metal and Its Alloys as Cause of Nickel Allergy

Jurij J. Hostýnek, Katherine E. Reagan, and Howard I. Maibach

CONTENTS

Abstract 100
4.1   Introduction 100
4.2   Analytical Methods for Nickel Detection 112
    4.2.1   Chemical Methods 112
        4.2.1.1   Dimethylglyoxime Spot Test 112
        4.2.1.2   Nitric Acid Spot Test 112
    4.2.2   Physical Methods 113
        4.2.2.1   Inductively Coupled Plasma-Atomic
                     Emission Spectroscopy (ICP-AES) 113
        4.2.2.2   Inductively Coupled Plasma-Mass
                     Spectrometry (ICP-MS) 113
        4.2.2.3   Atomic Absorption Spectrophotometry (AAS) 114
        4.2.2.4   Particle Induced X-Ray Emission (PIXE) 114
4.3   *In Vitro* Release of Nickel in Artificial Sweat and Other
    Physiologic Media.. 114
    4.3.1   Leaching Experiments Done on Metallic Objects
        Containing Nickel 116
4.4   Safe Limits of Exposure: Danish and European Union
    Nickel Legislation 120
4.5   *In Vivo* Nickel Release and Its Clinical Effects by Type of Exposure 121
    4.5.1   Skin Contact.. 121
    4.5.2   Pierced Skin: Systemic Induction of Nickel Allergy...................... 123
    4.5.3   Orthodontic Devices.. 124
    4.5.4   Orthopedic Implants.. 130
    4.5.5   Gastrointestinal Exposure 133
4.6   Discussion 135
4.7   Acknowledgment.. 137
References.. 137

ABSTRACT

We have reviewed the release of nickel ion from the metal or its alloys in contact with sweat and other potentially corrosive artificial or physiological media; the effects that can have on the human organism; methods of nickel analysis; and recommended limits of exposure, designed to avoid further, inadvertent sensitization among the population. In the endeavor to identify the most likely sources of nickel with which people come in contact, and through which they are likely to acquire nickel sensitivity, researchers have examined a variety of nickel-containing alloys and articles such as jewelry, medical devices, tools, and coins to determine release of nickel ion. For that purpose the materials were immersed in blood, serum, artificial sweat, or physiological saline, and the media analyzed for resulting nickel content. Their data show that a number of the alloys and consumer items tested release amounts of nickel sufficient to elicit allergic reactions in those sensitized, if not induce nickel allergic hypersensitivity (NAH) in the naive organism. The most corrosive of the media tested proved to be those that contain proteins, serum being the most aggressive. Protection through plating with noble metals proves to be only partially effective in preventing nickel ion release, due to imperfections in surface coating. Such plating of the nickel interliner in jewelry may wear off with use, exposing the base metal matrix to chemical attack. The proximity of nickel to other metals creates a local galvanic element that promotes nickel ion release in a corrosive environment, and degree of sulfurization of stainless steel also has a significant effect on such release. Piercing of the earlobes, which amounts to systemic exposure, seems to be the main etiological factor leading to high prevalence of NAH among the young. The increasing use of nickel-releasing alloys in orthodontic appliances and orthopedic implants, on the other hand, constitutes only a minor factor in the incidence of NAH in the population, and exposure of the young, naive organism to low-level, slow release of nickel ion appears to have a tolerizing effect.

4.1 INTRODUCTION

Due to its metallurgical characteristics, nickel is a component of most alloys used in metal objects with which people come into frequent contact: articles of common everyday use, as well as medical devices designed for prolonged, intimate contact with live tissue. According to epidemiologic studies, three types of exposure can be considered the principal etiological factors leading to primary (induction) or secondary (elicitation) nickel sensitivity:

- Intimate and prolonged skin contact with nickel-releasing costume jewelry, particularly when piercing of the skin is involved for the sake of embellishment with articles made of nickel-releasing metal, which may also constitute systemic sensitization as the key inductive effect
- Sustained and habitual contact with nickel-releasing metal objects, particularly if the skin is chronically irritated by exposure to harsh chemicals, as it occurs in the occupational setting
- Exposure of the organism to nickel releasing orthopedic devices, such as prostheses or pace makers

Nickel thus continues in the role of premier contact allergen in industrialized societies. While survey of the general population indicates the level of sensitization (sometimes expressed as metal intolerance) to be around 10% among women and 3% among men (Bangha and Elsner, 1996; Marks et al., 1998; Sertoli et al., 1999), a good part of those tested do not exhibit clinical signs of allergy, and such prevalence is not obvious. Many patch test positive patients can tolerate low nickel exposures, presumably due to either low bioavailability or low sensitization levels (Kieffer, 1979; Andersen et al., 1993).

Test results from dermatology clinics on patients with dermatitis, however, document higher levels. Incidence of NAH among those patients can run as high as 17.6% among women and 11.7% among men (Dickel et al., 1998).

When skin, mucous membranes (e.g., oral exposure), or live tissue (e.g., ear piercing) come in contact with nickel metal or nickel-containing alloys, nickel ions are released through the natural process of oxidation (corrosion), with the potential to penetrate the organism. The free nickel ions bear the risk of primary sensitization of a naive organism or elicitation of an immune reaction in a nickel-sensitized individual. Such a reaction can be:

- Immediate type, IgE-mediated skin, nasal and bronchial (type I, anaphilac-toid) reactions
- Delayed type, cell-mediated (type 4) reactions, manifest as allergic contact dermatitis or eczema
- Systemic allergic rections, to gastrointestinal, respiratory, parenteral, or implantation exposure, most commonly manifest as pompholyx
- Contact stomatitis or mucosal allergy: stomatitis, gingivitis, cheilitis, oral or lichenoid reactions, with episodic skin involvement

With the premier role of nickel as a sensitizer in industrialized countries, and the increasing prevalence of hypersensitivity among the occupational and general populations, an ongoing research effort into the causes leading to this public health problem and the possible methods of prevention has resulted in a large volume of scientific publications. The connection between cause and effect, the many aspects of morbidity, and the deeper immunological mechanisms involved have been addressed there.

The purpose of this review is to present a comprehensive picture of the literature published since the various aspects associated with exposure to nickel were reviewed by Maibach and Menné (1989). The present review focuses primarily on the aspects of mobilization of nickel in various physiological media and the effects that it can have on humans. Derived from metal alloys as they are encountered in tools, medical devices, everyday objects of use, and personal adornment, nickel ions potentially become biologically available. Also discussed are methods of analysis and recommended limits of exposure designed to avoid further, inadvertent sensitization among the population.

Data on nickel release are presented in Table 4.1.

TABLE 4.1
Release Rates of Nickel in Various Media, Including Synthetic Sweat

Author	Medium	Article	Nickel Leached	Comments
Bang Pedersen et al., 1974	Synthetic sweat: 0.1% Lactic acid 0.1% Urea pH 6.5 (NH$_4$OH)	Coins	96–137 µg/coin	24 h; ambient temp.
	Distilled water	Coins	15–49 µg/coin	do.
	Distilled water/sweat	Alloys	5 µg	do., 11.2 cm^2
Samitz and Katz, 1975	Physiologic saline	Prosthetic materials	10–98 ppm	20–22°C
		AISI 303	11 ppm	(1 ppm = 10 µg)
		AISI 316	<1 ppm	
	Sweat***	Prosthetic materials	<1–990 ppm	
		AISI 302	3 ppm	
		AISI 303	102 ppm	
		AISI 316	<1 ppm	
	Whole blood	AISI 316	<1 ppm	
		Prosth. materials	<1–174 ppm	
	Blood plasma	AISI 316	<1 ppm	
		Prosth. materials	10 ppm	
Katz and Samitz, 1975	Physiologic saline	Stainless steel objects	1.5–0.25 µg	7 days; r.t.
	1% Ivory® liquid		0.51–0.25 µg	
	1% Palmolive® liquid		0.48–1.19 µg	
	Synthetic sweat*		15.2–175 µg	
	Physiologic saline	Alloys	0–5.97 µg	2–10 cm^2
	1% Ivory liquid		0.37–41 µg	
	1% Palmolive liquid		0.33–1.00 µg	
	Synthetic Sweat*		1.8–51.1 µg	

Reference	Solution	Material	Amount	Conditions
Christensen and Möller, 1978	Physiologic saline	Coins	268–453 µg	2–10 cm²
	Synthetic sweat*		3348–5637 µg	
	Water	Stainless-steel saucepans		Boiling temp. 80 min, pH 3.2
		New	Mean 6.0 µg	pH 4–5
		New	Mean 12.4 µg	pH 2.3–3.5
		New	Mean 14.7 µg	pH 2–3
		Used	Mean 20.3 µg	pH 1.8–3.2
Menné and Solgaard, 1979	Synthetic sweat*	Danish kroner	409 µg/coin	24 h, 20°C
			691 µg/coin	24 h, 35°C
		Jeans buttons	<0.5–2.2 µg/button	24 h, 20°C
			<0.6–7.0 µg/button	24 h, 35°C
Brun, 1979	Water	Food preserves	0.05–1.5 mg/kg	1 h; boiling
		Stainless steel	0.15–1.7 mg/kg	
		Enamel	0.08–0.25 mg/kg	
		Stainless steel		
	Citric acid 0.1 M		0.33 mg/kg	
	Citric acid 0.01 M		0.05 mg/kg	
	Malic acid 0.1 M		0.25 mg/kg	
	Malic acid 0.01 M		Trace	
	Oxalic acid 0.1 M		9.5 mg/kg	
	Oxalic acid 0.01 M		3.2 mg/kg	
	Oxalic acid 0.001 M		Trace	
	Citric acid 0.1 M		0.08 mg/kg	
	Citric acid 0.01 M		Trace	

(continued)

TABLE 4.1 (CONTINUED)
Release Rates of Nickel in Various Media, Including Synthetic Sweat

Author	Medium	Article	Nickel Leached	Comments
	Malic acid 0.1 M		0.05 mg/kg	
	Malic acid 0.01 M		Trace	
	Oxalic acid 0.1 M		0.45 mg/kg	
	Oxalic acid 0.01 M		0.15	
	Oxalic acid 0.001 M		Trace	
Larsen and Brandrup, 1980	Synthetic sweat***	Buttons	<0.01–14.6 ppm/10 ml	24 h
Park and Shearer, 1983	0.05% NaCl	Stainless steel (AISI 304, AISI 303)		37°C
			40 µg	2 days
			125 µg ± 22	12 days
Fischer et al., 1984a	Synthetic sweat*	Earring studs and clasps		Room temp., 1 week pH 6.4
	Hypoallergenic	0.005 µg		
	Gold plated	0.04–25 µg		
	Silver plated	0.05–1.0 µg		
	Stainless	0.05–19 µg		
	Earring studs and clasps, unused			
	Stainless	0.06 µg		
	Gold plated	2.6–7.5 µg		
	Silver plated	0.05–0.1 µg		
Fischer et al., 1984b	Synthetic sweat*	White-gold discs	0.09–0.82 µg	Room temp., 1 week pH 6.4
		Rh plated discs	0.04–0.54 µg	30°C, 6 weeks pH 6.5
Menné et al., 1987a	Synthetic sweat*	Dermatitis-causing earrings		
		Safe alloys		

Reference	Solution	Material	Release	Conditions
Hemingway and Molokhia, 1987	Synthetic sweat:	Stainless	0.01 µg	
	0.3% NaCl	White gold	0.02 µg	
	0.1% NaSO$_4$	Ni-tin	0.1 µg	
	0.2% Urea	Sensitizing alloys		
	0.2% Lactic acid	Nickel-silver	20 µg	
	0.19% Glycerol trioleate	Ni-iron	65 µg	
	0.01% Na oleate	Ni, chemical	32 µg	
	0.019% Glycerol tristearate	Ni, chemical	40 µg	
	0.01% Na stearate	Ni, chemical	45 µg	
		Ni wire	1 µg/cm^2/150 min	30°C, pH 4.05
		Ni wire	3 µg/cm^2/150 min	30°C, pH 4.48
		Ni wire	12 µg/cm^2/150 min	30°C, pH 5.7
Emmett et al., 1988	Human plasma	Earrings	0.99 µg/cm^2	37°C, 2 days
			279 µg/cm^2	37°C, 7 days
	Physiologic saline		3.95 µg/cm^2	37°C, 2 days
			44 µg/cm^2	37°C, 7 days
	Synthetic sweat*		1.6 µg/cm^2	37°C, 2 days, pH 5.3
			103 µg/cm^2	37°C, 7 days, pH 5.3
			3.95 µg/cm^2	37°C, 2 days, pH 6.6
			11 µg/cm^2	37°C, 7 days, pH 6.6
			1.75 µg/cm^2	37°C, 2 days, pH 7.8
			4 µg/cm^2	37°C, 7 days, pH 7.8

(continued)

TABLE 4.1 (CONTINUED)
Release Rates of Nickel in Various Media, Including Synthetic Sweat

Author	Medium	Article	Nickel Leached	Comments
Santucci et al., 1988	Synthetic sweat*	Earring clips and clasps	49–103 µg	23°C, av. of 12 h
Gjerdet et al., 1991	Saliva	Orthodontic appliances	67.6 ng/ml	In vivo, immediate
			7.8 ng/ml	In vivo, after 3-week delay
			8.2 ng/ml	In vivo, with no appliance
Grimsdottir et al., 1992a	Physiologic saline	Orthodontic appliances	ND - 10.4 µg	23°C, 14 days
			ND - 7.6 µg	23°C, 7 days
Räsänen et al., 1993	Human plasma	Ear piercers	0.03–104.59 $\mu g/cm^2$/week	37°C
Kanerva et al., 1994	Synthetic sweat*	Rivets	<0.1–95 $\mu g/cm^2$/week	30°C, 7 days
		Earrings	0.8–165 do.	
		Necklace	6.4–62 do.	
		Watchband	<0.1–3.1 do.	
		Ring	216–435 do.	
		Rivets	<0.1–33 $\mu g/cm^2$	2nd to 3rd week
		Earrings	0.5–65	
		Necklace	1.1–3.1	
		Watchband	<0.1–1.9	
		Ring	40–108	
		Rivets	<0.1–8.6 $\mu g/cm^2$	4th to 6th week
		Earrings	1.2–15	
		Necklace	2.5–15	
		Watchband	<0.1–0.9	
		Ring	17–96	

Reference	Medium	Material	Ni release	Conditions
Haudrechy et al., 1994	Synthetic sweat**	Ni plated stainless	100 µg/cm²/week	pH 4.5, room temp.
		Stainless steel	<0.3 µg/cm²/week	
		AISI 304	<0.3 µg/cm²/week	
		AISI 316L	<0.3 µg/cm²/week	
		AISI 430	<0.3 µg/cm²/week	
		AISI 303	1.5 µg/cm²/week	
Bumgardner and Lucas, 1994	95% Minimum ess. Medium + 5% Fetal bovine serum	Dental alloys		37°C, 24 h
		Ni metal	400 ppm	
		Neptune™	100 ppb	
		Rexalloy™	259 ppb	
		Regalloy T™	200 ppb	
		Vera Bond™	225 ppb	
Bumgardner and Lucas, 1995	95% Minimum ess. Medium + 5% Fetal bovine serum	Dental alloys		37°C, 24 h
		Ni metal	>324.1 ppm	
		Neptune	1 ppb	
		Rexalloy	253 ppb	
		Regalloy T	200 ppb	
		Vera Bond	225 ppb	
		Ni metal	324.1 ppm	37°C, 48 h
		Neptune	150 ppb	
		Rexalloy	290 ppb	
		Regalloy T	225 ppb	
		Vera Bond	260 ppb	
		Ni metal	324.1 ppm	37°C, 72 h
		Neptune	190 ppb	
		Rexalloy	340 ppm	
		Regalloy T	290 ppb	
		Vera Bond	310 ppb	

(continued)

TABLE 4.1 (CONTINUED)
Release Rates of Nickel in Various Media, Including Synthetic Sweat

Author	Medium	Article	Nickel Leached	Comments
Kerosuo et al., 1995	Physiologic saline	Orthodontic appliances	ND - 2 µg	Static conditions
			0–2.5 µg	2 h, 23°C
			0.5–2 µg	2–26 h
			17.1 µg	2–8 days
				8 days (fixed appls.)
			44.3 µg	Dyn. conditions
				8 days
Flint and Packirisamy, 1995	Water	Foodstuffs in new S30400 SS saucepans	ND - 8 µg	4 min–2 h
				Boiling temp.
Haudrechy et al., 1997	Synthetic sweat**	Stainless steel		Room temp.
		AISI 303	1.4 µg/cm²/week	pH 4.5
		AISI 303	0.3 µg/cm²/week	pH 6.6
		AISI 304	0.2 µg/cm²/week	pH 4.5
		AISI 304L	0.11 µg/cm²/week	pH 4.5
		AISI 304L	<0.09 µg/cm²/week	pH 6.6
		AISI 304L + Ca	<0.09 µg/cm²/week	pH 4.5
		AISI 304L + Ca	<0.09 µg/cm²/week	pH 6.6
		AISI 304L + Cu	<0.09 µg/cm²/week	pH 4.5
		AISI 304L + Cu	0.29 µg/cm²/week	pH 6.6
Cortada et al., 1997	Artificial saliva (g/l): K_2HPO_4 0.2 KCl 1.2 KSCN 0.33 N_2HPO_4 0.26	Cr–Ni alloy	50 ng/ml	37°C, 15 days, pH 6.7

Accominotti et al., 1998

NaCl 0.70
NaHCO$_3$ 1.50
Urea 1.50
Lactic acid to pH 6.7
Water

Menu #1 in:		
Glass	155 µg/kg	pH 8.7
Stainless steel 436	88 µg/kg	
Stainless steel 304	11.2 µg/kg	
do. - polished	131 µg/kg	
Menu #2 in:		
Glass	62 µg/kg	pH 7.5
Stainless steel 436	85 µg/kg	
Stainless steel 304	75 µg/kg	
do. - polished	65 µg/kg	
Menu #3 in:		
Glass	22 µg/kg	pH 7.5
Stainless steel 436	38 µg/kg	
Stainless steel 304	22 µg/kg	
do. - polished	24 µg/kg	
Menu #4 in:		
Glass	86 µg/kg	pH 8.5
Stainless steel 436	91 µg/kg	
Stainless steel 304	98 µg/kg	
do. - polished	78 µg/kg	
Menu #5 in:		
Glass	93 µg/kg	pH 8
Stainless steel 436	67 µg/kg	
Stainless steel 304	93 µg/kg	
do. - polished	84 µg/kg	

(continued)

TABLE 4.1 (CONTINUED)
Release Rates of Nickel in Various Media, Including Synthetic Sweat

Author	Medium	Article	Nickel Leached	Comments
		Menu #6 in:		
		Glass	20 µg/kg	pH 8
		Stainless steel 436	14 µg/kg	
		Stainless steel 304	21 µg/kg	
		do. - polished	18 µg/kg	
		Menu #7 in:		
		Glass	91 µg/kg	pH 8.5
		Stainless steel 436	65 µg/kg	
		Stainless steel 304	75 µg/kg	
		do. - polished	70 µg/kg	
		Menu #8 in:		
		Glass	16 µg/kg	pH 8
		Stainless steel 436	10 µg/kg	
		Stainless steel 304	18 µg/kg	
		do. - polished	19 µg/kg	
		Menu #9 in:		
		Glass	8 µg/kg	pH 7
		Stainless steel 436	17 µg/kg	
		Stainless steel 304	17 µg/kg	
		do. - polished	21 µg/kg	
		Menu #10 in:		
		Glass	28 µg/kg	pH 7.5
		Stainless steel 436	27 µg/kg	
		Stainless steel 304	33 µg/kg	
		do. - polished	17 µg/kg	

		pH 8
Menu #11 in:		
Glass	75 µg/kg	
Stainless steel 436	42 µg/kg	
Stainless steel 304	54 µg/kg	
do. - polished	43 µg/kg	
Tools	0.11–36 µg/cm^2/kg	
Synthetic sweat****		pH 6.5, 30°C, 1 week

Lidén et al., 1998

4.2 ANALYTICAL METHODS FOR NICKEL DETECTION

4.2.1 CHEMICAL METHODS

The most commonly used general procedures in analytical chemistry are based on colorimetry, whereby a metal is complexed with an organic molecule to yield a characteristic color.

4.2.1.1 Dimethylglyoxime Spot Test

The dimethylglyoxime (DMG) test is one such colorimetric method commonly used in analytical inorganic chemistry to detect the presence of nickel (Feigl, 1958) and a method designated to quantitate nickel release on metal surfaces as a potential source of NAH. The test is rapid and easily performed for screening purposes, accurate to approximately 10 ppm (0.001% or 2.1 μg Ni/g) (Wall, 1992). That semiquantitative test is based on complexation of nickel (II) ions with DMG in ammoniacal solution, yielding a pink-colored solution or precipitate, followed by addition of hydrogen peroxide to reduce the possibility of false-positive reactions, since silver, manganese, iron, and cobalt ions also give colored precipitates with this reagent.

As used in dermatology, the DMG test verifies the presence of (bioavailable) nickel in materials suspected of causing nickel allergy in patients (Marks and DeLeo, 1992). False-negative test results have been noted, however; materials did not give a color reaction, yet NAH patients reacted on intimate and prolonged skin contact with the tested alloy (Menné et al., 1987c). In case of suspected false-negative reaction, the material surface is etched with strong acid to penetrate possible patina of passive surface film (oxidized metal) prior to application of DMG and ammonia; the presence of nickel in the bulk of the material is thus revealed, but not necessarily the presence of nickel that may become bioavailable on simple skin contact (Cavelier et al., 1985).

4.2.1.2 Nitric Acid Spot Test

Recent research by Haudrechy and Kanerva into allergenic potential of nickel-containing consumer goods, where the DMG and synthetic sweat tests were the methods of choice, correlated those test results with patch tests using the same materials. Some resulting discrepancies have led these same researchers to question the accuracy and validity of the DMG test for the safety assessment of stainless steels (Haudrechy et al., 1994; Haudrechy et al., 1997; Kanerva et al., 1994). When the DMG test is applied to the analysis of certain grades of stainless steel, the test appears to be negative, and only on addition of hydrochloric acid does the coloration appear. When peroxide is added, however, that coloration may disappear again, indicating that complex formation has occurred between DMG and iron, and not nickel.

To yield a reliable reading in the analysis of stainless steels in particular, with the purpose of detecting their allergenic potential on skin contact, differentiation is necessary between high- and low-sulfur steels, since only the former were shown to release harmful amounts of nickel. For that purpose, use of 3N HNO_3 is recommended as an alternative to the DMG tests; it is applied as a drop and left on the metal surface for 5 minutes. A black coloration indicates the presence of a high quantity of sulfur in the alloy, sufficient indication for the presence of leachable nickel and thus of allergenic potential (Haudrechy et al., 1994).

4.2.2 PHYSICAL METHODS

Going beyond conventional chemical analysis, physical methods afford sensitivities in metal detection that are lower by several orders of magnitude, often reaching below the ppb level. Adapted to monitoring of toxic elements in biological substrates, such as tissues or body fluids, such sensitivity is essential for the assessment of risk to humans from environmental and occupational exposures to toxic metals without the need to resort to radionuclides. Thus monitoring of nickel levels in skin and body fluids by physical methods can provide adequate estimates of dose absorbed, indicating the need for corrective intervention.

4.2.2.1 Inductively Coupled Plasma-Atomic Emission Spectroscopy (ICP-AES)

ICP-AES permits detection of metals at the trace amount level, obviating the use of radioisotopes (Dipietro et al., 1988; Parsons et al., 1983). For the detection of nickel, the current quantitation limit falls in the 5 to 10 ppb (μg/L) range, a factor of five above the true instrumental detection limit as defined by the Environmental Protection Agency (U.S.) (EPA, 1986).

Quantitative detection of metals is accomplished by ionization of elements in inductively coupled argon plasma maintained by the interaction of a radio frequency field and ionized argon gas. In a sample aerosol (e.g., a vaporized metal salt solution) atoms and ions are activated at 6000°C to an unstable energy state, and as they revert to their ground state they emit light of characteristic wavelength and intensity that can be measured.

4.2.2.2 Inductively Coupled Plasma-Mass Spectrometry (ICP-MS)

ICP-MS is a technique that is applicable to μg/l (ppb) concentrations of a large number of elements in aqueous medium upon appropriate sample preparation of biological materials. Reliability of the method for elemental analysis is based upon multilaboratory performance compared with that of either furnace atomic absorption spectroscopy or ICP-AES. Normal instrument detection limit for nickel can be anticipated at 0.5 ppb.

The method measures ions produced by a radio-frequency inductively coupled plasma. The compound to be analyzed, present in liquid form, is nebulized and the resulting aerosol transported by argon gas into the plasma torch. The ions produced are entrained in the plasma gas and introduced, by means of a water-cooled interface, into a quadrupole mass spectrometer. The ions produced in the plasma are sorted according to their mass-to-charge ratios and quantified with a channel electron multiplier (EPA, 1986).

4.2.2.3 Atomic Absorption Spectrophotometry (AAS)

AAS with Zeeman background correction is the reference method accepted by the International Union of Pure and Applied Chemistry (IUPAC) and the International Agency for Research on Cancer (IARC) for trace element analysis (Brown et al., 1981).

The method is based on absorption of radiation energy by free atoms, characteristic for each element. In an atomizer, thermal energy (air-acetylene flame) converts the analyte to free atoms. In the ground state they absorb resonance radiation from a light source that emits characteristic radiation, i.e., the spectrum of the analyte element, whereby an electron transitions from the ground state to one of the empty orbitals at a higher energy level. A portion of this light is thus attenuated by such resonance absorption in the probe. A photomultiplier detector measures the change in radiation intensity and converts it into an absorbance signal. There is a linear relationship between absorbance and the concentration of the analyte. The technique is intrinsically specific, since the atoms of a particular element absorb radiation only of their own characteristic wavelength (Reynolds, 1970).

AAS is the most common technique for nickel analysis in biological fluids. The sample to be analyzed is digested in acid, the nickel then either chelated with ammonium tetramethylene dithiocarbamate, the chelate extracted with 4-methyl-2-pentanone, and the nickel in the extract measured by AAS, or the initial acid solution analyzed as such by AAS directly (Sunderman, 1989). Currently the detection limit for nickel by AAS in body fluids (urine, serum) is 0.4 to 0.05 ppb (Sunderman, 1993).

4.2.2.4 Particle Induced X-Ray Emission (PIXE)

Particle induced x-ray emission analysis with a proton microprobe allows the determination of trace elements in epidermal strata prepared by cryosection (Cullander et al., 2000). In PIXE a proton beam activates an atomic electron, lifting it into a higher orbital. When an outer shell electron falls back to fill the vacancy created, the transition is measured as the emission of an x-ray photon characteristic of the excited atom. The method with an elemental sensitivity approaching 0.1 mg/kg (0.1 ppm) is also useful in bulk analysis of alloys with multi-element detection capability, and in spatial analysis to localize elements present in a sample (Johansson and Campbell, 1988). Using this analytical method, Forslind et al. (1985) and Malmqvist et al. (1987) have been able to localize nickel in the superficial strata of human skin, with a spacial resolution of 3 μm by 15 μm and a detection limit of about 30 ppm. The concentration of nickel following exposure to a nickel solution was found to be highest in the outer parts of the epidermis, mainly in the outermost stratum corneum.

4.3 *IN VITRO* RELEASE OF NICKEL IN ARTIFICIAL SWEAT AND OTHER PHYSIOLOGIC MEDIA

Analytical results on leaching rates for nickel from various alloys and objects in a variety of biological media are presented in Table 4.1.

Definition and thereby reconstitution of human sweat in absolute terms is not feasible because of variability in its composition and pH. Gender differences are marked, and fluctuations occur due to environmental as well as subjective, endocrine factors. Most striking are changes in composition due to the rate of sweat secretion. Sodium and chloride content, one decisive factor in the corrosivity of sweat, is low under quiescent conditions due to the reabsorption (conservation) mechanism before sweat reaches the ostium of the sweat duct (Cage and Dobson, 1965). Sodium ion level can be as low as 1.7 meq/l and chloride ion 2.8 meq/l (Grice et al., 1975). As sweating rate increases, that control mechanism is overwhelmed and the salt concentration can rise, approximating or even exceeding that in plasma (Guyton, 1991).

Other significant components of sweat — urea, lactic acid, and potassium ions — also increase at high rates of secretion, and their concentrations can reach the levels in plasma (Guyton, 1991).

Another factor defeating the attempt to standardize artificial sweat is the phenomenon experienced by a group of individuals, referred to as "rusters," who exude palmar sweat of inordinately high rate and low pH, resulting in a pronounced corrosive action on metal surfaces (Jensen, 1979). Variability of sweat pH was measured as pH 2.1 to pH 6.9 (Haudrechy et al., 1997).

Values of the main components of sweat are listed in Table 4.2, the levels representing approximations only, however, which are subject to variation due to environmental and individual temperature, diet, age, gender, etc.

Leaching or release of nickel from metal objects in contact with bodily fluids is a continuous variable which is difficult to predict with accuracy. Aside from immediate environmental factors, the microenvironment within the particular alloy is a principal determinant, due to the action of electromotive forces generated by the presence of a multitude of possible accompanying metals (Cavelier et al., 1985). Denture and orthodontic materials, for example, may feature as many as 5 to 20 metals. Review of published data on corrosion shows that release rates, as determined through leaching tests, do not correlate with Ni content in an alloy (Flint, 1998). Other metals in immediate proximity form a galvanic element (or pile), whereby an electron current flows from the more electro-negative (e.g., nickel) to the more

TABLE 4.2
Mean Levels of Eccrine Sweat Components in meq

Sodium	Men	51.9 meq/l
	Women	36.5 meq/l
Potassium	Men	7.5 meq/l
	Women	10.0 meq/l
Chloride		29.7 meq/l
Urea		260–1220 mg/l
Lactic acid		360–3600 mg/l
Amino acids		270–2590 mg/l
Ammonia		60–110 mg/l

Source: Geigy Scientific Tables, 7th Ed., 1975.

electro-positive one (e.g., Cu), resulting in oxidation or solution ("corrosion") of the more electro-negative metal. Thus whether and how much nickel can be extracted will depend on the immediate surrounding materials (metals) present in the alloy.

4.3.1 LEACHING EXPERIMENTS DONE ON METALLIC OBJECTS CONTAINING NICKEL

Model solubilization studies by Samitz and Katz (1975) show that levels of up to 99 ppm of nickel are released from a 2 to 5 cm^2 surface area of (unspecified) stainless steel prostheses, suture wires, and screws on immersion in physiological saline, sweat, or blood plasma for one week at room temperature.

Elicitation of nickel allergic reactions upon handling (or swallowing) of coinage has been repeatedly reported (Bettley, 1971; Black, 1972; Ewing and Miller, 1991; Gilboa et al., 1988; Gollhausen and Ring, 1991; Husain, 1977; Kanerva et al., 1998; Lacroix et al., 1979; Preininger, 1934; Räsänen and Tuomi, 1992; Rothman, 1930; van Ketel, 1985), and nickel release by the action of sweat has been measured for coins of different origins (Bang Pedersen et al., 1974; Katz and Samitz, 1975; Menné and Solgaard, 1979). Also the accelerated leaching of nickel from coins and metal buttons in distilled water and synthetic sweat at elevated temperatures was determined in those two studies by Katz and by Menné. Refer to Table 4.1 for details.

Comparative tests simulating corrosion of implant metals *in vitro* demonstrated that the electrochemical process of oxidation in the presence of enzymes, proteins, and other components of actual serum is accelerated in comparison to straight physiological saline. Corrosion testing of implants thereby becomes more relevant for *in vivo* conditions when it is conducted in a proteinaceous medium (whole blood, serum, saliva) (Brown and Merritt, 1980; Samitz and Katz, 1975) as opposed to testing in standard saline solution (Grimsdottir, 1992a; Kerosuo, 1995).

Upon critical review of published patch test results, of the effects of exposure to nickel occurring in the work environment, and evaluation of typical consumer exposure, Menné (1994) concluded that induction of NAH was not likely below a threshold release concentration of 0.5 µg/cm^2/week from consumer products, or elicitation at concentrations of <0.1 to 1 µg/cm^2 under occlusion, or 15 µg/cm^2 nonoccluded. The irritated skin of hypersensitive individuals might react to 0.5 ppm nickel (0.0075 mg/cm^2). These conclusions were based primarily on the following data reviewed in his paper.

Primary sensitization (induction) was seen in 9% of a cohort of 172 volunteers on repeated occluded exposure to 25% NiCl$_2$ in 0.1% SLS (over unspecified lengths of time), and further prolonged exposure increased that sensitization rate (Vandenberg and Epstein, 1963). The highest sensitization rate of 50% was reached with 10% induction concentration and 2.5% eliciting concentration when using nickel sulfate (Kligman, 1966). Industrial or occupational exposure ranging from 2 to 6% to 10 to 30% solutions were seen to result in correspondingly elevated rates of sensitization. Larsen and Bandrup (1980) suggest that levels of nickel released from clothes accessories are 100 to 1000 times higher to induce NAH than would occur in already sensitized individuals. Thus primary sensitization will not be likely from exposure of healthy, intact skin to nickel released from objects of everyday use.

Only the high concentrations of nickel found in solutions of industrial use carry such risks.

An approach to measure threshold levels for reactivity is the application on the skin of metal disks (7 mm diameter, 0.4 mm thickness) of known nickel release in sweat under standard conditions, illustrated by Fischer et al. (1984b). All 18 patients thus reacted positively to at least one of the white-gold disks of 2.5 to 15% nickel content, releasing 0.09 to 0.82 µg Ni/week. There was no correlation between nickel content and nickel release. Analysis of used and unused studs, clasps, and earrings showed that they all released nickel to some degree upon one-week storage in synthetic sweat, and neither gold nor silver plating prevented this. Nickel release ranged from 0.005 to 442 µg/object/week. Nickel-sensitive women wearing these studs and clasps showed reactions to objects that released <0.5 µg/object/week.

The corrosion resistance of various nickel-containing materials was measured by Randin (1988) in oxygenated artificial sweat (perspiration): Ni, CuNi 25 (coin alloy), NiAl (colored intermetallic compounds), tungsten carbide + Ni (hard metal), white gold (jewelry alloy), FN42 and Nilo Alby K (controlled expansion alloys), and NiP (electroless nickel coating) are in an active state and dissolve as measured by corrosion current density (no numerical nickel data given). By contrast, austenitic stainless steels, TiC + Mo2C + Ni (hard metal), NiTi (shape-memory alloy), Hastelloy X (superalloy), Phydur (precipitation hardening alloy), PdNi and SnNi (nickel-containing coatings) are in a passive state and may pit only under certain extreme conditions.

Bioavailability of nickel from metal alloy samples and metal objects designed for prolonged skin contact was measured in a number of studies. First, Menné and Maibach (1987) compared the analytical sensitivity of the dimethylglyoxime (DMG) stick test with energy dispersive x-ray and Zeeman atomic absorption spectrometry. While the DMG stick test will identify most nickel-releasing alloys, exceptions would still point to provocation tests or patch tests in suspected cases of NAH. Flame atomic absorption analysis for the metal upon immersion in synthetic sweat was compared with results from the DMG test (Kanerva et al., 1994). Out of ten samples studied, only small amounts (<0.5 µg/cm^2/week) were released from two samples, and the DMG test was negative. From five samples, more than 0.5 µg/cm^2/week was released, and the DMG test was positive. For three samples, however, the DMG test was negative, though the flame atomic absorption spectrometry test showed considerable nickel release (up to 165 µg/cm^2/week). Therefore, although the DMG test can be used as a first-line test for determining nickel release, also some DMG-negative metal materials can possibly induce nickel sensitization, and should not be advertised as safe in this respect (Menné et al., 1987b).

In a study by Haudrechy et al. (1994), the release of nickel from nickel-plated materials and various grades of stainless steel in artificial sweat was investigated systematically in a study of standard alloys: low-sulfur stainless steel grades like AISI 304, 316L, or 430 (S ≤ 0.007%) released less than 0.03 µg/cm^2/week of nickel in acid artificial sweat and elicited no reactions in patients already sensitized to nickel. In contrast, nickel metal or nickel-plated samples released around 100 µg/cm^2/week of Ni, and high-sulfur stainless steel (AISI 303, with approximately

0.3% sulfur added) released about 1.5 μg/cm^2/week in artificial sweat. Applied as patch tests on patients sensitized to nickel, the latter metals elicited positive reactions in 96% and 14% of the patients, respectively. The authors concluded that low-sulfur stainless steels like AISI 304, 316L, or 430, even though containing Ni, should not elicit nickel contact dermatitis, while metals having a mean corrosion resistance like the high-sulfur stainless steel (AISI 303) or nickel-plated steel should be avoided. The determining characteristic was the corrosion resistance in chloride media, which, for stainless steels, is connected, among other factors, to sulfur content. Also suggested is replacing the DMG test, which can give false negative readings on stainless steels, with the nitric acid spot test, which allows identification of low-sulfur-containing steels.

The question remained open concerning the grades with an intermediate sulfur content, around 0.03%. Subsequently Haudrechy et al. (1997) performed three tests: leaching experiments, DMG and HNO$_3$ spot tests, and clinical patch tests. However, only stainless steels were tested: a low-sulfur AISI 304 and high-sulfur AISI 303 as references and three grades with a sulfur content around 0.03%: AISI 304L, AISI 304L with added Ca, and AISI 304L+Cu. Leaching experiments showed that the four grades of stainless steel with a sulfur content of less than 0.03% released less than 0.5 μg/cm^2/week in acid sweat while the resulfurized AISI 303 released around or more than 0.5 μg g/cm^2/week. This was explained by the poorer corrosion resistance of the resulfurized grade. Yet all grades had the same negative reaction to the DMG test, which demonstrates again its lack of sensitivity. In contrast, the HNO$_3$ spot test distinguished AISI 303 from the nonresulfurized grades. Clinical patch tests again showed that some patients (4%) were intolerant to AISI 303, while none was intolerant to the other grades. This study confirms that nonresulfurized stainless steels (S ≤ 0.03%) like Ni-containing 304 and 304L should not elicit Ni contact dermatitis, while the resulfurized grades such as AISI 303 or nickel-plated steel (S > 0.1%) should be avoided. Leaching, DMG test, and nitric acid spot tests showed that 304 and 316 grades released low levels of nickel (<0.5 μg/cm^2/week) and gave negative DMG and spot tests. Ni-plated steels and AISI 303 released higher levels of nickel (>0.5 μg/cm^2/week) and showed positive DMG and spot tests. Thus, Ni-containing 304 and 316 steels should not induce contact dermatitis, while 303 should be avoided. A reliable nitric acid spot test is proposed to distinguish this grade from other stainless steels.

Different alloys used in orthodontics were studied by Grimsdottir et al. (1992a) to determine whether nickel and chromium will be released from these alloys when stored in physiologic saline. Face-bows, brackets, molar bands, and arch wires were analyzed. Most of the different parts in the face-bows, brackets, and molar bands were similar to conventional 18/8 stainless steel. Except for the wires, most appliances included a variable amount of silver solder, the highest found in face-bows. After 14 days in 0.9% sodium chloride, the largest amount of nickel and chromium was leached from face-bows and the least from arch wires. Soldered stainless steel face-bows seemed to be very susceptible to corrosion. The release of nickel seemed to be related to both the composition and the method of manufacture of the appliances, but the release was not proportional to the nickel content.

Four commercially available nickel–chromium alloys used in orthodontry, Neptune™, Rexalloy™, Regalloy T™, and Vera Bond™, were tested as to their corrosion behavior using Auger electron microscopy, and corrosion resistance was put in relation with the surface characteristics of the alloys, which have a bearing on corrosivity. The alloys were chosen in order to compare a possible effect that the presence of beryllium in the alloy may have on surface characteristics and corrosion resistance. Neptune and Rexalloy are free of beryllium; the other two contain low levels of the element. Corrosivity was tested in culture conditions at 37°C, conditions chosen to make comparisons with further planned cell culture studies possible. In this investigation, Neptune had the best corrosion characteristics of the Ni-Cr dental casting alloys evaluated; together with Rexalloy it exhibited the more smooth and featureless surface. Vera Bond and Regalloy T, both containing Be, had etched appearances and severe pitting, and showed accumulation of corrosion products (Bumgardner and Lucas, 1993).

Bumgardner and Lucas (1994) further evaluated the dental alloys Neptune, Rexalloy, Regalloy T, and Vera Bond for their suitability as dental restorative materials, by an electrochemical corrosion test and the cytotoxicity of the resulting metal ion release in culture media. Pure nickel metal released on the order of 400 ppm nickel in cell culture media, compared with 100 to 255 ppb from the four Ni-Cr dental casting alloys. Particularly the comparison of the effect of beryllium as a component of the dental alloys Regalloy T and Vera Bond on their corrosion resistance with nonberyllium, nickel base alloys revealed increased corrosivity due to the presence of Be. All alloys demonstrated decreased corrosion rates in cold solution sterilized samples in complete cell culture media. The viability of human gingival fibroblast cell cultures was not affected by metal ions released from any of the nickel alloys tested.

The release of metal ions from nickel-chrome casting alloys was investigated in incremental three-dimensional cell culture tests, again by Bumgardner and Lucas (1995). Metal ion release was correlated to changes in cellular morphology, viability, and proliferation. Morphology and viability were not affected by the alloys' corrosion products, but cellular proliferation did decrease. Analysis of nickel levels showed that, of four dental alloys tested (Rexalloy, Regalloy T, Vera Bond, and Neptune), Neptune released the lowest amount of nickel and also caused the smallest decrease in cellular proliferation. Pure nickel samples released greater than 324 ppm nickel over the 24 to 72 h tests. These levels are 1000 times greater than those determined from the commercial alloys. All alloys released increasing amounts of nickel ions at successive test intervals.

The metallic ion release in oral implants with superstructures of different metals and alloys used in clinical dentistry was determined by Cortada et al. (1997) in an artificial saliva environment at 37°C. The measurements of the ion release were performed by means of the Inductively Coupled Plasma Mass Spectrometry technique. The titanium oral implant coupled with a chromium–nickel alloy released a high quantity of ions, while the implant coupled with the titanium superstructure presents a low value of ion release.

The amount of nickel ions liberated from various metal objects, including metal fashion accessories, orthopedic implants and orthodontic appliances, and its effect in biological systems, have been determined in several model experiments as well as *in vivo* measurements. Nickel release data are summarized in Table 4.1.

4.4 SAFE LIMITS OF EXPOSURE: DANISH AND EUROPEAN UNION NICKEL LEGISLATION

In view of the increasing incidence of NAH noted in most industrialized countries where epidemiology is conducted, based on clinical experience and investigations of reactivity to nickel alloys, dermatologists in Europe have elaborated regulatory standards that would limit nickel present or released from commonplace metal items of direct and prolonged contact, in order to minimize the risk of induction or elicitation of nickel allergy (Avnstorp et al., 1990; Lidén et al., 1996; Menné, 1994; Menné et al., 1987a; Menné et al., 1987b). The intent was to remove the most sensitizing nickel alloys from direct and prolonged skin contact by the consumer, but still make it possible for industry to continue its use of low nickel-releasing stainless steels and white-gold alloys.

Nickel release from items designed for prolonged use coming in direct contact with the skin was evaluated in a differentiated approach, based on two benchmarks:

- Levels known to rarely cause NAH or elicit allergic reactions, such as low sulfur stainless steel or white gold (Fischer et al., 1984a; Kanerva and Aitio, 1997; Menné et al., 1987a; Menné et al., 1987b)
- Levels commonly inducing and eliciting nickel dermatitis (Haudrechy et al., 1994; Haudrechy et al., 1997; Menné, 1994; Menné and Calvin, 1993)

Based on the results of such research (Menné and Rasmussen, 1990), legislation was introduced in Denmark in 1991, and subsequent to verification that such a maximum threshold is appropriate, a standard analytical methodology that includes analysis of nickel release from objects stored in artificial sweat to ascertain observance was adopted by the European Union (EU) in the European Nickel Directive in 1994 (EU, 1994; Lidén et al., 1996). Intended to reduce the prevalence of sensitization (primary prevention) and recurring dermatitis in the sensitized population (secondary prevention), the legislation states that nickel may not be used (a) in post assemblies used during epithelization unless they are homogenous and the concentration of nickel is less than 0.05%; (b) in products intended to come into direct and prolonged contact with the skin, such as earrings, necklaces, watch straps, or zippers, if the nickel release is greater than 0.5 µg Ni/cm^2/week; and (c) in coated products under (b), unless the coating is sufficient to ensure that nickel release will not exceed 0.5 µg Ni/cm^2/week after 2 years of normal use (EU, 1994). Standard methods to implement the control of the three parts that make up the regulation are in place and have been agreed upon, and in different countries of the EU the legislation is now in force.

The threshold thus mandated should prevent contact dermatitis in most sensitized subjects, albeit some nickel-allergic individuals are still expected to react even to levels of 0.05 µg Ni/cm^2/week (Fischer et al., 1984b; Gawkrodger, 1996).

4.5 *IN VIVO* NICKEL RELEASE AND ITS CLINICAL EFFECTS BY TYPE OF EXPOSURE

The etiology of NAH can involve several types of exposure and routes of penetration: intimate skin contact, systemic absorption through piercing of live tissue, presence of orthodontic devices or orthopedic implants, or intake with food or drink. Sensitization through systemic exposure in particular typically becomes manifest through periodically recurring vesicular, palmar eczema known as pompholyx, a clinical form never elicited by dermal (external) contact (Möller, 1993).

The widely accepted diagnostic test for NAH is the skin patch test. In most instances reviewed, the patch procedures shared similarities, but may not have been identical. Application was mainly for 48 h with nickel sulfate — with either the Al-test® or Finn Chamber® — and readings at 48, 72, or 96 h. Most followed the International Contact Dermatitis Research Group (ICDRG) or related reading scales that required a minimum of erythema and edema for allergic morphology considerations (ICDRG, 1988).

4.5.1 SKIN CONTACT

A broad range of nickel-containing objects and coatings used in jewelry, watches, and clothes were patch tested in 100 nickel-sensitive subjects and in 20 nickel-negative controls by Lidén et al. (1996). Three nonplated stainless-steel alloys tested caused no patch-test reaction. Nickel interliners under gold, silver, or chromium plating, as well as silver and some white-gold alloys, caused positive patch-test reactions. Ear ornaments, wrist watches, and buttons were the objects most frequently causing dermatitis. Half the nickel-sensitive participants suspected that they had been sensitized before the age of 20. These results have been used as the basis for developing clinically relevant analytical methods for nickel release in the EU Nickel Directive (EU, 1994) regulation aimed at the prevention of nickel allergy.

The levels of incidental nickel encountered in objects of daily use were found to lie below 5 ppm, not representing a risk of eczematous reaction even in sensitized individuals, as such exposure is brief (Basketter et al., 1993). In a single open application on the forearm of 51 nickel-sensitive subjects, over an observation period of 2 to 3 days none reacted to 100 ppm of an aqueous nickel solution, indicating a threshold for casual open exposure to lie above that level (Menné and Calvin, 1993).

In the application of nickel alloy disks, the release rate of metal ions determined in synthetic sweat at 0.5 µg Ni/cm^2/week appeared to represent a threshold value, having induced only weak reactions if any in nickel-sensitive subjects (Menné et al., 1987b).

Twelve subjects sensitive to nickel were patch tested with serial dilutions of $NiSO_4$ in petrolatum and water. The provocation thresholds of nickel producing reactions in those patients ranged from 0.47 µg (0.01%) to 5.2 µg (2.5%) in petrolatum and higher in aqueous solutions (Emmett et al., 1988).

Cavelier et al. (1985) inquired into the reactivity to nickel-containing objects habitually coming into intimate contact with the skin of nickel-sensitive individuals, such as is realized with metal fasteners on clothing items. In the first experiment, analysis by x-ray energy dispersion and the DMG spot test was performed for nickel on 57 metal clothing objects containing nickel but not alloys. Reactivity was then tested in 22 NAH patients by skin contact with a variety of items and patch testing with nickel-plated discs of gold/copper/cadmium and chromium of varying thickness. Reactivity to nickel was observed if the metal was at all part of the objects tested. The study led to the conclusions:

- Lack of dermatitis in NAH individuals can be achieved only if no nickel is used in objects such as those that were investigated in the study, although nickel-containing alloys were not tested in this study. The DMG test is not sufficiently sensitive to analyze for nickel release at levels that will still elicit reactions in those sensitized to nickel.
- Nickel-containing objects intended for long-term, intimate skin contact can be plated effectively only with chromium, a metal more electronegative than nickel, if such plating is heavier than one micron; at lighter plating, due to (unavoidable) fissures in the surface layer, chromium will act as a pile, resulting in dissolution of the passivated chromium and thus remove the anticorrosive layer.
- Protective plating of nickel-containing alloys can be achieved by use of highly electropositive (noble) metals such as gold, silver, platinum, or palladium, if plating is heavier than 5 µm. This is due to the imperfections in the surface of deposited metal; permeation of such layers through fissures will only favor corrosion (dissolution) of the more electronegative nickel.

Reaction of 13 patients sensitized to one or more metals was tested by Cavelier et al. (1989) with various metallic discs kept in contact with the skin over 48 h. Reactivity was observed for all samples, although application of a protective layer of bright copper greatly reduces the occurrence of untoward reactions. Reaction or the variability in reactivity to different manufactured metal samples of nickel–cobalt alloy, chromium, or chromium-plated cobalt were also tested in nine individuals positive to patch testing with nickel sulfate (5% in petrolatum) or to nickel sulfate and cobalt chloride. Five patients sensitive to nickel only did not react to all metal samples, except for the nickel–cobalt alloy in three cases; three patients allergic to nickel and cobalt reacted to all the metal samples. Four of the five patients allergic only to nickel failed to react to cobalt metal samples only.

In order to assess the "angry back" phenomenon in adjacent patch test sites in the range of 300 to 0.01 µg nickel sulfate hexahydrate/cm^2, patch testing using nickel sulfate under occlusion (T.R.U.E. TEST®) was conducted on the back of 72 nickel-sensitive patients randomly selected from two dermatology clinics in Denmark and Sweden by Andersen et al. (1993). Ten patches of differing dilutions and two placebos were left in place for 48 h; reaction was read at 96 h: 64 subjects responded to 0.1 to 300 µg Ni/cm^2 (threshold). Such a range in response, even in this homogenous cohort, is an indication of the individual variation in susceptibility to sensitization and in the allergenic reactivity of nickel. Statistics did not show evidence of "angry back" phenomenon in this study. However, some placebos in nickel-sensitives and nickel patches in controls also showed a positive reaction.

The potential threshold for evoking a reaction to nickel on contact of irritated skin with that ubiquitous metal was investigated through the hand-immersion experiment on a cohort of volunteers with NAH. Upon exposure twice daily to a surfactant solution containing various concentrations of nickel, there was no evidence of elicitation reactions up to a nickel concentration of 0.1 ppm (Allenby and Goodwin, 1983). No reaction was seen in another hand-immersion study at a 1 ppm nickel concentration twice daily for 23 days on the skin of four sensitized volunteers following pretreatment with SDS (Allenby and Basketter, 1994). In another threshold study by the same authors, the minimal eliciting concentration on SDS-pretreated skin of nickel-sensitized individuals was 0.5 ppm under occlusion (Allenby and Basketter, 1993).

Jewelry of 500 patients at a dermatology clinic was tested by Ingber et al. (1997) using the DMG test for nickel release, in addition to the jewelry of 32 female nickel patch test positive patients. The 32 patients were also screened by questionnaire for hand eczema and atopy. Watches, watchstraps, and earrings gave the most common positive DMG test results; 59.3% of the NAH patients presented with hand eczema, versus 15.4% of patients with nonnickel contact dermatitis. Earlobe dermatitis was present in 84.3%, and more than 80% were atopic.

Lidén et al. (1998) investigated nickel released from hand-held tools over one week in artificial sweat (Lidén et al., 1998). Nickel values ranged from 0.11 to 0.12 $\mu g/cm^2/week$ for multi-purpose pliers and socket wrenches, to 56 $\mu g/cm^2/week$ for bit holders. They conclude that limits for release of nickel as had been defined in the EU Directive by the Committee for Standardization may not be suitable for industrial materials and tools. Indeed, the EU regulation applies only to items intended to remain in close skin contact over prolonged periods of time.

Finally, Lidén et al. (1998) also determined the release in artificial sweat of nickel and various other precious and nonprecious metal ions from alloys used in industry to fabricate jewelry. Analysis of material typically used in the manufacture of jewelry was singled out for corrosion analysis to account for the fact that metals in contact with other metals, as in alloys, exhibit variable corrosion characteristics due to the variable galvanic effects prevailing. The one alloy containing nickel (white-gold solder also containing gold, silver, copper, and zinc) released 0.09 μg $Ni/cm^2/wk$.

4.5.2 PIERCED SKIN: SYSTEMIC INDUCTION OF NICKEL ALLERGY

For purposes of the present review, piercing of the ears and other sites on the human integument, a practice becoming increasingly popular, is not considered to be equivalent to epicutaneous contact. Perforating the skin to anchor metallic objects involves exposure to alloys that may contain various amounts of nickel. In particular this involves post assemblies introduced during epithelization of the wound caused by piercing, objects that remain in place for extended periods. Such traumatization may be considered equivalent to systemic dosing. Human plasma is the most aggressive physiological medium for dissolving nickel, e.g., from earrings (Emmett et al., 1988). Corrosion of the foreign object in this microenvironment may release components into the organism, some of which can then act as allergens. As a rule, literature refers to such objects used for personal adornment as costume jewelry, implying that they are made of inexpensive metallic materials potentially releasing high levels of nickel. In many cases, costume jewelry is plated with nickel, which may release nickel ions upon direct and prolonged contact with the skin. It was established, however, that higher-grade, gold-plated jewelry, and even some objects made of noble metal alloys that contain nickel and other metals to impart the appropriate metallurgical properties to them, may release nickel ions with intimate and prolonged contact. It is ultimately not the percentage in metal composition of alloys, for example those containing base metals such as nickel, that determines the rate of ion release; it is the microstructure of the alloy and the proximity of electropositive and electronegative metals that result in corrosion and ion release due to electrogalvanic effects (Cavelier et al., 1985; Flint and Packirisamy, 1995; Grimsdottir et al., 1992b). In gold-plated earrings, for instance, Ishikawaya et al. (1997) determined that the nickel interliner beneath the gold plating becomes exposed with use, with the potential to induce NAH. Scanning electron microscopy and x-ray microanalysis of the surface of both used or unused gold-plated jewelry revealed that the gold surface is defective, that is, not continuous, exposing the underlying nickel, which is then subject to corrosion and may release nickel ion on tissue contact.

In Denmark, NAH prevalence among women suspected to be a consequence of skin piercing now reaches 12.2% in the group aged 15 to 34 years (Nielsen and Menné, 1992). Such an elevated incidence of sensitization in the young finds confirmation in a Spanish study involving children up to the age of 14 (Sevila et al., 1994). Patch testing of patients in a dermatology clinic there resulted in 101 cases with a positive allergic contact dermatitis (ACD) reaction to at least one allergen, of which 57 (54.4%) were considered relevant. Among these, 21 tested positive to nickel. Such an increasing trend is attributed to the increase in the use of costume jewelry, often involving perforation of the skin on various parts of the body, or the intimate and prolonged contact with buttons, rivets, and other types of metallic fasteners on garments. In Japan, where ear piercing is also becoming increasingly popular, a study involving 377 dermatology patients compared occurrence of dermatitis due to diverse metal allergies, and identified ear piercing as a definite risk factor: rate of hypersensitivity to nickel (patch tested with 5% nickel sulfate) was 38.3% in patients with pierced ears, versus 25.6% of patients without (Nakada and Iijima, 1996).

4.5.3 ORTHODONTIC DEVICES

The release of ions from nickel (as well as other metals) present in orthodontic devices such as crowns, bands, brackets, wire retainers, and bridgework, is due to electrochemical corrosion occurring in microenvironments of varying composition (Cavelier et al., 1985; Flint, 1998). The oral cavity in particular provides exceptional conditions for this process, due to a combination of endogenous and exogenous factors (Gjerdet et al., 1991). The products of corrosion may then be taken up either through the oral mucosa directly, or by the soft tissues of the GI tract (Trombelli et al., 1992). Transported by blood throughout the organism, reaction products with endogenous proteins are deposited in various organs and tissues, and can elicit an allergic reaction in specific target organs such as the skin (Bergman et al., 1980).

Having observed several cases of multiple sensitivities to metals following restorative dentistry, Koch and Balmer (1995) coined the term "dental restoration metal intolerance syndrome" to describe the condition.

Blood analysis of patients receiving orthodontic treatment in particular showed that biodegradation of appliances had no measurable effect on nickel blood levels (Bishara et al., 1993).

Even though the extensive use of base-metal alloys has been of major concern to the dental profession, the relatively few case reports attributing hypersensitivity reactions of the skin to nickel in particular fail to substantiate this concern (Staerkjaer and Menné, 1990). In NAH reports where sensitization is confirmed by patch testing, clinical expression of sensitization due to orthodontic appliances (and to orthopedic implants as well), is the exception, and oral mucosal involvement is even rarer (Jones et al., 1986). This latter phenomenon has been explained by the apparent requirement for higher antigen concentrations to engender intraoral reaction, due to coating (passivation) of the mucosa by salivary glycoproteins, differences in permeability of the skin and oral mucosa, and differences in concentration of dendritic cells in the two membranes (Magnusson et al., 1982; Nielsen and Klaschka, 1971; Spiechowicz et al., 1984; Staerkjaer and Menné, 1990; Wilson and Gould, 1989).

Allergy to gold-based dental restorations is being reported with increasing frequency (Aro et al., 1993; Fisher, 1992; Fregert et al., 1979; Izumi, 1982; Koch and Bahmer, 1995; Marcusson, 1996; Mongkolnam, 1992; Mountcastle et al., 1986; Namikoshi et al., 1990; Schöpf et al., 1970; Stenman and Bergman, 1989; Wiesenfeld et al., 1984). Also, palladium-based alloys used in orthodontic appliances are increasingly being associated with cases of stomatitis and oral lichenoid reactions, aside from positive patch test reactions (Gebhardt and Geier, 1996; Downey, 1989; Marcusson, 1996; Nakayama and Imai, 1982; Richter, 2001; van Loon et al., 1984). It seems to occur mainly in patients who have high sensitivity to nickel (Guerra et al., 1988; van Loon et al., 1984; Wataha and Hanks, 1996).

All casting alloys, including titanium, seem to have a potential for eliciting adverse reactions in hypersensitive patients due to release of antigenic metal ions in the oral corrosive environment, and the recommendation to substitute allergenic nickel in prostheses with palladium or titanium may not yield the benefits hoped for. In an investigation of 311 patients referred to a German dental clinic for verification of suspected allergy, 13% were confirmed by Tschernitschek et al. (1998) as sensitized to various denture base materials. The remarkable result of patch testing was the preponderance of palladium positives for the period 1995–97 over all other metals tested (11), with 12 Pd positives versus 6 Ni positives. This represents a reversal in ranking when compared with the extended period 1982–97, where the overall incidence was 24 for Ni compared to 19 for Pd. New in that survey was also titanium hypersensitivity, with two cases testing positive.

Conversely, induction of tolerance may be a possible benefit of the use of intraorally placed alloys. In nonsensitized individuals, oral antigenic contacts to nickel and chromium may induce tolerance rather than sensitization, particularly if such exposure occurs at an early age. In a dermatology department in Belfast, records showed that orthodontic treatment preceding ear piercing reduced the occurrence of NAH from 36 to 25% (Todd and Burrows, 1989). When wearing dental braces preceded ear piercing, NAH was significantly reduced, as resulted from a retrospective review of records from 2176 patients attending 9 European patch test clinics: in female patients with pierced ears 25% versus 39%; in males 7% versus 22% (van Hoogstraten et al., 1991). Kerosuo et al. (1996) investigated the frequency of NAH in 700 adolescents in function of orthodontic treatment with metallic appliances and ear piercing, among other criteria by way of skin patch testing and patient history. None of the girls outfitted with orthodontic appliances prior to ear piercing was sensitive to nickel, while 35% of the girls having had ears pierced prior to orthodontic treatment were sensitized. Immersed in a 0.05% sodium chloride solution, a level typical for saliva, at 37°C such appliances released an average of 40 µg total (soluble and precipitated) Ni per day, 125 µg ± 22 for 4 quadrants of appliances over 12 days. This appears as a minor factor in relation to an average dietary intake of up to 500 µg/day (Park and Shearer, 1983).

Nickel release from orthodontic appliances was investigated in 0.9% physiologic saline over the extended period of 14 days. The amounts leaked ranged between none from archwires, to 10.4 µg from face-bows. These levels found were not proportional to the Ni content of the appliances (Grimsdottir et al., 1992a). Other metals present in the alloys appear to have a bearing on metal corrosion and release, depending on the electromotive gradients in the local galvanic elements (Cavelier et al., 1985).

Intraoral corrosion and release of nickel was recorded by Gjerdet et al. (1991) in a study of 34 patients outfitted with fixed orthodontic appliances. The levels of nickel in the saliva of 6 patients sampled within hours of placement of the appliances in the mouth were significantly elevated, versus levels detected prior to treatment (median of 67.6 ng/ml vs. 8.2 ng/ml; $p < 0.05$; range of 0.0 to 200 ng/ml before appliances), but decreased again dramatically at 3 weeks posttreatment, to 7.8 ng/ml, not statistically significant from pretreatment. These findings may be due to the fact that the oral environment can passivate the metal surface through formation of an oxide layer formed in the oral environment, a phenomenon observed also by others (Edie et al., 1981). The investigators note, however, that such modification in corrosion dynamics is again subject to highly individual variables, as described by the wide variations in nickel levels recorded in the above study by Gjerdet.

The biocompatibility of a high-gold alloy (Iropal W), two low-gold alloys (Argenco 9 and Gold EWL-G), one palladium alloy (Argipal), two palladium–silver alloys (Argenco 23 and EWL-G), one chrome–nickel alloy (Wiron-88), two chrome–cobalt alloys (Wironium and Wirocast) and a 22-carat-gold alloy were evaluated histopathologically in rats for their suitability as dental alloys by Kansu and Aydin, by subcutaneous implantation. The metal discs were implanted for 15, 30, or 60 days in 111 rats, 7 samples for each test period. The most vigorous toxic reactions were seen with the chrome–nickel alloy samples (Wiron-88), according to all histopathology criteria. The high score exhibited by Wiron-88 is attributed to the 65% nickel content of the alloy. The mildest toxic response was recorded with the 22-carat-gold alloy. The high-gold alloy and the palladium groups showed reactions similar to that of 22-carat gold. The low-gold group and the palladium–silver alloys had scores falling between the basic metal alloy and the precious metal alloy groups (Kansu and Aydin, 1996a). Those metal alloys were also examined for relevance as to the allergenic potentials, by skin patch tests with the corresponding metal salts on humans by Kansu and Aydin. This was done since significant correlation exists between reactivity to metal salts and the metallic form in respective alloys (Richter, 2001), depending on the amount of metal ion released from the alloy under relevant conditions. Sixty subjects (ages 17 to 23) were divided in 3 groups of 20, based on the criteria: (1) history of severe metal allergy; (2) moderate metal allergy; (3) no metal allergy known. Based on skin patch test results with nickel sulfate, potassium dichromate, silver nitrate, cobalt nitrate, copper sulfate, palladium chloride, platinum chloride, and gold chloride, nickel sulfate produced the most vigorous allergic response, while gold chloride showed the least of all. Also the number of positives was highest to nickel sulfate in all 3 groups tested. The authors conclude that patch testing is generally indicated in patients with a history of metal allergy to avoid elicitation of reactions by exposure to inappropriate materials (Kansu and Aydin, 1996b). Moffa et al. (1977), Blanco-Dalmau et al. (1984) and Morris (1987) had come to similar conclusions in their earlier work.

Nickel and chromium concentrations were investigated in saliva of patients with different types of fixed appliances by Kerosuo et al. (1997). Saliva samples were collected from 47 orthodontic patients, ages 8 to 30 years. Four samples from each subject were collected: (1) before insertion of the appliance, (2) 1 to 2 days after, (3) 1 week after, and (4) 1 month after insertion of the appliance. Although a considerable variation in individual concentrations of both nickel and chromium in the saliva was observed, no significant differences were found between the no-appliance samples and the samples obtained after insertion of the appliances in the same patient. The results suggest that nickel and chromium concentrations of saliva are not significantly affected by fixed orthodontic appliances during the first month of treatment. Several studies in large and small cohorts of dental patients have been conducted to investigate the role of oral exposure to nickel containing restorative materials. These are reviewed here, together with reports of anecdotal observations.

Higher concentrations of the allergen appear to be required for the elicitation of reactions in the oral mucosa than those leading to involvement of the skin (Magnusson et al., 1982; Nielsen and Klaschka, 1971). In a controlled study (n = 10) involving subjects with skin reactions to nickel and positive nickel patch tests, prosthetic appliances containing as much as 66% Ni caused no adverse general or oral clinical or histological reactions over exposure times of up to 40 months.

With the purpose of observing whether sensitized subjects outfitted with a nickel-removable prosthesis would exhibit any manifestations of NAH, a population of 100 dental patients (50 women, 50 men) were subjected to a preoperative test for NAH by Jones et al. (1986) using a standard patch test. Inserts were put into 10 patients: 5 had positive patch test reactions, and 5 were patch-test negative. The metal insert consisted of Ticonium, an alloy of 70% nickel, 16% chromium, 2% aluminum, and 0.5% beryllium, and Vitallium™, an alloy that contains no nickel. The incidence of initial NAH was significant: 20% for women and 2% for men. However, none of the test subjects showed reactivity to nickel alloyed with chromium in the intraoral prostheses. Possibly the chromium metal alloyed with the nickel reduces the release of nickel ions in the oral environment. The authors conclude that patients with a history of NAH are not necessarily prevented from successfully wearing a nickel-containing dental prosthesis.

A study conducted by Staerkjer and Menné (1990) with 1085 girls outfitted with orthodontic devices shows that even patients with NAH are not at greater risk of developing allergic reactions of the oral mucosa when wearing an intraoral appliance.

Bishara et al. (1993) studied accumulation of nickel in blood following orthodontic therapy, involving 18 females and 13 males, ages 12 to 38, treated for malocclusions. Orthodontic therapy using appliances made of nickel–titanium did not result in a significant or consistent increase in the blood levels of nickel. The amounts of nickel and chromium metal released in the oral environment due to corrosion over the 5 months of the study lay significantly below the average dietary intake (Bishara et al., 1993; Park and Shearer, 1983). Statistical analysis of the results was not deemed appropriate in Bishara's study because the majority of nickel blood levels lay below the limit of detection.

In a study by Koppenburg et al. (1988) involving 472 orthodontic patients and the analysis of their case histories, including immunotoxicological aspects, the conclusion is also reached that, while symptoms of a preexisting hypersensitivity to nickel may be amplified by salivary corrosion of dental (nickel containing) steel as it is used in banding and bracketing in orthodontics, induction of NAH through exposure of the oral mucosa is not likely.

While NAH does not necessarily result in adverse oral reactions on exposure to nickel-containing dental alloys, nevertheless an indirect causal relationship was demonstrated repeatedly between allergic reactions of the immediate or delayed type and nickel-releasing appliances, since oral and generalized symptoms cleared completely upon removal of orthodontic appliances (España et al., 1989; Guimaraens et al., 1994; Kerosuo and Kanerva, 1997; Romaguera et al., 1989; Temesvári and Racz, 1988; Trombelli et al., 1992; Veien et al., 1994). In a comparison of two distinct cohorts it resulted that allergy to $NiSO_4$ was significantly higher among dental patients (22%) than in eczematous subjects (17%) (Marcusson, 1996).

In a survey by Blanco-Dalmau et al. (1984), the prevalence of NAH among 403 students, faculty, and employees in a dental clinic was 28.5% patch-test positives to 5% nickel sulfate. Prevalence was significantly higher in women than men: 31.9% of the women tested were positive and 20.7% of the men, for a total of 115 patients, representing a significant difference between the two genders ($p < 0.05$).

Other publications report onset and remission from NAH symptoms of the immediate type: impaired respiratory function and excematous skin, or of delayed, cell-mediated type characterized by stomatitis, "burning mouth syndrome" (Guerra et al., 1993; Kanerva et al., 1995), erythema, edema, and erosions, ulceration of the oral mucosa, generalized dermatitis, in function of presence and removal of dental devices, respectively, as mentioned below. These observations would point to such devices as causative in the occurrence of clinically relevant nickel allergy.

A female patient developed gingivostomatitis and ulceration after having a metal dental prosthesis fitted; this disappeared after removal of the prosthesis, which contained 74 to 78% nickel. Patch testing had shown positivity to nickel only, out of 21 allergens (Romaguera et al., 1989). Days after implantation of nickel-containing prostheses, a female patient developed generalized wheals. Patch tests were strongly positive to nickel (and cobalt), and at 24 h there was a positive reaction to nickel on intradermal testing. On oral administration of nickel sulfate, the patient developed itching of the skin without visible eruption, generalized wheals, and lower-limb and eyelid oedema. After removal of the prostheses, however, the patient remained free of skin lesions for more than 2 years (España et al., 1989). In 3 girls ages 13 to 18 with NAH, removal of dental plates correlated with disappearance of the symptoms of hypersensitivity (Temesvári and Racz, 1988). Removal of orth-odontic appliances (stainless-steel bracket, arch bands, and stainless-steel wiring) provided complete clearance of dermatitis due to nickel hypersensitivity in a 23-year-old woman (Trombelli et al., 1992). In a patient with vesicular hand eczema and a positive patch test to nickel, an orthodontic appliance was suspected to be the causative agent. Dermatitis cleared completely upon removal of the appliance and replacement with acrylic material (Veien et al., 1994). When the dental brace (con-taining 8% nickel) was removed, dermatitis cleared in a 17-year-old girl who patch tested positive to nickel sulfate (Wilson and Gould, 1989).

With recent efforts toward improving orthodontic materials, such as stainless steel which in those applications customarily contained 8 to 12% nickel and other materials, nickel-titanium alloys with as much as 74 to 78% nickel (Romaguera et al., 1989) are being adopted. It has been suggested that the use of titanium in these alloys improves performance and lessens allergenicity (Bass et al., 1993). These still contain as much as 70% nickel, however. What appears as incidence of *de novo* sensitization due to long-term orthodontic therapy using the so-labeled titanium wire was described by Bass et al. (1993). In a prevalence and longitudinal study of 29 patients, 5 were Ni patch test positive prior to orthodontic therapy, but the number rose to 7 at 3 months posttreatment. The two newly sensitized patients both had received Ni–Ti wire with stainless steel brackets. There was no clinical allergic response in those patients, however. Pure titanium wire free of nickel is available, to be sure, but is seldom used as it has insufficient tensile strength.

In the Department of Oral Diagnosis, University of Umea (Sweden), 151 patients were tested with the standard series of dental materials (Axéll et al., 1983) in an investigation of potential side-effects of dental materials (Stenman and Bergman, 1989). Twelve persons in this group had oral mucosal changes of different types, pointing to allergic reactions. Of the 151 patients, 39 women and 7 men had positive skin reactions to one or more of the substances used in patch testing with the standard test series of dental materials. The majority of the positive reactions were related to metals; 21 (14%) among them to nickel, 20 of them women, and 1 man. A number of positive reactions to organic test substances were also noted.

Patch testing of a battery of 35 dental test substances was performed in 24 patients with visible lichenoid oral mucosal lesions and in 24 patients with "burning mouth syndrome" (BMS) without visible lesions (Skoglund and Egelrud, 1991). Positive reactions to nickel sulfate patches were found in 21% (5 of 24) of the patients with BMS, as opposed to 3% (1 of 24) of the patients with lichenoid lesions. This difference was also statistically significant. Although metallic nickel is a rare component in dental restorations, the oral mucosa is daily exposed to nickel through food and water intake. Total removal of nickel from the environment of the patient can therefore be hard to accomplish.

The orthodontic studies noted, although epidemiologic and lacking the vigor of placebo-controlled observation, fit in with the experience of Lowney (1968) of inducing tolerance by oral exposure. The literature on induction of tolerance is beyond the scope of this review.

Following surgery to correct mandibular misalignment, a patient developed "burning mouth syndrome" at the site of the mandibular osteotomy. This patient also had had earlier adverse reactions to stainless-steel wire used in previous osteotomy that had to be removed because of similar symptoms, bringing relief from the allergic reaction. Removal of the mandibular wires resulted in elimination of the symptoms from the mandibular region as well. The patient's dermatologic tests confirmed allergy to nickel as well as to other substances (Guyuron and Lasa, 1992).

Vilaplana et al. (1994) patch tested 66 patients, who were referred by dermatologists and odontologists, for suspected adverse reactions to prostheses. In addition to the T.R.U.E. TEST, the Standard Series and Chemotechnique's dental screening series, a specially prepared test series of 16 metals was used for that investigation into the role of metal alloys in allergic reactions to dental materials. ACD or adverse reactions of the oral mucous membranes due to dental prostheses were more frequent than expected. The three top allergens found to give positive reactions on patch testing, in order of frequency (number in males in parentheses) were salts of nickel 21 (1), cobalt 10 (2) and dichromate 5 (2).

The case is reported of a nickel-sensitive patient who demonstrated loss of alveolar bone after the placement of crowns with a high nickel content. The authors recommend that the history of metal sensitivity be evaluated before placement of crowns which contain nonprecious alloys (Bruce and Hall, 1995).

Hay and Ormerod (1998) described severe oral and facial allergic reaction in a patient with extensive oral dental restoration presenting with allergy to six metals (confirmed by patch test), nickel among them. Use of the term "dental restoration metal intolerance syndrome" is suggested, and also patch-testing patients suspected of metal hypersensitivity prior to dental restoration.

4.5.4 ORTHOPEDIC IMPLANTS

Leaching of nickel from metallic prostheses such as total joint replacements, pacemakers, or plates and screws implanted subcutaneously potentially leads to elicitation of allergic nickel contact dermatitis in patients allergic to nickel (Evans et al., 1974; Kubba et al., 1981; Landwehr and van Ketel, 1983; Laugier and Foussereau, 1966). Cutaneous reactions to such immune response due to orthopedic implants (eczematous dermatitis, urticaria, or bullous reactions) are difficult to categorize (i.e., induction versus elicitation reactions) because it is often difficult to establish a cause-and-effect relationship between implant and clinical dermal event. While the allergenic potential of materials such as nickel or cobalt is well established, also the preexisting immunological state of a patient is difficult or impossible to ascertain. Review of cutaneous involvement as consequence of orthopedic (or orthodontic) implants shows that rarely do reports mention presurgical patch testing to determine the preexisting immune status of patients (Kubba et al., 1981).

Trace concentrations of nickel may be liberated from implants such as joint prostheses, plates and screws for fractured bones fabricated from stainless steel or Vitallium, all containing varying percentages of nickel, cobalt chromium, and molybdenum, or from nickel–cadmium battery pacemakers which contain up to 35% nickel (Menné et al., 1987b). Model solubilization studies by Samitz and Katz (1975) show that ppm levels of nickel are released from stainless-steel prostheses materials AISI 302, 303, 316 (2 to 5 cm^2 surface area) on immersion in physiological saline, sweat, or blood plasma for one week at room temperature (details in Table 4.1).

In most earlier cases, metal sensitization due to implanted joint replacements was correlated with loosening or mechanical failure of the prostheses; mechanical attrition of the loose parts articulating against each other leads to increased solubilization of the alloy components (Elves et al., 1975) and cell and bone necrosis due to inflammation can lead to loosening of the implant (Cortada et al., 1997). The risk of sensitization to nickel and other heavy metals used in artificial joints appears to be diminishing now, however, thanks to the development of improved materials and safer alloys, which minimize mechanical failure and abrasion through metal-to-metal contact (Török et al., 1995).

Metallic orthopedic implants, particularly those of the dynamic type such as full joint replacements, are subject to corrosion due to electrogalvanic effects (Brown and Merritt, 1980) and to mechanical wear as it occurs in articulating (dynamic) joints. Metal constituents are thereby liberated that potentially can trigger immune reactions (Török et al., 1995). The occurrence of metal sensitivity was evaluated by Merritt and Brown in 164 patients with orthopedic implants having implants removed, by measuring the *in vitro* lymphocyte migration inhibition factor (LIF) as an indicator of antigen-stimulated T cells.

Lymphocytes activated by an encounter with an antigen (a cell-mediated immune reaction) move through the blood and lymphatic circulation. Such migration explains why immunologic reactions acquire a systemic character, producing a generalized response causing release of cytokines, even though contact with antigen may occur only locally (internally through ion release from prostheses, or epicutaneously with an environmentally occurring antigen, such as nickel ions). Presence of LIF released by sensitized lymphocytes can be tested for by incubation with specific antigen, and LIF can then be assayed by purifying polymorphonuclear leukocytes from the blood and placing them in agarose. Cell migration is measured at 18 to 24 h, the relative areas of migration are determined, and the amount of inhibition of leukocyte migration calculated. The *in vitro* LIF test makes the determination of the state of sensitivity possible (preexisting, acquired, or none), on patients prior to implantation or after removal. The outcome of the test shows that the patient either does not produce LIF (a "nonmigrator," i.e., is not sensitive to the metal, or produces LIF to the metal salt, is sensitized). In case the patient shows no cell migration, including in the (positive) cell migration control test with PHA (phyto haemagglutinin, a T cell mitogen which can also trigger cell functions and lymphokine production), then the test is inconclusive.

In a study by Merritt and Brown (1981), of the 164 patients (all with metallic implants) tested for LIF, 61 (37%) were "nonmigrators." In the cases where blood samples were analyzed after implant removal, cell migration was reestablished in two to six weeks and gave a positive LIF test. Based on the outcome of their study, the authors came to the conclusion that in view of the frequency of orthopedic surgery the problem due to allergic sensitization is minor. The condition of failing cell migration by the LIF test may prove to be a valuable adjunct in patient diagnosis. The authors also suggest that, after careful search for other causes, the implant should be suspected and its removal be considered. Individuals who are skin test negative may still be reacting to the metal implant because of the presence of antibody or of deep-tissue–metal complexes antigenically distinct from skin–metal complexes. The use of the LIF test has been recommended to detect adverse reactions in sensitive individuals and in those reacting to the presence of an implant.

The choice of implant should be based on release of metal ion rather than on composition. The use of alternative alloys should be discouraged until their acceptability in regard to function, biocompatibility, and nonsensitizing qualities has been documented by groups such as the Biocompatibility Section of the ASTM Committee F-4 on Medical and Surgical Materials and Devices. Some patients are or may become sensitized to implant constituents and react to the implant. Animal studies (in rabbits and guinea pigs) indicate that such reactions are likely to involve the accumulation of inflammatory cells at the implant site, with eventual necrosis leading to implant loosening. The manifestation of the reaction *in vivo* will depend on the localization of the metal ion to which the host is reacting. Ions released from the corroded implant may spread throughout the body, leading to systemic reactions. The main focus of the reaction then may not be at the site of implant or skin contact, but the foreign body may still be its cause (Merritt and Brown, 1981).

It has been suggested by Kubba et al. (1981) and Merritt and Brown (1981) that there is an immunologic cross- or co-reaction between metal–protein complexes of nickel and cobalt. Thus, the use of cobalt–chrome alloys, considered as an alternative to (nickel-containing) stainless steel, will not necessarily avoid future problems in a nickel-sensitive subject. In the selection of implant materials, traditional materials should be replaced only when function, biocompatibility, and immunological characteristics have been certifed by competent institutions such as the Biocompatibility Section of the ASTM Committee F-4 on Medical and Surgical Devices.

The use of metallic heads articulating with metallic cups for total hip replacements was reviewed critically by Merritt and Brown (1996) for immunological and toxicological safety, as the alloys contain immunogenic metals such as nickel, cobalt, and chromium. Particular focus was directed to the release and biologic fate of those metal species liberated through corrosion and wear. For cobalt–chromium alloys, amount of metal ions liberated appears to be well tolerated by the biologic system. Nickel and cobalt ions are rapidly transported from local tissues to the blood and rapidly eliminated in the urine. Increases observed in urinary nickel levels are small and transient. Chromium, however, is stored in tissues and red blood cells, and is eliminated more slowly.

Blood nickel concentrations in patients with stainless-steel hip prostheses of the metal-to-plastic type were analyzed by Linden et al. (1985) by means of electrothermal atomic absorption spectrophotometry, in serum and whole-blood specimens from 13 patients 9 to 15 years after hip replacement. In 12 of the 13 patients, nickel concentrations in serum and whole blood did not differ significantly from those of 30 healthy controls. One patient was seen to have elevated nickel levels in serum and blood, attributed to renal insufficiency. X-ray examinations did not reveal alterations in bone structure in the area of the implants. The study shows that patients with stainless-steel hip prostheses of the metal-to-plastic types do not develop hypernickelemia in the absence of corrosion.

Lyell et al. (1978) observed that life-threatening peri-prosthetic intolerance developed with two successive nickel-containing mitral-valve prostheses in a patient allergic to nickel. Neither prosthesis had been implanted satisfactorily. The nickel-free replacement prosthesis appeared satisfactory 22 months after insertion. It was unclear if allergy to nickel was involved in the failure of the earlier prostheses.

When a female patient was diagnosed with an abdominal aortic aneurysm, endoluminal repair was performed by insertion of a self-expanding endograft. Three weeks later the patient suffered a severe episode of erythema and eczema, and patch testing was positive to nickel and cobalt. Analysis of the endograft revealed a content of 55% nickel and 21% titanium (Giménez-Arnau et al., 2000).

In the attempt to resolve inconsistencies in the results of previous studies addressing trace metal concentrations in body fluids of patients with knee or hip replacement surgery, Ni (Co and Cr) concentrations in serum and urine were determined in a group of patients after total knee or hip replacement with porous-coated prostheses, selected to avoid metal-to-metal contact. Trace metal analyses were done by electrothermal atomic absorption spectrophotometry. Subjects in group A were healthy controls, subjects in group B had prostheses fabricated of Ti-Al-V alloy, subjects in group C prostheses made of Co-Cr alloy. Although nickel levels in the two types of alloys were <0.2% and <0.1% (by weight), respectively, one or two days after surgery nickel in serum and urine specimens from both groups were elevated 11-fold compared with preoperative values, diminishing again by two weeks. The postoperative levels of nickel noted in blood and urine are possibly due to metal release from the drills, scalpels, cutting jigs, and drilling jigs, or it may represent a previously unrecognized pathophysiological response to surgical stress, similar to disturbances noted in nickel metabolism observed in patients with other pathological conditions (Sunderman et al., 1989).

4.5.5 GASTROINTESTINAL EXPOSURE

Induction of NAH by the oral route appears unlikely. The elicitation of a systemic dermal reaction in those already sensitized may occur, however, when they are exposed to soluble nickel species released from cooking utensils or certain foods (Accominotti et al., 1998; Brun, 1979; Flint and Packirisamy, 1995). Water faucets, often nickel plated, may release nickel, adding to oral exposure. It is also thought likely that nickel released from orthodontic devices by intraoral corrosion, reviewed earlier, bind to and thus activate lymphocytes via the gastrointestinal tract (Hutchinson, 1975; Veien, 1989; Burrows, 1992; Sinigaglia, 1994), enter the bloodstream, and preferentially concentrate on a specific organ, such as the skin, rather than by direct penetration through the oral mucosa. A state of NAH may thus be maintained by nickel ions of various origins that are ingested, eliciting immunologic reactions of both the immediate (urticaria) and delayed type (eczema), and may be a factor contributing to a state of chronic, unremitting sensitization. This dietary effect has been demonstrated by Cronin et al. (1980) by controlled exposure of nickel-sensitized eczematous patients to a soluble nickel salt in their diet. The cutaneous reaction following ingestion showed a dose-dependent response: only a few reacted to a bolus dose below 1.25 mg nickel ion (as nickel sulfate), but nearly all react to amounts over 2.5 mg Ni. Such exposure elevates serum levels and increases urinary excretion. In four female patients presenting with chronic hand eczema and periodic vesicular eruptions, levels of urinary nickel excretion were directly correlated with the outbreak of vesicles (Menné and Thorboe, 1976).

Urinalysis is seen to be the most practical indicator of chronic exposure to nickel and nickel compounds, and was used in controlled experiments to demonstrate the opposite effect: a nickel-poor diet resulted in reduced urinary excretion of the metal and alleviated symptoms of dermatitis in allergic subjects, commensurate with the degree of sensitization (Burrows, 1992; Veien et al., 1993a; Veien et al., 1993b).

Nickel intake is almost unavoidable through the normal human diet, since the element occurs in most plants, being especially concentrated in plant seeds (Schroeder et al., 1962). Nuts and cocoa beans, for example, are reported to contain as much as 5 to 10 mg Ni/kg (Ellen et al., 1978), which may explain the frequently voiced complaint of "allergy to nuts." The mechanism of adaptation to low doses of antigen was demonstrated by Santucci et al. (1988). When a group of 25 nickel-sensitive females was given 10 mg nickel sulfate in a single dose, 18 experienced flare-ups. However, when 15 days later 17 of the 25 patients were given gradually increasing doses over 3 months (month 1 = 0.67 mg Ni/day; month 2 = 1.34 mg Ni/day; month 3 = 2.24 mg Ni/day), 14 ended the trial without flare-ups. The majority thus were able to adapt and finally showed no clinical reaction to continuing oral administration of the allergen. Challenge by patch test or incidental dermal exposure, however, produced an unchanged allergic reaction as observed before the study. That was taken as an indication of intestinal adaptivity, rather than a build-up of immunological tolerance. Role and impact of dietary nickel in nickel-sensitive patients has been investigated by Veien in dietary-depletion studies. Reducing nickel intake by half by adhering to a low-nickel diet, such restriction generally improves, but does not cure, clinical manifestations of NAH; only approximately 50% of patients with eczema involved in that program showed marked improvement of the hypersensitivity state (Veien, 1989).

Rate of nickel release from alloys is dependent on both pH (Accominotti et al., 1998; Christensen and Moller, 1978; Emmett et al., 1988; Haudrechy et al., 1997; Hemingway and Molokhia, 1987) and temperature (Menné and Solgaard, 1979).

Nickel is released in appreciable amounts (up to 38.7 μg Ni) from (used) stainless-steel cooking utensils at the low pH prevailing with certain foods. In an experiment by Christensen and Möller (1978) using boiling water at varying pH, Ni amounts released correlated inversely with the pH of the water (lower release at higher pH), with a maximum mean value of 20.3 μg released in 80 min. at boiling temperatures and at a pH of 3.2. In cooking experiments with various foods and natural organic acids, oxalic acid was seen as the most aggressive in releasing Ni from steel cooking utensils, releasing up to 9.5 mg Ni/l when boiling a 0.1 M solution for 1 h (Brun, 1979).

In an extensive program preparing standard household recipes in 19 Cr/9 Ni stainless-steel cooking utensils, Flint and Packirisamy (1995) showed that the contribution of nickel in the diet is negligible. In the worst-case scenario, where nickel release was measured in the processing of acid fruits, the amount released in new pans first used amounted to approximately one fifth of the normal daily intake for the average person (around 200 µg).

Accominotti et al. (1998) analyzed the release of nickel (and chromium) levels after cooking 11 standard menus in different grades of stainless-steel utensils. Those values were compared with those obtained by cooking in glassware (yielding Ni levels intrinsic in the foodstuff). The authors conclude that, while significant differences exist between the release of metal, depending on the materials used in food preparation, the levels of nickel release as measured by atomic absorption spectrometry are low (highest for vegetable preparation) when compared with the metal levels contained in the menus. They conclude that there is no advantage for nickel-sensitive patients in switching to materials other than good quality stainless steel.

Cases have been documented in which adverse reactions occurred as a consequence of swallowed nickel coins. Lacroix et al. (1979) described a widespread eczematous (allergic) reaction in a child 18 h after it had swallowed a Canadian quarter. After surgical removal of the coin, erythema markedly subsided, and 6 days later the child was free of dermatitis. Serum nickel levels were determined in a child that presented with generalized nickel dermatitis after having swallowed a Canadian nickel (Ewing and Miller, 1991). Twenty-four hours after ingestion, serum nickel levels were 20.2 µg/l (normal 0.2 to 3.0 µg/l). They returned to normal again after the (severely corroded) coin had been removed via endoscopy.

4.6 DISCUSSION

Considerable data on the release of nickel on contact with skin and other tissues from all types of alloys used in the manufacture of items of everyday use and medical applications have become available, the investigations undoubtedly prompted by the perceived risk of NAH to public health. Not only sweat and inflammatory exudates are factors in solubilizing nickel; also serum, apparently the most aggressive medium acting in specific circumstances such as ear piercing, can play a decisive role on the path towards systemic immunization. This motivated the special requirement contained in the EU Nickel Regulation as to the permissible level of nickel (<0.05%) in materials intended for skin piercing (EU, 1994). This virtually mandates use of nickel-free materials for such applications. The remaining part of the EU Nickel Directive is based on release of nickel (<0.5 µg/cm^2/week) for articles in direct and prolonged contact with the skin.

Results from the many studies conducted to clarify the causal relationship between exposure and risk for NAH induction or elicitation due to the introduction of extraneous materials in the human organism can lead to conflicting conclusions. The issues investigated are complicated by numerous objective and subjective factors; note that each investigator seeks the answers to a question, but isn't always able to control the biologic variables. Also, the literature must be "normalized" for dose: some provide data in percentages, others in molarity. In essence, reducing the data to mass per unit area (e.g., µg/cm^2) offers ease of extrapolation in those publications. Such a review therefore does not permit drawing definitive conclusions, as apparent contradictory findings on the subject abound in the literature. Also, the fact that a reaction to nickel may not appear immediately, but months or years following first contact with the allergen, makes it difficult to project a focused picture correlating cause and effect (Marzulli and Maibach, 1976).

The risk assessment of the presence of nickel at any level in items intended for intimate, long-term contact with the skin seems to depend on the particular cohort involved in such studies. This appears due to the wide range of susceptibility to sensitization seen in the population, as well as the unknown release of nickel ion from the material in contact with corrosive materials. Some studies suggest that for human-health reasons the release of nickel in items coming into direct and prolonged contact should be closely monitored (Cavelier et al., 1988; Cavelier et al., 1985).

While data on dermal absorption of the Ni (II) ion are scant, even less is known about its penetration through mucous membranes. A number of elicitation and systemic reactions have been claimed as a consequence of oral exposure to dental materials, although such claims are generally poorly documented. The clinical data available suggests that the overall risk is low for patients who are not nickel hypersensitive prior to such exposure, and some authors even categorically reject the occurrence of nickel allergic reactions to dental alloys (Barrière et al., 1979; Spiechowicz et al., 1984). A patient with NAH prior to orthodontic treatment may in rare cases show adverse reactions induced by restorative materials. In young patients, the slow, sustained release of nickel from orthodontic appliances may even induce tolerance to nickel if they are not hypersensitive at the start of such exposure (Todd and Burrows, 1989; van Hoogstraten et al., 1991; Kerosuo et al., 1996). A major confounding factor determining the outcome of the many studies may be the large variety in nickel-bearing alloys that are the focus of a particular investigation. Electropositivity of the metals associated with nickel will create a galvanic element generating an electric current from the electronegative element (metal) to the electropositive and thus determine rate and extent of nickel release, particularly in a corrosive environment (Cavelier et al., 1985; Grimsdottir et al., 1992a; Lidén et al., 1998; Morgan and Flint, 1989).

NAH is becoming a minor component of complications in orthopedic surgery, thanks to the development of improved materials and safer alloys, which minimize mechanical failure and the incidence of abrasive metal-to-metal contact (Török et al., 1995). While the number of implants inserted is large, the incidence of clinically relevant metal sensitivity complications is small. There is not substantial-enough evidence to date to suggest that the orthopedic surgeon should alter the usual implant protocol because a patient is sensitive to a metal. Follow-up monitoring for long-term compatibility is indicated, however, for any type of adverse reactions.

Current *in vitro* release data offers an excellent start toward understanding the aspect of percutaneous penetration and NAH potential. Investigation of the other contributing factors should increase our insight, possibly leading to successful interventions that might decrease sensitization. The excellent data currently available could thus be appropriately refined using technological advances leading to insights that mimic the clinical-biological situation existing for man and potentially resulting in NAH.

A practical and natural sequence of events could be:

- Exposure of metal objects to a more clinically relevant biological medium
- Definition of the nickel ion load in the SC

- Correlation of SC load with percutaneous penetration
- Correlation of percutaneous penetration with elicitation of NAH

This sequence may then provide the possibility for clinical intervention and ultimately decrease the elicitation of NAH.

At this point it is not clear to what degree exposure to traditional metallic dental restoration materials has a bearing on the frequency of NAH. However, such hypersensitivity might be expected to increase with certain recent advances in materials technology, which, as an instance, brought the customary average of 8% nickel in stainless steel for such applications to 70% nickel in Ni–Ti in orthodontic wire. It is not content, but release of nickel ion from alloys, that needs to be considered. With the increase in NAH reported (Blanco-Dalmau et al., 1984; Angelini, 1989; Kiec-Swierczynska, 1990a; Kiec-Swierczynska, 1990b; Kiec-Swierczynska, 1996; Mattila, 2001), regulation of maximum permissible nickel release from metallic objects of daily use appears justified from the public-health point of view. Release from metal objects has been sufficiently researched to allow the conclusion that a likely possibility of breaking the increasing NAH incidence lies in marketing or using metal items for personal metal adornment with minimal release of nickel. Such an improving trend could be documented most recently by Johansen et al. (2001) in a Danish population, following implementation of the Danish regulation on nickel release.

The quality of the data reviewed represents state of the science at the time these studies were performed; subsequent advances in analytical chemistry and physical detection methods applicable to biological materials, such as inductively coupled plasma atomic emission spectroscopy and mass spectroscopy, permit highly reliable analyses of contamination and release concentrations down to the ppm and even to the ppb level for most heavy metals, including nickel. With the graded patch data now available, the ppm level is clinically relevant in terms of NAH elicitation (Andersen et al., 1993). Previous limitations can now be technically dealt with without the need to resort to nucleotides.

4.7 ACKNOWLEDGMENT

We gratefully acknowledge the financial support by the Nickel Producers Environmental Research Association (NiPERA) toward this review project.

REFERENCES

Accominotti, M. et al., Contribution to chromium and nickel enrichment during cooking of foods in stainless steel utensils, *Contact Dermatitis*, 38, 305–310, 1998.

Allenby, C.F. and Goodwin, B.F., Influence of detergent washing powders on minimal eliciting patch test concentrations of nickel and chromium, *Contact Dermatitis*, 9, 491–499, 1983.

Allenby, C.F. and Basketter, D.A., An arm immersion model of compromised skin. II. Influence on minimal eliciting patch test concentrations of nickel, *Contact Dermatitis*, 28, 129–133, 1993.

Allenby, C.F. and Basketter, D.A., The effect of repeated open exposure to low levels of nickel on compromised hand skin of nickel allergic subjects, *Contact Dermatitis*, 30, 135–138, 1994.

Andersen, K.E. et al., Dose-response testing with nickel sulphate using TRUE test in nickel-sensitive individuals, *Br. J. Dermatol.*, 129, 50–56, 1993.

Angelini, G. and Veña, G.A., Allergia da contatto al nickel. Considerazioni su vecchie e nuove acquisizioni, *Bollettino di Dermatologia Allergologica e Professional*, 4, 5–14, 1989.

Aro, T. et al., Long-lasting allergic patch test reaction caused by gold, *Contact Dermatitis*, 28, 276–281, 1993.

Avnstorp, C., Menné, T., and Maibach, H.I., Contact allergy to chromium and nickel, in *Immunotoxicity of Metals and Immunotoxicology*, Dayan, A.D., Ed., Plenum Press, New York, 1990, pp. 83–91.

Axéll, T. et al., Standard patch test series for screening of contact allergy to dental materials, *Contact Dermatitis*, 9, 82–84, 1983.

Bang Pedersen, N. et al., Release of nickel from silver coins, *Acta Derm. Venereol. (Stockh.)*, 54, 231–234, 1974.

Bangha, E. and Elsner, P., Sensitizations to allergens of the European standard series at the Department of Dermatology in Zurich 1990–1994, *Dermatology*, 193, 17–21, 1996.

Barrière, H. et al., Allergie aux détergents et allergie au nickel, *Ann. Dermatol. Vénérol.*, 106, 33–37, 1979.

Basketter, D.A. et al., Nickel, cobalt, and chromium in consumer products: a role in allergic contact dermatitis?, *Contact Dermatitis*, 28, 15–25, 1993.

Bass, J.K., Fine, H., and Cisneros, G.J., Nickel hypersensitivity in the orthodontic patient, *Am. J. Orthodont. Dentofac. Orthop.*, 103, 280–285, 1993.

Bergman, M., Bergman, B., and Söremark, R., Tissue accumulation of nickel released due to electrochemical corrosion of non-precious dental casting alloys, *J. Oral Rehab.*, 325–330, 1980.

Bettley, F.R., Nickel coin dermatitis, *Contact Dermatitis Newsl.*, 9, 198, 1971.

Bishara, S.E., Barrett, R.D., and Moustafa, I.S., Biodegradation of orthodontic appliances. Part II. Changes in the blood level of nickel, *Am. J. Orthodont. Dentofac. Orthop.*, 103, 280–285, 1993.

Black, H., Dermatitis from nickel and copper in coins, *Contact Dermatitis Newsl.*, 12, 326–327, 1972.

Blanco-Dalmau, L., Carrasquillo-Alberty, H., and Silva-Parra, J., A study of nickel allergy, *J. Prosthet. Dent.*, 52, 116–119, 1989.

Brasch, J. and Geier, J., Patch test results in schoolchildren. Results from the Information Network of Departments (IVDK) and the German Contact Dermatitis Research group (DKG), *Contact Dermatitis*, 37, 286–293, 1997.

Brasch, J., Geier, J., and Schnuch, A., Differentiated contact allergy lists serve in quality improvement, *Hautarzt*, 49, 184–191, 1998.

Brown, S.A. and Merritt, K., Electrochemical corrosion in saline and serum, *J. Biomed. Mat. Res.*, 14, 173–179, 1980.

Brown, S.S. et al., IUPAC reference method for analysis of nickel in serum and urine by electrothermal atomic absorption spectrophotometry, *Clin. Biochem.*, 14, 295–302, 1981.

Bruce, G.J. and Hall, W.B., Nickel hypersensitivity-related periodontitis, *Compendium of Continuing Education in Dentistry*, 178, 180–184, 1995.

Brun, R., Nickel in food: the role of stainless-steel utensils, *Contact Dermatitis*, 5, 43–45, 1979.

Bumgardner, J.D. and Lucas, L.C., Surface analysis of nickel-chromium dental alloys, *Dent. Mat.*, 9, 252–259, 1993.

Bumgardner, J.D. and Lucas, L.C., Corrosion and cell culture evaluations of nickel-chromium dental castings, *J. Appl. Biomat.*, 5, 203–213, 1994.

Bumgardner, J.D. and Lucas, L.C., Cellular response to metallic ions released from nickel-chromium dental alloys, *J. Dent. Res.*, 74, 1521–1527, 1995.

Cage, G.W. and Dobson, R.L., Sodium secretion and reabsorption in the human eccrine sweat gland, *J. Clin. Invest.*, 44, 1270–1276, 1965.

Cavelier, C., Foussereau, J., and Massin, M., Nickel allergy: analysis of metal clothing objects and patch testing to metal samples, *Contact Dermatitis*, 12, 65–75, 1985.

Cavelier, C. et al., Nickel allergy: tolerance to metallic surface-plated samples in nickel-sensitive humans and guinea pigs, *Contact Dermatitis*, 19, 358–361, 1988.

Cavelier, C. et al., Allergy to nickel or cobalt: tolerance to nickel and cobalt samples in man and in the guinea pig allergic or sensitized to these metals, *Contact Dermatitis*, 21, 72–78, 1989.

Christensen, O.B. and Möller, H., Release of nickel from cooking utensils, *Contact Dermatitis*, 4, 343–346, 1978.

Cortada, M. et al., Metallic ion release in artificial saliva of titanium oral implants coupled with different metal superstructures, *Bio.-Med. Mat. Eng.*, 7, 213–220, 1997.

Cronin, E., Di Michiel, A.D., and Brown, S.S., Oral challenge in nickel-sensitive women with hand eczema, in *International Conference on Nickel Toxicology, Swansea, Wales*, Brown, S.S. and Sunderman, F.W., Eds., Academic Press, London, 1980, pp. 150–152.

Cullander, C. et al., A quantitative minimally invasive assay for the detection of metals in the stratum corneum, *J. Pharm. Biomed. Anal.*, 22, 265–279, 2000.

Dickel, H. et al., Patch testing with a standard series, *Dermatosen*, 46, 234–243, 1998.

Dipietro, E.S. et al., Comparison of an inductively coupled plasma-atomic emission spectrometry method for the determination of calcium, magnesium, sodium, potassium, copper and zinc with atomic absorption spectroscopy and flame photometry methods, *Sci. Total Environ.*, 74, 249–262, 1988.

Edie, J.W., Andreasen, G.F., and Zaytoun, M.P., Surface corrosion of nitinol and stainless steel under clinical conditions, *Angle Orthodontry*, 51, 319–324, 1981.

Ellen, G., van den Bosch-Tibbesma, G., and Douma, F.F., Nickel content of various Dutch foodstuffs, *Z. Lebensm. Unters. Forsch.*, 166, 145–147, 1978.

Emmett, E.A. et al., Allergic contact dermatitis to nickel: Bioavailability from consumer products and provocation threshold, *J. Am. Acad. Dermatol.*, 19, 314–322, 1988.

España, A. et al., Chronic urticaria after implantation of 2 nickel-containing dental prosthesis in a nickel-allergic patient, *Contact Dermatitis*, 21, 204–206, 1989.

Evans, E.M., Walex, S., and Freeman, M.A.R., Metal sensitivity as a cause of bone necrosis and loosening of the prosthesis in total joint replacement, *J. Bone Joint Surg.*, 56B, 626–642, 1974.

Ewing, S. and Miller, R., Generalized nickel dermatitis in a 6-year-old boy as a result of swallowing a Canadian nickel, *J. Am. Acad. Dermatol.*, 25, 855–856, 1991.

Fischer, T. et al., Contact sensitivity to nickel in white gold, *Contact Dermatitis*, 10, 23–24, 1984a.

Fischer, T. et al., Nickel release from ear piercing kits and earrings, *Contact Dermatitis*, 10, 39–42, 1984b.

Fisher, A.A., Possible combined nickel and gold allergy, *Am. J. Contact Dermat.*, 3, 52, 1992.

Flint, G.N., A metallurgical approach to metal contact dermatitis, *Contact Dermatitis*, 39, 213–221, 1998.

Flint, G.N. and Packirisamy, S., Systemic nickel: the contribution made by stainless-steel cooking utensils, *Contact Dermatitis*, 32, 218–224, 1995.

Forslind, B. et al., Recent advances in x-ray microanalysis in dermatology, *Scanning Electron Microsc.*, Part 2, 687–695, 1985.

Fregert, S., Kollander, M., and Poulsen, J., Allergic contact stomatitis from gold dentures, *Contact Dermatitis*, 5, 63–64, 1979.

Gawkrodger, D.J., Nickel dermatitis: how much nickel is safe?, *Contact Dermatitis*, 35, 267–271, 1996.

Gilboa, R., Al-Tawil, N.G., and Marcusson, J.A., Metal allergy in cashiers: an in vitro and in vivo study for the presence of metal allergy, *Acta Derm. Venereol. (Stockh.)*, 68, 317–324, 1988.

Giménez-Arnau, A. et al., Metal-induced generalized pruriginous dermatitis and endovascular surgery, *Contact Dermatitis*, 43, 35–40, 2000.

Gjerdet, N.R. et al., Nickel and iron in saliva of patients with fixed orthodontic appliances, *Acta Odont. Scand.*, 49, 73–78, 1991.

Gollhausen, R. and Ring, J., Allergy to coined money: nickel contact dermatitis in cashiers, *J. Am. Acad. Dermatol.*, 25, 365–369, 1991.

Grice, K. et al., An evaluation of Na, Cl and pH ion-specific electrodes in the study of the electrolyte contents of epidermal transudate and sweat, *Br. J. Dermatol.*, 92, 511–518, 1975.

Grimsdottir, M.R., Gjerdet, N.R., and Hensten-Pettersen, A., Composition and in vitro corrosion of orthodontic appliances, *Am. J. Orthodont. Dentof. Orthop.*, 101, 525–532, 1992a.

Grimsdottir, M.R., Hensten-Pettersen, A., and Kullmann, A., Cytotoxic effect of orthodontic appliances, *Eur. J. Orthodont.*, 14, 47–53, 1992b.

Guerra, L. et al., Sensitization to palladium, *Contact Dermatitis*, 19, 306–307, 1988.

Guerra, L. et al., Role of contact sensitizers in the "burning mouth syndrome," *Am. J. Contact Dermat.*, 4, 154–157, 1993.

Guimaraens, D., Gonzales, M.A., and Condé-Salazar, L., Systemic contact dermatitis from dental crowns, *Contact Dermatitis*, 30, 124–125, 1994.

Guyuron, B. and Lasa, C.I., Jr., Reaction to stainless steel wire following orthognathic surgery, *Plast. Reconstr. Surg.*, 89, 540–542, 1992.

Haudrechy, P. et al., Nickel release from nickel-plated metals and stainless steel, *Contact Dermatitis*, 31, 249–255, 1994.

Haudrechy, P. et al., Nickel release from stainless steels, *Contact Dermatitis*, 37, 113–117, 1997.

Hay, I.C. and Ormerod, A.D., Severe oral and facial reaction to 6 metals in restorative dentistry, *Contact Dermatitis*, 38, 216, 1998.

Hemingway, J.D. and Molokhia, M.M., The dissolution of metallic nickel in artificial sweat, *Contact Dermatitis*, 16, 99–105, 1987.

Husain, S.L., Nickel coin dermatitis, *BMJ*, 2, 998, 1977.

ICDRG, Revised European standard series, *Contact Dermatitis*, 19, 391, 1988.

Ingber, A., Klein, S.K., and David, M., The nickel released from jewelry in Israel and its clinical significance, *Contact Dermatitis*, 39, 195–197, 1997.

Ishikawaya, Y., Suzuki, H., and Kullavanija, P., Exposure of nickel in used and unused gold-plated earrings: a study using scanning electron microscopy and x-ray microanalysis, *Contact Dermatitis*, 36, 1–4, 1997.

Izumi, K., Allergic contact gingivostomatitis due to gold, *Arch. Dermatol. Res.*, 272, 387–391, 1982.

Jensen, O., "Rusters." The corrosive action of palmar sweat. II. Physical and chemical factors in palmar hyperhidrosis, *Acta Derm. Venereol. (Stockh.)*, 59, 139–143, 1979.

Johansen, J. et al., Changes in the pattern of sensitization to common contact allergens in Denmark between 1985–86 and 1997–98, with a special view to the effect of preventive strategies, *Br. J. Dermatol.*, 142, 490–495, 2001.

Johansson, S.A.E. and Campbell, J.L., *PIXE: A Novel Technique for Elemental Analysis*, John Wiley & Sons, New York, 1988.

Kanerva, L. and Aitio, A., Dermatotoxicological aspects of metallic chromium, *Eur. J. Dermatol.*, 7, 79–84, 1997.

Kanerva, L. et al., Nickel release from metals, and a case of allergic contact dermatitis from stainless steel, *Contact Dermatitis*, 31, 299–303, 1994.

Kanerva, L., Estlander, T., and Jolanki, R., Dental problems, in *Practical Contact Dermatitis*, McGraw-Hill, New York, 1995, pp. 397–432.

Kanerva, L., Estlander, T., and Jolanki, R., Bank clerk's occupational allergic nickel and cobalt contact dermatitis from coins, *Contact Dermatitis*, 38, 217–218, 1998.

Katz, S.A. and Samitz, M.H., Leaching of nickel from stainless steel consumer commodities, *Acta Derm. Venereol. (Stockh.)*, 55, 113–115, 1975.

Kerosuo, H. et al., Nickel allergy in adolescents in relation to orthodontic treatment and piercing of ears, *Am. J. Orthodont. Dentofac. Orthoped.*, 109, 148–154, 1996.

Kerosuo, H., Moe, G., and Hensten-Pettersen, A., Salivary nickel and chromium in subjects with different types of fixed orthodontic appliances, *Am. J. Orthodont. Dentofac. Orthoped.*, 111, 595–598, 1997.

Kiec-Swierczynska, M., Occupational dermatoses and allergy to metals in Polish construction workers manufacturing prefabricated building units, *Contact Dermatitis*, 23, 27–32, 1990a.

Kiec-Swierczynska, M., Allergy to chromate, cobalt and nickel in Lodz 1977–1988, *Contact Dermatitis*, 22, 229–231, 1990b.

Kiec-Swierczynska, M., Occupational allergic contact dermatitis in Lodz: 1990–1994, *Occup. Med.*, 46, 205–208, 1996.

Kieffer, M., Nickel sensitivity: relationship between history and patch test reaction, *Contact Dermatitis*, 5, 398–401, 1979.

Kligman, A.M., The identification of contact allergens by human assay. 3. The maximization test: a procedure for screening and rating contact sensitizers, *J. Invest. Dermatol.*, 47, 393–409, 1966.

Koch, P. and Bahmer, F.A., Oral lichenoid lesions, mercury hypersensitivity and combined hypersensitivity to mercury and other metals: histologically-proven reproduction of the reaction by patch testing with metal salts, *Contact Dermatitis*, 33, 323–328, 1995.

Koppenburg, P. et al., Die kieferothopädische Apparatur-ein Schritt zur Sensibilisierung gegen Metalle?, *Fortschritte in der Kieferothopaedie*, 49, 62–69, 1988.

Kubba, R., Taylor, J. S., and Marks, K.E., Cutaneous complications of orthopedic implantations, *Arch. Dermatol.*, 117, 554–560, 1981.

Lacroix, J., Morin, C.L., and Collin, P.-P., Nickel dermatitis from a foreign body in the stomach., *J. Pediat.*, 95, 428, 1979.

Landwehr, A.J. and van Ketel, W.G., Pompholyx after implantation of a nickel-containing pacemaker in a nickel-allergic patient, *Contact Dermatitis*, 9, 147, 1983.

Larsen, F.S. and Brandrup, F., Nickel release from metallic buttons in blue jeans, *Contact Dermatitis*, 6, 298–299, 1980.

Laugier, P. and Foussereau, J., Les dermites allergiques à distance provoquées par le matériel d'osthéosynthèse, *Gazette Médicale de France*, 73, 3409–3418, 1966.

Lidén, C., Menné, T., and Burrows, D., Nickel-containing alloys and platings and their ability to cause dermatitis, *Br. J. Dermatol.*, 134, 193–198, 1996.

Lidén, C. et al., Nickel release from tools on the Swedish market, *Contact Dermatitis*, 39, 127–131, 1998.

Lim, J.T.E. et al., Changing trends in the epidemiology of contact dermatitis in Singapore, *Contact Dermatitis*, 26, 321–326, 1992.

Linden, J. V. et al., Blood nickel concentrations in patients with stainless-steel hip prostheses, *Ann. Clin. Lab. Sci.*, 15, 459–464, 1985.

Lowney, E.D., Immunologic unresponsiveness to a contact sensitizer in man, *J. Invest. Dermatol.*, 51, 411–417, 1968.

Lyell, A., Bain, W.H., and Thomson, R.M., Repeated failure of nickel-containing prosthetic heart valves in a patient allergic to nickel, *Lancet*, 2, 657–659, 1978.

Magnusson, B. et al., Nickel allergy and nickel-containing dental alloys, *Scand. J. Dent. Res.*, 90, 163–167, 1982.

Maibach, H.I. and Menné, T., Eds., *Nickel and the Skin: Immunology and Toxicology,* CRC Press, Boca Raton, FL, 1989.

Malmqvist, K.G. et al., The use of PIXE in experimental studies of the physiology of human skin epidermis, *Biol. Trace Element Res.*, 12, 297–308, 1987.

Marcusson, J.A., Contact allergies to nickel sulfate, gold sodium thiosulfate and palladium chloride in patients claiming side-effects from dental alloy components, *Contact Dermatitis*, 34, 320–323, 1996.

Marks, J.C. and DeLeo, V.A., *Contact and Occupational Dermatology*, Mosby Year Book, St. Louis, 1992.

Marks, J.G. et al., North American Contact Dermatitis Group patch test results for the detection of delayed-type hypersensitivity to topical allergens, *J. Am. Acad. Dermatol.*, 38, 911–918, 1998.

Marzulli, F.N. and Maibach, H.I., Contact allergy: predictive testing in man, *Contact Dermatitis*, 2, 1–17, 1976.

Mattila, L. et al., Prevalence of nickel allergy among Finnish university students, *Contact Dermatitis*, 44, 218–223, 2001.

Menné, T. and Solgaard, P., Temperature-dependent nickel release from nickel alloys, *Contact Dermatitis*, 5, 82–84, 1979.

Menné, T. and Rasmussen, K., Regulation of nickel exposure in Denmark, *Contact Dermatitis*, 23, 57–58, 1990.

Menné, T. and Maibach, H.I., Reactions to systemic exposure to contact allergens: systemic contact allergy reactions (SCAR), *Immunol. Allergy Pract.*, 9, 373–385, 1987.

Menné, T. et al., Patch test reactivity to nickel alloys, *Contact Dermatitis*, 16, 255–259, 1987a.

Menné, T. et al., Evaluation of the dimethylglyoxime stick test for the detection of nickel, *Dermatosen*, 35, 128–130, 1987b.

Menné, T. and Calvin, G., Concentration threshold of non-occluded nickel exposure in nickel-sensitive individuals and controls with and without surfactant, *Contact Dermatitis*, 29, 180–184, 1993.

Menné, T., Quantitative aspects of nickel dermatitis. Sensitization and eliciting threshold concentrations, *Sci. Total Environ.*, 148, 275–281, 1994.

Menné, T. and Thorboe, A., Nickel dermatitis — nickel excretion, *Contact Dermatitis*, 2, 353–354, 1976.

Merritt, K. and Brown, S.A., Distribution of cobalt chromium wear and corrosion products and biologic reactions, *Clinical Orthopaedics and Related Research*, 329 Suppl., S233–243, 1996.

Merritt, K. and Brown, S.A., Metal sensitivity reactions to orthopedic implants, *Int. J. Derm.*, 20, 89–94, 1981.

Moffa, J.P., Beck, W.D., and Hoke, A.W., Allergic response to nickel containing dental alloys, *J. Dent. Res.*, 56B, Abst. No. 107, 1977.

Möller, H., Yes, systemic nickel is probably important! (letter), *J. Am. Acad. Dermatol.*, 28, 511–513, 1993.

Mongkolnam, P., The adverse effects of dental restorative materials–a review, *Austr. Dent. J.*, 37, 360–367, 1992.

Morgan, L.G. and Flint, G.N., Nickel alloys and coatings: release of nickel, in *Nickel and the Skin: Immunology and Toxicology*, Maibach, H.I. and Menné, T., Eds., CRC Press, Boca Raton, FL, 1989, p. 49.

Morris, F.H., Veterans administration cooperative studies project no. 147. IV. Biocompatibility of base metal alloys, *J. Prosthet. Dent.*, 58, 1–4, 1987.

Mountcastle, E.A., James, W.D., and Rodman, O.G., Allergic contact stomatitis to a dental impression material (letter), *J. Am. Acad. Dermatol.*, 15, 1055–1056, 1986.

Nakada, T. and Iijima, M., Metal allergy, *Jpn. Med. J.*, 3756, 37–42, 1996.

Namikoshi, T. et al., The prevalence of sensitivity to constituents of dental alloys, *J. Oral Rehab.*, 17, 377–381, 1990.

Nielsen, C. and Klaschka, F., Teststudien an der Mundschleimhaut bei Ekzemallergikern, *Deutsche Zahn, Mund und Kieferheilkunde*, 57, 201–218, 1971.

Nielsen, N.H. and Menné, T., Allergic contact sensitization in an unselected Danish population. The Glostrup Allergy Study, Denmark, *Acta Derm. Venereol. (Stockh.)*, 72, 456–460, 1992.

Park, H.Y. and Shearer, T.R., In vitro release of nickel and chromium from simulated orthodontic appliances, *Am. J. Orthod.*, 84, 156–159, 1983.

Parsons, M.L., Major, S., and Forster, A.R., Trace element determination by atomic spectroscopic methods-state of the art, *Appl. Spectrosc.*, 37, 411–418, 1983.

Preininger, T., Überempfindlichkeit gegen Nickelgeld, *Dermatol. Wochenschr.*, 99, 1082–1084, 1934.

Randin, J. P., Corrosion behavior of nickel-containing alloys in artificial sweat, *J. Biomed. Mat. Res.*, 22, 649–666, 1988.

Räsänen, L. and Tuomi, M., Diagnostic value of the lymphocyte proliferation test in nickel contact allergy and provocation in occupational coin dermatitis, *Contact Dermatitis*, 27, 250–254, 1992.

Reynolds, R.J. and Aldous, K., Eds., *Atomic Absorption Spectroscopy: A Practical Guide*, Barnes & Noble, New York, 1970.

Richter, G., Ergebnisse und Probleme mit Dentallegierungen im Epikutantest, *Occup. Environ. Dermatol.*, 49, 5–12, 2001.

Romaguera, C., Grimalt, F., and Vilaplana, J., Contact dermatitis from nickel: an investigation of its sources, *Contact Dermatitis*, 19, 52–57, 1988.

Romaguera, C., Vilaplana, J., and Grimalt, F., Contact stomatitis from a dental prosthesis, *Contact Dermatitis*, 21, 204, 1989.

Rothman, S., Überempfindlichkeit gegen Hartgeld, *Dermatol. Wochenschr.*, 90, 98–99, 1930.

Samitz, M.H. and Katz, S.A., Nickel dermatitis hazards from prostheses, *Br. J. Dermatol.*, 92, 287–290, 1975.

Santucci, B. et al., Nickel sensitivity: effects of prolonged oral intake of the element, *Contact Dermatitis*, 19, 202–205, 1988.

Schöpf, E., Wex, O., and Schulz, K.H., Allergische Kontaktstomatitis mit spezifischer Lymphocytenstimulation durch Gold, *Hautarzt*, 21, 422–424, 1970.

Schroeder, H.A., Balassa, J.C., and Tipton, I.H., Abnormal trace metals in man — chromium, *J. Chronic Dis.*, 15, 941–964, 1962.

Sertoli, A. et al., Epidemiological survey of contact dermatitis in Italy (1984–1993) by GIRDCA, *Am. J. Contact Dermat.*, 10, 18–30, 1999.

Sevila, A. et al., Contact dermatitis in children, *Contact Dermatitis*, 30, 292–294, 1994.

Skoglund, A. and Egelrud, T., Hypersensitivity reactions to dental materials in patients with lichenoid oral mucosal lesions and in patients with burning mouth syndrome, *Scand. J. Dent. Res.*, 99, 320–328, 1991.

Spiechowicz, E. et al., Oral exposure to a nickel-containing dental alloy of persons with hypersensitive skin reactions to nickel, *Contact Dermatitis*, 10, 206–211, 1984.

Staerkjaer, L. and Menné, T., Nickel allergy and orthodontic treatment, *Eur. J. Orthodont.*, 12, 284–289, 1990.

Stenman, E. and Bergman, M., Hypersensitivity reactions to dental materials in a referred group of patients, *Scand. J. Dent. Res.*, 97, 76–83, 1989.

Sunderman, F.W., Jr., Biological monitoring of nickel in humans, *Scand. J. Worker Environ. Health*, 19 (Suppl. 1), 34–38, 1993.

Sunderman, F.W., Jr., Chemistry, analysis and monitoring, in *Nickel and the Skin: Immunology and Toxicology*, Maibach, H.I. and Menné, T., Eds., CRC Press, Boca Raton, FL, 1989, pp. 2–8.

Sunderman, F.W. et al., Cobalt, chromium and nickel concentrations in body fluids of patients with porous-coated knee or hip prostheses, *J. Orthop. Res.*, 7, 307–315, 1989.

Temesvári, E. and Racz, I., Nickel sensitivity from dental prosthesis, *Contact Dermatitis*, 18, 50–51, 1988.

Todd, D.J. and Burrows, D., Nickel allergy in relationship to previous oral and cutaneous nickel contact, *Ulster Med. J.*, 58, 168–171, 1989.

Török, L. et al., Investigation into the development of allergy to metal in recipients of implanted hip prostheses: a prospective study, *Eur. J. Dermatol.*, 5, 294–295, 1995.

Trombelli, L. et al., Systemic contact dermatitis from an orthodontic appliance, *Contact Dermatitis*, 27, 259–260, 1992.

Tschernitschek, H., Wolter, S., and Korner, M., Allergien auf Zahnersatzmaterialien, *Dermatosen*, 46, 244–248, 1998.

van Hoogstraten, I.M.W. et al., Reduced frequency of nickel allergy upon oral nickel contact at an early age, *Clin. Exp. Immunol.*, 85, 441–445, 1991.

van Ketel, W.G., Occupational contact with coins in nickel-allergic patients, *Contact Dermatitis*, 12, 108, 1985.

van Loon, L.A.J. et al., Contact stomatitis and dermatitis to nickel and palladium, *Contact Dermatitis*, 11, 294–297, 1984.

Vandenberg, J.J. and Epstein, W.L., Experimental nickel contact sensitization in man, *J. Invest. Dermatol.*, 41, 413–416, 1963.

Veien, N.K., Systemically induced eczema in adults, *Acta Derm. Venereol. (Stockh.)*, 147 (Suppl), 12–55, 1989.

Veien, N.K., Hattel, T., and Laurberg, G., Low nickel diet: an open, prospective trial, *Am. Acad. Dermatol.*, 29, 1002–1007, 1993a.

Veien, N.K., Hattel, T., and Laurberg, G., Systemically aggravated contact dermatitis caused by aluminium in toothpaste, *Contact Dermatitis*, 28, 199–200, 1993b.

Veien, N.K. et al., Stomatitis or systemically-induced contact dermatitis from metal wire in orthodontic materials, *Contact Dermatitis*, 30, 210–213, 1994.

Veien, N. et al., Dental implications of nickel hypersensitivity, *J. Prosth. Dent.*, 56, 507–509, 1986.

Vilaplana, J., Romaguera, C., and Cornellana, F., Contact dermatitis and adverse oral mucous membrane reactions related to the use of dental prostheses, *Contact Dermatitis*, 30, 80–84, 1994.

Wall, L.M., Spot tests and chemical analysis for allergen evaluation, in *Textbook of Contact Dermatitis*, Rycroft, R.J.G. et al., Eds., Springer-Verlag, Heidelberg, 1992. pp. 277–285.

Wataha, J.C. and Hanks, C.T., Biological effects of palladium and risk of using palladium in dental casting alloys, *J. Oral Rehab.*, 23, 309–320, 1996.

Wiesenfeld, D. et al., Allergy to dental gold, *Oral Surg.*, 57, 158–160, 1984.

Wilson, A.G. and Gould, D.J., Nickel dermatitis from a dental prosthesis without buccal involvement, *Contact Dermatitis*, 21, 53, 1989.

5 Skin Absorption of Nickel and Methods to Quantify Penetration

Jurij J. Hostýnek, Katherine E. Reagan, and Howard I. Maibach

CONTENTS

Abstract 147
5.1   Introduction 148
5.2   Qualitative Observations 149
5.3   Quantitative Methods and Permeation Data 153
    5.3.1   *In Vitro* Dermal Absorption 154
    5.3.2   *In Vivo* Percent Dose Absorbed 155
    5.3.3   The "Disappearance Method" 156
    5.3.4   Predictive Models 157
    5.3.5   Data on Nickel Absorption 157
5.4   Summary, Conclusions, and Criticism 159
5.5   Outlook 161
Acknowledgment 161
References 161

ABSTRACT

Literature on qualitative and quantitative data of nickel absorbed through human or animal skin and its appendages *in vitro* or *in vivo* presents studies conducted using several experimental methods. Values for permeability coefficients (Kps), a yardstick permitting comparison of nickel salts in relation to other (metal) compounds, are rarely reported as such (an exception is nickel chloride [Emilson et al., 1993]) and for the present purpose are derived whenever possible by interpretation of the (often incomplete) experimental data. The "best number" for the *in vitro* Kps of nickel compounds gleaned from the literature is on the order of 10^{-6} cm/h. Also reported here are the Kps for four nickel salts determined in our laboratory through isolated human stratum corneum, measured for the first time under steady-state conditions. Using micro-diffusion cells and analysis by inductively coupled plasma mass spectroscopy, the values derived range from 5.2 to 8.5×10^{-7} cm/h.

5.1 INTRODUCTION

Aside from endogenous factors in the target organism, skin permeation is determined by the physicochemical parameters and reactivity of permeants (Barry, 1983; Scheuplein and Blank, 1967; Scheuplein and Blank, 1971). Based on experience with the therapeutic action of dermatologicals, we anticipate ready skin penetration by lipophilic compounds. But it is counterintuitive that polar structures such as water or electrolytes, e.g., salts in aqueous solution, should also penetrate to a significant degree. For water and other hydrophilic, charged molecules, however, including several metal compounds, this could be observed also, not in the least based on morbidity due to skin exposure to such xenobiotics. That process, though, proceeds at an average of two to three orders of magnitude slower than the penetration of small-molecular-weight, lipophilic nonelectrolytes (Hostýnek et al., 1993). Reactions observed in the skin of hypersensitive individuals following frequent occupational contact or experimental exposure to allergenic metals such as nickel (Gilboa et al., 1988; Hegyi and Gasparik, 1989; Husain, 1977; Kaaber et al., 1987; Kanerva et al., 1998; Kanerva et al., 1994; Preininger, 1934; Rothman, 1930) are an indication of their diffusion through the stratum corneum (SC).

Numerous compounds commonly used in consumer and personal-care products bear an electron charge: quats (antimicrobials), betaines (surfactants) or salts of aluminum, zirconium, lead, zinc or mercury (antiperspirants, hair colorants, disinfectants, etc.). That such charged molecules may penetrate the skin was formerly disregarded, mainly due to lack of radioisotopes or analytical methods sufficiently sensitive to detect low levels of penetration. Metal isotopes and modern microanalytical methods now do provide ample evidence for ready permeation through the structures of the skin and its appendages (Potts et al., 1992). Uptake of zwitterionic surfactants has been measured *in vivo* (Bucks et al., 1993) and *in vitro* (Ridout et al., 1991). Finally, allergic sensitization as detected with patch testing using metal-releasing objects also provides evidence for the facile violation of the SC barrier. (Cavelier et al., 1985; Cavelier et al., 1989; Lidén et al., 1996; Menné et al., 1987; Haudrechy et al., 1994) Conventionally, skin diffusivity is described by the permeability coefficient K_p — a flux value, normalized for concentration, that represents the rate at which the chemical penetrates the skin. A wide range of experimental techniques has been used *in vivo* and *in vitro* to measure dermal absorption of nickel compounds; the results, when the data permit, are presented here as K_p values describing the flux of individual compounds through animal or human skin. The K_p is derived by Fick's law of diffusion (Fick, 1855) from flux measurements through a biological barrier under conditions of steady state (J_{ss}), *in vitro*, from an infinite reservoir of the compound, through a biological barrier, and normalized for the concentration (C) applied: $J_{ss} = K_p \Delta C$. Expressed as depth of diffusion per unit of time (here in cm/h), it provides a basis for comparison of the relative absorption rates of diverse chemicals. When the permeant is applied from aqueous solution, it also represents the method by which numerous compound-specific penetration data currently available have been generated. While the K_p is the best descriptor of membrane penetration characteristic for those materials that do conform with Fick's law of diffusion, data, particularly on the absorption of nickel, have rarely been collected in a manner permitting direct deduction of these values. Also, percutaneous diffusion characteristics of nickel salts do not meet the criteria of so-called Fickian behavior due to nickel's high electrophilicity, making it likely to bind to skin components, retarding its migration through the skin and resulting in the formation of depots. Nevertheless, because Kp is the most convenient parameter for comparison of percutaneous penetration kinetics, its value is estimated whenever literature results are amenable to appropriate transformation. Human skin absorption data for nickel is compiled in Table 5.1.

5.2 QUALITATIVE OBSERVATIONS

Nickel shows a special affinity for keratin encountered in SC cells, which has a retarding effect on skin penetration rates (Alder et al., 1986; Cotton, 1964; Ermolli et al., 2001; Fullerton and Hoelgaard, 1988; Samitz and Katz, 1976; Santucci et al., 1998). Thus absorption through the appendages (sweat ducts, follicles, and sebaceous glands) appears to proceed at a faster rate than transcellularly (Wells, 1956). When applied on the skin, certain nickel salts thus also require considerable induction (lag) times before measurable penetration is observed (24 to 90 h) due to binding to cellular and intercellular components (Bennett, 1984; Ermolli et al., 2001; Fullerton et al., 1988; Fullerton et al., 1986). Such binding to epidermal and dermal tissue is also responsible for establishing depots of the metal in the epidermis, which functions as a local reservoir for xenobiotics. Such binding to tissue, reversible or irreversible, allows compounds to partition into the protein or lipid phases of the various dermal strata (Ermolli et al., 2001; Fullerton et al., 1986; Kolpakov, 1963; Samitz and Katz, 1976; Spruit et al., 1965) and for purposes of risk assessment represents one of the imponderables of skin-penetration studies with nickel and similar electrophilic compounds.

In penetration through the appendages, nickel appears to be sequestered by chelation, primarily by urocanic acid and histidine occurring in human sweat. Proposed as one of the functions of such components of sweat is the sequestration of nickel and other potentially toxic xenobiotics from the body, as well as the prevention of their absorption (Mali et al., 1964). Nickel absorption studies of nickel on powdered SC showed that the metal binds preferentially to carboxyl groups, rather than amino groups (Samitz and Katz, 1976), although Santucci arrived at the opposite conclusion (Santucci et al., 1998). Sustained exposure to nickel metal dust in the industrial setting can induce dermatitis collectively described as "nickel rash": papules, erythema, and vesicles progressing to weeping eczema resulting from release of nickel ion (Bulmer and Mackenzie, 1926). These effects seen in the epidermal tissues all confirm the ability of the metal ion to penetrate beyond the SC.

Autoradiography of human skin exposed *in vitro* to $^{63}NiCl_2$ revealed that nickel accumulated within 1 h in the hair shafts besides depositing in the SC (Lloyd, 1980). After 4 h the basal and suprabasal epidermal cells were also labeled. Incubation of homogenized human epidermis with nickel chloride solutions indicated establishment of an equilibrium depending on the nickel concentration in the incubation medium (Fullerton and Hoelgaard, 1988). Such reversible binding to constituents of the skin is consistent with the observation *in vivo* that the epidermis can function as a dynamic nickel reservoir (Samitz and Katz, 1976).

TABLE 5.1
Human Skin Permeation by Nickel Compounds *in Vitro*

Compound (Membrane)	Temperature (°C)	Concentration	Vehicle	Time (h)	$10^4 \cdot Kp$ (cm/h)	Ref.
$^{63}NiSO_4$ (epidermis)	37	100 mM	Saline	24	0.1	Samitz and Katz, 1976
		100 mM		90	0.03	
		10 mM		24	0.03	
		10 mM		90	0.03	
		1 mM		24	0.04	
		1 mM		90	0.07	
		2 mM	Sweat	1	0.3	
		2 mM		5	0.02	
$NiCl_2$ (f. th., not occluded)	37	1.32 mg/ml	Water	144	0.034	Fullerton et al., 1986
(f. th., occluded)					0.53–2.3	
$NiSO_4$ (f. th., occluded)					0.03	
$NiCl_2$ (f. th.)	37	0.62%	Hydrogel	48	<0.045	Fullerton et al., 1988
		1.25%			0.13	

$^{63}NiCl_2$ (f. th.)	22	2.5%			0.16	Emilson et al., 1993
		5%			0.37	
	40	0.62%		96	0.045	
		1.25%			0.088	
		2.5%			0.13	
		5%			0.29	
	60	5%	Distilled water	18	0.55	
		5%			1.2	
		5%			1.4	
$NiSO_4$ (stratum corneum)	37	1%	Water	96	0.0085	Tanojo et al., 2001
$NiCl_2$ (stratum corneum)	37	1%	Water	96	0.0068	
$Ni(NO_3)_2$ (stratum corneum)	37	1%	Water	96	0.0016	
$Ni(OAc)_2$ (stratum corneum)	37	1%	Water	96	0.0010	

Note: f. th. = full-thickness skin.

The effect of the counter ion (e.g., chloride, sulfate), concentration, and occlusion on the percutaneous absorption rate and on the irritation potential of nickel salts as indicators of penetration has been demonstrated in human skin *in vivo* and *in vitro*. The irritation potential was determined by application under occlusion on healthy volunteers, and irritancy was evaluated by objective measurement with the laser Doppler technique. Comparison of equimolal concentrations showed a clear dose–response relationship, whereby nickel chloride and nickel nitrate were more irritating than nickel sulfate; 0.30 *M* aq. nickel chloride and nickel nitrate caused erythema, while lower concentrations (0.01 to 0.10 *M*) did not affect skin blood flow, a measure of irritation (Wahlberg, 1996). Applied as a chloride, nickel permeates at 50 times the rate of the sulfate. Occlusion may increase skin penetration by xenobiotics up to tenfold, as observed by Feldmann and Maibach (1965) and Maibach and Feldman (1994) and almost 20-fold by nickel chloride (Fullerton et al., 1986). Under all experimental conditions, induction times (time elapsed before permeant becomes detectable in the receptor phase) were substantial: 50 h for the chloride under occlusion (Fullerton et al., 1986) and 90 h for the sulfate (Samitz and Katz, 1976).

In order to visualize the depth-concentration profile of nickel as it transits the SC, and with the expectation of gaining insight into the mode of penetration through the microcosmos of the skin, the standard protocol of sequential tape stripping of the exposed skin (Pinkus, 1951; Rougier et al., 1986) was implemented in our laboratory on human volunteers exposed to a number of nickel salts (Hostýnek et al., 2001a).

Following single open application at levels of 0.001 to 1% of the metal in methanol as the chloride, sulfate, nitrate, and acetate salts over 30 min to 24 h on the skin of volunteers, the application sites (volar forearm and intrascapular region) were tape stripped 20 times and analyzed for metal content by inductively coupled plasma mass spectroscopy (ICP-MS).

In order to obtain an accurate, quantitative picture of the actual permeant depth concentration gradient, analytical results from individual strip analysis must be normalized for the mass of SC removed with each tape strip. While mean thickness and number of cell layers of the SC vary inter- and intraindividually with anatomical site, investigations demonstrated that, after the first two to three strips, for a given skin site and test subject each subsequent tape strip removed the same amount of SC, down to approximately the twentieth strip ($r^2 = 0.99$) (Schwindt et al., 1998). This allows establishing a realistic permeant concentration profile in function of strip number for the interval of third to twentieth strip directly from analysis data.

The concentration-versus-depth profiles obtained using this method confirmed the diffusion characteristic of nickel, as described earlier by others (Fullerton et al., 1988; Fullerton et al., 1986). The four nickel salts followed similar patterns in their SC diffusion, leading to the following conclusions:

- Accumulation of nickel in the SC increased as a function of exposure time; i.e., the concentration gradient between the superficial and deeper layers of the SC increases commensurately with duration of exposure.
- While the concentration gradients of metal retained in the SC vary with counter ion, anatomical site, dose, and exposure time, for all variables

tested the profiles converge toward nondetectable levels (<7 ppb) beyond the fifteenth tape strip, independent of these parameters. The only notable exception is the concentration profile of nickel applied as the nitrate, which remains constant at 1% of dose from the third through the twentieth strip. The nitrate was also found to be the most lipophilic of the four nickel salts, determined by solubility in n-octanol at saturation. This may explain the limited but steady diffusion of the nitrite occurring through the lipophilic medium of the intercellular lipid bilayer.

The steep initial concentration gradient observed for all four nickel salts confirmed earlier observations of surface reservoir formation. In-depth intracellular diffusion of nickel ion through human SC occurs to a minimal degree, and only after considerable lag times of 50 to 90 h (Bennett, 1984; Fullerton et al., 1988; (Fullerton et al., 1986; Samitz and Katz, 1976). Such accumulation of nickel in the uppermost layers of the SC was also visualized using proton-induced x-ray emission (micro-PIXE) analysis. (Forslind et al., 1985; Malmqvist et al., 1987). These results allow us to reach the following conclusions:

- The counter ion in nickel salts plays a major role in their passive diffusion through the SC, suggestive of ion pairing.
- Since mass balance calculations documented that, particularly at higher concentrations (1%), up to 35% of the applied dose remained unaccounted for, the metal may choose the alternate, shunt pathway for diffusion to a significant degree, an observation also made using autoradiography or Micro-PIXE analysis (Bos et al., 1985; Lloyd, 1980; Odintsova, 1975). In this context it is important to note that by tape stripping of the SC, hair follicles are not removed, whereby significant amounts of the nickel applied may elude detection (Finlay and Marks, 1982; Finlay et al., 1982).

Ready dissolution of nickel metal on contact with the skin (*in vivo*) was also demonstrated in a model experiment applying nickel powder on the skin of human volunteers under occlusion. Sequential tape stripping of the application site after increasing periods of occlusion, starting at 5 min, showed the presence of nickel in depth to the level of the glistening layer, in an increasing mode with elapsed time, penetration continuing after the tenth strip at a constant rate. The experiment helps to illustrate the ready oxidation of nickel metal to form the soluble (diffusible) ion, presumably penetrating along the intercellular route (Hostýnek et al., 2001b).

5.3 QUANTITATIVE METHODS AND PERMEATION DATA

Different *in vitro* and *in vivo* methods are available for measuring skin diffusivity, and mathematical descriptions of dermal absorption toward formulation of predictive algorithms have been developed as well.

5.3.1 *In Vitro* Dermal Absorption

The *in vitro* method uses diffusion cells, whereby the permeant in the donor cell at a concentration C is detected in time intervals in the receptor cell allowing measuring the flux J. It is the preferred method for reliable deterivation of the permeation coefficient Kp, used to predict and optimize absorption characteristics of drugs for medical use.

Kp was adopted as a benchmark to characterize diffusivity of chemicals through biological membranes; it serves to describe the flux value Jss of xenobiotics through human skin. It is determined under conditions of steady state, *in vitro*, from a virtually infinite reservoir in the donor compartment, to a receptor compartment where concentration C remains close to zero (by constant solvent removal), and normalized for concentration. Expressed as depth of diffusion per unit of time (here in cm/h), the Kp provides a basis for comparison of the absorption rates of diverse chemicals, and when the permeant is applied from aqueous solution, it also represents the method by which most compound-specific penetration data currently available in the literature has been generated.

In vitro permeation studies are more reproducible than the *in vivo* approach, as they can be performed under controlled conditions using controllable parameters. Several static and flow-through *in vitro* diffusion cell designs have been developed for various purposes, representing the compartments inside and outside the body (Bronaugh and Stewart, 1985; Cooper, 1984; Franz, 1975; Gummer et al., 1987; Tiemessen et al., 1988).

In a characteristic arrangement, in the flow-through version the membrane (excised skin) is placed between the two cells, secured by an O ring. The top chamber receives an adequate volume of penetrant in solution, a temperature-controlled bottom chamber with continually circulating solution removes the penetrating amounts on the receptor side of the membrane, and a sampling port withdraws fractions at specific time intervals for analysis. The solute migrates by passive diffusion from the fixed higher concentration medium in the donor chamber into the less concentrated solution in the receptor chamber.

A newly designed diffusion cell of the two-chambered, flow-through type was used in our laboratory for monitoring permeation profiles and to determine the Kp for several nickel salts through human excised skin. (Tanojo et al., 1997). The new design allows application of the permeant in the donor compartment at finite or infinite dose, automated sampling, and maintenance of ideal sink conditions. The unique design optimizes acceptor–membrane contact by transporting the contents of the acceptor chamber through a spiral channel, eliminating stagnant domains in the compartment and ensuring optimal sink conditions and adquate mixing in the acceptor compartment.

According to Fick (1855), the steady-state penetration flux Jss per unit path length is proportional to the concentration gradient ΔC (or C, if receptor phase is constantly removed) and to the penetrant's permeation constant Kp. When the diffusion of permeant has reached a constant value (steady-state flux Jss), Fick's First Law of Membrane Diffusion allows the calculation of the permeation coefficient according to the equation: $Jss = Kp \cdot C$.

The *in vitro* technique is easily standardized and allows the determination of Kp through skin as long as the barrier properties are not affected by either permeant or carrier solvent. That implies that the permeant may not react with barrier material, i.e., change barrier permeability with time. Since a number of heavy metals are reactive with epidermal protein to some degree, however, this somewhat prejudices the general validity of Kp values. Nickel has a particular affinity for keratin, which slows its penetration rate (Wells, 1956; Alder et al., 1986; Cotton, 1964; Ermolli et al., 2001; Fullerton and Hoelgaard, 1988; Menczel et al., 1985; Samitz and Katz, 1976; Santucci et al., 1998). Still, following the initial delay (lag time) in permeation, as is observed under the dynamic conditions of the diffusion experiment, steady flux Jss is attained through the membrane, which permits calculation of Kp. Expressing depth of permeation per unit of time (here in cm/h), human penetration data currently available for nickel, including those acquired in our own laboratory, are presented in Table 5.1.

A problem inherent in the *in vitro* approach as reported in the literature is the lack of total dose accountability, as often in experiments reported the results are based on the quantity of permeant found in the receptor phase of the *in vitro* system only, disregarding material retained in the SC. At steady-state flux, rate of penetration can be estimated, but the question of final body burden resulting from exposure remains unanswered. Residual permeant may subsequently diffuse further, eluding the risk-assessment effort. Retention in the SC, forming a depot in a dynamic equilibrium and thus potentially reversible, was shown to occur with nickel (Alder et al., 1986; Fullerton et al., 1986; Samitz and Katz, 1976; Santucci et al., 1998). In our *in vitro* experiment conducted using human SC with four nickel salts we also analyzed the membrane for such residual permeant (Tanojo et al., 2001).

5.3.2 *In Vivo* Percent Dose Absorbed

It appears important that, whenever possible, absorption data be determined *in vivo*, in man or primates, for as accurate a risk assessment as possible. Human studies are the "gold standard" with which all other results should be evaluated. In this fashion uncertainties associated with the use of cadaver skin or adjustments for species variation are avoided. One principal *in vivo* methodology, using human volunteers or monkeys, was developed by Feldmann and Maibach, (1969; 1970; 1974) and is the most applied *in vivo* method for the determination of skin absorption. It yields a large part of all data so far available on skin penetration by drugs and pesticides, as it appears a valid alternative to the "disappearance" approach (see below). In the latter, any radioactive label retained in the body, or excreted via another route, will not be detected in the urine or feces.

In human studies, after topical application of the permeant the plasma levels of test compounds are low, usually falling below assay detection, and so it becomes necessary to use radiolabelled chemicals. In principle, the compound labeled with carbon-14 or tritium, or a metal nuclide, is applied to the skin in a minimal volume of a volatile solvent that is left to evaporate, and the total amount of radioactivity excreted is then determined. The amount retained in the body is corrected for by determining the amount of radioactivity excreted following parenteral administration of the test compound. According to Feldmann and Maibach the following expression to correct for nonassayed radioactivity (RA) applies: % absorbed = total RA after topical dosing × 100/total RA after parenteral dosing. The resulting radioactivity value is then expressed as the percent of the applied dose absorbed. Fick's postulates for membrane diffusion are not met there since a concentration of the penetrant cannot be defined, and neither is a steady-state equilibrium reached with this method; thus a permeability coefficient characterizing the compound cannot be calculated. Nevertheless, together with the toxicity of a chemical, the percent of a substance absorbed is the second factor critical for risk assessment; conducted in a vehicle relevant to human exposure and at realistic dose levels it gives a measure for human exposure and an indication of the amount potentially absorbed in (the worst) case of total body immersion.

In practice, a known amount of the test substance is applied to the skin; for absorption of the compound to mimic real-life exposure it is applied at the "in use" concentration; the site of application is left unprotected as the site of application should be relevant to the anticipated exposure; mostly, though, the skin area is covered with a rigid plastic shield, left in place for the duration of exposure to avoid mechanical loss of substance through abrasion. Duration of exposure will depend on the objectives of the study. At the end of the exposure period, the skin is washed to remove unabsorbed compound, and may be subjected to tape stripping to remove SC that has absorbed the test material. Skin washings and strips should be analyzed for compound as well as parent compound (metabolites) residing in the SC. Over the entire duration of the experiment, blood, urine, expired air, and feces may be collected at regular intervals for subsequent analysis for the presence of test compound or metabolites. Timing of blood sampling will depend on the pharmacokinetics of the chemical applied, i.e., on the movement of the dose, closely tracked from the start, along the ascending portion of the concentration curve, and several times before and after the apparent peak concentration. Urine sampling at intervals over the daytime should be documented as to timing and volume.

5.3.3 THE "DISAPPEARANCE METHOD"

An indirect method to measure absorption involves monitoring the loss (disappearance) of radioactive compound following its application on the surface, and the appearance of radioactivity in the excreta following the topical application of a labeled compound. The total radioactivity in the excreta is a mixture of the parent compound and any labeled metabolites that may result from metabolism of the parent in the skin and in the body. The method can involve single-point measurement, or continuous or periodic monitoring of compound uptake.

The method has been used extensively with radiolabelled metal salts, primarily by Wahlberg (1965a). To measure the loss of material from the skin surface over time, the guinea pig is the model mostly used *in vitro* and *in vivo*, with a limited number of experiments conducted on human skin *in vitro*. Consistently using that technique, Wahlberg and co-workers studied a dozen metal salts for their skin diffusivity. Although the data on skin disappearance were obtained over relatively short exposure times, the results are valuable as benchmarks, allowing at least partial validation of other measurements. The method has been used by others, also to investigate skin penetration of nickel through human skin. To make up for the overall paucity of data on skin absorption by nickel ion, those values are included in the table in a separate column.

A limitation in this approach lies in the fact that once the applied compound has penetrated beyond detection, its further fate remains inscrutable, especially since the application of radioactive material on man is limited for ethical reasons. Especially in the case of nickel, the depth of penetration through the epidermis remains unknown. Also, nickel is subject to some form of homeostatic control, and is known to reversibly form deposits in the skin (Fullerton et al., 1986). Thereby even recovery in excreta may not afford a relevant mass balance. Advantages of this method are that it requires small amounts of active formulation (at pharmacologically insignificant concentrations), it is inexpensive, relatively rapid, and applicable in clinical studies.

5.3.4 PREDICTIVE MODELS

Scheuplein and coworkers formulated an anatomically based description of the skin penetration process (Scheuplein, 1965; Scheuplein and Blank, 1971) based on Fick's concept of permeability of biological membranes expressed as Kp, the permeability coefficient (Fick, 1855). Under the hypothesis that permeation of the SC barrier proceeds via the intercellular (interlamellar) lipid bilayers, Scheuplein et al. reduced the process to two determinants for skin diffusion by chemical compounds: size and polarity. These are expressed as molecular weight and octanol-water partition coefficient P, used to calculate Kp (as opposed to deriving it through *in vitro* experimentation). Under observance of ideal conditions required by Fick, this theoretical approach was used by different authors to formulate predictive algorithms for diffusivity of organic nonelectrolytes, arriving at varying degrees of correlation with actually measured permeation constants (Bunge et al., 1994; Kasting et al., 1987; Potts and Guy, 1992; Potts and Guy, 1995). The attempt to apply a mathematical approach to metal compounds thus far has failed, however, due to the idiosyncratic properties and behavior of metals in general, and nickel in particular: oxidation states, metabolism (change in ionic charge in transit through the dermal strata), ionic radius, electropositivity, redox potential, hydration state, homeostasis, regulating effect of metallothioneins, counter ion, pH, polarity, and polarizability (Hostýnek et al., 1998).

5.3.5 DATA ON NICKEL ABSORPTION

A major factor affecting reliability of percutaneous absorption data is the methodology used. Different methods expectedly lead to different results. Hardly have any two investigators used the same approach (see Table 5.1).

Despite its prominent role as an allergen, reports on quantitative percutaneous absorption of nickel are infrequent, and *in vivo* experiments in humans involve few subjects. In the first such report, with an eye on the comparison of normal and hypersensitive individuals, Nørgaard (1955) demonstrated the absorption of nickel through normal human skin using the "disappearance method." The radiation from protected, dried aqueous deposits of $^{57}NiSO_4$ (12 to 100 µg Ni) on the skin at several body sites decreased by 61% in 41 h. Since the half-value thickness of skin for ^{57}Ni is 0.3 mm and the epidermis is about 0.1 mm, measured radiation will not be reduced to the degree observed in these experiments until the ^{57}Ni has passed through the epidermis and entered the dermis, where it can be transported by blood or lymph. In other words, the decrease in measured radiation corresponds to absorption of nickel through dermis and epidermis. Results comparing absorption in nickel-sensitive individuals were the same as those conducted with normal individuals (Nørgaard, 1955).

In a subsequent demonstration that nickel can be absorbed, Nørgaard (1957) applied ^{57}Ni (unspecified compound) to two rabbits and two guinea pigs. After 24 h the kidneys, liver, urine, and blood of all the animals were radioactive. No quantitative information was given. Since the application sites had been treated with a calcium thioglucolate depilatory, however, these experiments are not completely satisfactory for demonstrating absorption by normal, untreated skin.

Another, similar *in vivo* guinea-pig experiment (Lloyd, 1980) established that measurable nickel, 0.005% and 0.009% of 40 µCi $^{63}NiCl_2$, reached the plasma and urine, respectively, within 4 h. After 12 and 24 h the amounts rose to 0.05 to 0.07% in plasma and 0.21 to 0.51% in urine. The washed skin at the site of application retained much more ^{63}Ni: 5.3% after 24 h, and 53 to 59% in the "nonhomogenizable" skin, but neither recovery of nickel in the washes, nor amounts of nickel detected in whole-body count were reported.

Diffusion of 2 µCi of $NiSO_4$ (0.001, 0.01, 0.1 M) through heat-separated human epidermis was slow (Samitz and Katz, 1976). After 17 h only one of the six diffusion cells yielded measurable nickel, and after 90 h that spanned two more sampling times, two of the six cells at no time presented measurable nickel in the receptor chamber. Permeability coefficients (diffusion area not reported), estimated from measured amount of nickel, were $0.03 \times 10^{-4} - 0.1 \times 10^{-4}$ cm/h. The authors note that five nonionic detergents as 2% solutions carrying the ^{63}Ni "do little to enhance the diffusion of nickel."

The *in vitro* percutaneous fluxes of 1.32 mg nickel as the chloride and sulfate through full-thickness human skin were compared by Fullerton et al. (1986). After lag times of about 50 h in experiments lasting 144 to 239 h, occluded $NiCl_2$ entered the receptor fluid about 5 to 40 times more rapidly than (a) $NiSO_4$, (b) $NiCl_2$ with added Na_2SO_4 or (c) $NiSO_4$ with added NaCl. Solutions (b) and (c) had identical ionic activities, and the Ni^{++} and Cl^- concentrations were the same as for the $NiCl_2$ solution. Without occlusion, the permeation of nickel decreased by more than 90%. Nickel in the skin tissue at the end of the experiments (calculated as the difference between the applied nickel and sum of the nickel in the receptor solution plus the nickel recovered by washing the skin) was also greater after exposure to pure $NiCl_2$ than to sulfate-containing solutions. These results are in agreement with cited patch test results wherein occlusion and the use of nickel chloride rather than nickel sulfate are more likely to produce positive reactions in patients. Estimated permeability coefficients after the lag time were $0.5 \times 10^{-4} - 15 \times 10^{-4}$ cm/h for pure $NiCl_2$ and $0.03 \times 10^{-4} - 0.2 \times 10^{-4}$ cm/h in the presence of sulfate.

Subsequently additional, similar *in vitro* experiments explored the effect of six hydrogels as vehicles for $NiCl_2$ and of petrolatum for both $NiCl_2$ and $NiSO_4$ (Fullerton et al., 1988). Petrolatum was the poorest vehicle for $NiCl_2$ and for $NiSO_4$. The sulfate, again a poorer penetrant than the chloride, yielded no detectable nickel in the receptor phase after 96 h.

Because skin reactions due to nickel salts are common, it appears interesting to measure their diffusivity through the SC, a main barrier of the skin. Advanced diffusion system and analytical techniques available now make possible a better measurement of permeant flux, as compared to earlier experiments. In our laboratory Tanojo et al. (1997) isolated human SC by trypsinization of dermatomed cadaver leg skin. The diffusion system included diffusion cells with a spiral line. Pure water was used as acceptor solution. Aqueous solutions of nickel salts — $Ni(NO_3)_2$, $NiSO_4$, $NiCl_2$ and $Ni(-OOCCH_3)_2$ at 1% Ni^{2+} concentration — were used as the donor solution, in 400 μl/cell. The receptor fluid was collected as four-hour fractions up to 96 h after the application of the donor solutions. The nickel concentration in the receptor fluid was analyzed using inductively coupled plasma mass spectrometry. From the flux data at steady state, the permeability coefficients of the four nickel salts were calculated to:

$$Ni(NO_3)_2 \ 5.24 \pm 1.64 \times 10^{-7} \text{ cm/h } (n = 7)$$

$$NiSO_4 \ 8.52 \pm 5.50 \times 10^{-7} \text{ cm/h } (n = 3)$$

$$NiCl_2 \ 6.81 \pm 1.19 \times 10^{-7} \text{ cm/h } (n = 4)$$

$$Ni(-OOCCH_3)2 \ 5.20 \pm 1.05 \times 10^{-7} \text{ cm/h } (n = 4)$$

These results showed a relatively slow permeation of nickel salts across human SC. This might be the first report of the permeation of nickel using SC and agrees with earlier experiments conducted using the full-thickness human skin *in vitro* (Fullerton et al., 1986). A different penetration pathway and mechanism of diffusion needs to be invoked to explain the facile and widespread sensitization reactions in humans reported from contact with the metal and its salts. Direct and prolonged skin contact with nickel-releasing objects alone can also elicit dermatitis in sensitized individuals due to ease of oxidation on skin contact to yield diffusible ion (Bumgardner and Lucas, 1995; Haudrechy et al., 1994; Haudrechy et al., 1997; Lidén et al., 1998; Santucci et al., 1989), constituting an important factor in the pathogenesis of nickel allergy (Husain, 1977; Kanerva et al., 1998; Kanerva et al., 1994). Nickel ions resulting from oxidation on the skin *in vivo* thus may penetrate via the shunt pathway more rapidly, in contrast to slow transcellular diffusion as measured *in vitro* by us and others.

5.4 SUMMARY, CONCLUSIONS, AND CRITICISM

Compiling a significant compendium of relevant data on percutaneous absorption of metals is challenging due to the paucity of robust experimental results. In gathering data on skin penetration of metals, most attempts to deal with this phenomenon in a quantitative manner seems to meet with serious technical obstacles that discourage investigators from further pursuits. This becomes evident from the fact that experimental data are extremely limited, with the exception of Wahlberg's extensive investigations of metals absorption, which unfortunately excluded nickel (Wahlberg, 1965a, 1965b, 1965c, 1968a, 1968b, 1968c, 1970; Wahlberg and Skog, 1962, 1963). Experiments performed by others have followed most disparate procedures. Some experimental difficulties have now been overcome by the relatively recent availability of most metals in their radioactive form, and refined analytical techniques that permit trace detection of xenobiotics in tissue to determine disposition of metals in the organism in particular.

Our own *in vitro* experiments, conducted on human SC with a recently developed, optimized micro-diffusion cell, confirm the minute order of magnitude of nickel ion diffusion (Tanojo et al., 2001).

With data so far available, a realistic assessment of nickel penetration through skin appears handicapped by several difficulties. The route(s) of permeation is (are) essentially unknown and can only be inferred. While nickel undeniably penetrates — witness the ease with which it elicits allergic reactions — experimental attempts to quantify actual degree of penetration give minute and variable values. Most striking are the long induction (lag) times seen *in vitro*, and ultimately the difficulty in finding a significant level in the receptor phase. Lag times measured are on the order of 50 to 90 h, the observed permeability coefficients on the order of 10^{-6} to 10^{-5} cm/h, which approximates the counter-current rate of corneocyte desquamation (Bunge et al., 1994). Thus part of the applied dose that binds to tissues in the skin is eventually lost by exfoliation (calculation based on 10 μm thickness and shedding of one SC layer per day).

The apparent paradox of insignificant (transcellular or intercellular) diffusion measured with nickel salts on the one hand, and clinical evidence of sensitization rates and epidemiology on the other, pointing to facile nickel ion penetration of the SC to the depth of live tissue, particularly from contact with the metal, invites an explanation. At this point, based on recent data generated in our laboratory (Hostýnek et al., 2001a; Hostýnek et al., 2001b), we postulate the intercellular lamellar bilayers as an alternate route of diffusion of lipophilic nickel soaps, formed with endogenous fatty acids on the surface of the skin.

It appears unlikely that analysis of data obtained for nickel so far will allow conclusions applicable to metal compounds in general, since different mechanisms of diffusion appear to operate for different metals and categories of compounds. Much of the ambiguity involves the fact that experimental data are limited and the experiments performed have followed different procedures. No consistency can be found, making comparisons across studies difficult. Current flux data, generated with varying techniques, is highly discrepant. *In vitro* data with human skin shows barely discernible penetration (Fullerton et al., 1988; Fullerton et al., 1986); disappearance measurements on the other hand suggest up to two thirds absorption (Nørgaard, 1955). Further complicating this situation, diverse animal-model data (*in vivo* and *in vitro*) are interspersed among corresponding measurements made using excised human skin or *in vivo* in man. Incongruities can be avoided by implementing standardized experimental protocols, and interpretation of data could become possible by reporting results that cover all relevant experimental details. Reliable *in vitro* permeation rates for nickel could thus be determined by applying a donor reservoir of virtually "infinite" dose, by collecting the receptor phase in short time intervals, and by extending collection times over several days, a procedure adopted in our own recent diffusion experiments (Tanojo et al., 2001).

Reporting of *in vivo* data identifying precisely area of skin exposure, and recently available, highly accurate methods of analysis (e.g., for nickel) in biological materials by ICP-MS or ICP-AES analysis, adapted to determine ppb levels of the metal in skin strips (Hostýnek et al., 2001a; Hostýnek et al., 2001b; Tanojo et al., 2001) or excreta (Templeton et al., 1994) could further fill in existing data gaps.

5.5 OUTLOOK

Current limitations in clarifying the true fate of nickel diffusing into the SC and beyond should become surmountable by improved analytical techniques currently available, such as the ICP-MS method described. This method allows detection of nickel to levels of 7 ppb in substrates such as skin (SC) strips, making the use of radio isotopes unnecessary for purposes of material recovery and balance in diffusion experiments. The standard protocol of tape stripping thus becomes available for examining the surface penetration of nickel through human SC *in vivo* in detailed and accurate fashion. Following single open applications, a concentration profile can be established through the different biological compartments.

Demonstrating the detailed pathways of diffusion in this manner will provide the basis for formulating appropriate methodologies for intervention in the population at risk. Further work is planned to investigate the rate of penetration of nickel soaps (fatty acid compounds) through the SC, with the hypothesis that such soaps are more diffusible than the free nickel ion.

ACKNOWLEDGMENT

We gratefully acknowledge the financial support by the Nickel Producers Environmental Research Association (NiPERA) toward this review project.

REFERENCES

Alder, J.F. et al., Depth concentration profiles obtained by carbon furnace atomic absorption spectrometry for nickel and aluminium in human skin, *J. Anal. At. Spectrom,.* 1, 365–367, 1986.

Barry, B.W., Basic principles of diffusion through membranes, in *Dermatology Formulations*, Swarbrick, J., Ed., Marcel Dekker, New York, 1983, p. 49.

Bennett, B.G., Environmental nickel pathways to man, in *Nickel in the Human Environment: Proceedings of a Joint Symposium Held at the International Agency for Research on Cancer, Lyon, France, 8–11 March 1983*, Sunderman, F.W. and Aitio, A., Eds., Oxford University Press, New York, 1984, pp. 487–495.

Bos, A.J. et al., Incorporation routes of elements into human hair; implications for hair analysis used for monitoring, *Sci. Total Environ.*, 42, 157–169, 1985.

Bronaugh, R.L. and Stewart, R.F., Methods for in vitro percutaneous absorption studies. IV. The flow-through diffusion cell, *J. Pharm. Sci.*, 74, 64–67, 1985.

Bucks, D.A.W. et al., Uptake of two zwitterionic surfactants into human skin in vivo, *Toxicol. Appl. Pharmacol.*, 120, 224–227, 1993.

Bulmer, F.M.R. and Mackenzie, E.A., Studies in the control and treatment of nickel rash, *Industrial Hyg.*, 8, 517–527, 1926.

Bumgardner, J.D. and Lucas, L.C., Cellular response to metallic ions released from nickel-chromium dental alloys, *J. Dent. Res.*, 74, 1521–1527, 1995.

Bunge, A.L., Flynn, G.L., and Guy, R.H., Predictive model for dermal exposure assessment, in *Water Contamination and Health*, Wang, R.G.M., Ed. Marcel Dekker, New York, 1994, pp. 347–373.

Cavelier, C., Foussereau, J., and Massin, M., Nickel allergy: analysis of metal clothing objects and patch testing to metal samples, *Contact Dermatitis*, 12, 65–75, 1985.

Cavelier, C. et al., Allergy to nickel or cobalt: tolerance to nickel and cobalt samples in man and in the guinea pig allergic or sensitized to these metals, *Contact Dermatitis*, 21, 72–78, 1989.

Cooper, E.R., Increased skin permeability for lipophilic molecules, *J. Pharm. Sci.*, 73, 1153–1156, 1984.

Cotton, D.W.K., Studies on the binding of protein by nickel, *Br. J. Dermatol.*, 76, 99–109, 1964.

Emilson, A., Lindberg, M., and Forslind, B., The temperature effect on in vitro penetration of sodium lauryl sulfate and nickel chloride through human skin, *Acta Derm. Venereol.*, 73, 203–207, 1993.

Ermolli, M. et al., Nickel, cobalt and chromium-induced cytotoxicity and intracellular accumulation in human hacat keratinocytes, *Toxicology*, 159, 23–31, 2001.

Feldmann, R.J. and Maibach, H.I., Penetration of C-14 hydrocortisone through normal skin — the effect of stripping and occlusion, *Arch. Dermatol.*, 91, 661–666, 1965.

Feldmann, R.J. and Maibach, H.I., Percutaneous penetration of steroids in man, *J. Investigative Dermatol.*, 52, 89–94, 1969.

Feldmann, R.J. and Maibach, H.I., Absorption of some organic compounds through the skin of man, *J. Investigative Dermatol.*, 54, 399–404, 1970.

Feldmann, R.J. and Maibach, H.I., Percutaneous penetration of some pesticides and herbicides in man, *Toxicol. Appl. Pharmacol.*, 28, 126–132, 1974.

Fick, A.E., On liquid diffusion, *Philos. Mag.*, 10, 30–39, 1855.

Finlay A. and Marks, R., Determination of corticosteroid concentration profiles in the stratum corneum using skin surface biopsy technique, *Br. J. Dermatol.*, 107, 33, 1982.

Finlay, A.Y., Marshall, R.J., and Marks, R., A fluorescence photographic photometric technique to assess stratum corneum turnover rate and barrier function in vivo, *Br. J. Dermatol.*, 107, 35–42, 1982.

Forslind, B. et al., Recent advances in x-ray microanalysis in dermatology, *Scanning Electron Microsc.*, Part 2, 687–695, 1985.

Franz, T.J., Percutaneous absorption: on the relevance of in vitro data, *J. Investigative Dermatol.*, 64, 190–195, 1975.

Fullerton, A. et al., Permeation of nickel salts through human skin in vitro, *Contact Dermatitis*, 15, 173–177, 1986.

Fullerton, A., Andersen, J.R., and Hoelgaard, A., Permeation of nickel through human skin in vitro — effect of vehicles, *Br. J. Dermatol.*, 118, 509–516, 1988.

Fullerton, A. and Hoelgaard, A., Binding of nickel to human epidermis in vitro, *Br. J. Dermatol.*, 119, 675–682, 1988.

Gilboa, R., Al-Tawil, N.G., and Marcusson, J.A., Metal allergy in cashiers: an in vitro and in vivo study for the presence of metal allergy, *Acta Derm. Venereol. (Stockh.)*, 68, 317–324, 1988.

Gummer, C.L., Hinz, R.S., and Maibach, H.I., The skin penetration cell: an update, *Int. J. Pharmaceutics*, 40, 101–104, 1987.

Haudrechy, P. et al., Nickel release from nickel-plated metals and stainless steel, *Contact Dermatitis*, 31, 249–255, 1994.

Haudrechy, P. et al., Nickel release from stainless steels, *Contact Dermatitis*, 37, 113–117, 1997.

Hegyi, E. and Gasparik, J., The nickel content of metallic threads in an Indian shawl, *Contact Dermatitis*, 21, 107, 1989.

Hostýnek, J.J. et al., Metals and the skin, *Crit. Rev. Toxicol.*, 23, 171–235, 1993.

Hostýnek, J.J. et al., Human skin penetration by metal compounds, in *Dermal Absorption and Toxicity Assessment*, Roberts, M.S. and Walters, K.A., Eds., Marcel Dekker, New York, 1998, pp. 647–668.

Hostýnek, J.J. et al., Human stratum corneum adsorption of nickel salts: investigation of depth profiles by tape stripping in vivo, *Acta Derm. Venereol. (Suppl.)*, 212, 11–18, 2001a.

Hostýnek, J.J. et al., Human stratum corneum penetration by nickel: in vivo study of depth distribution after occlusive application of the metal as powder, *Acta Derm. Venereol. (Suppl.)*, 212, 5–10, 2001b.

Husain, S.L., Nickel coin dermatitis, *Br. Med. J.*, 2, 998, 1977.

Kaaber, K. et al., Some adverse effects of disulfiram in the treatment of nickel-allergic patients, *Dermatosen in Beruf und Umwelt*, 35, 209–211, 1987.

Kanerva, L. et al., Nickel release from metals, and a case of allergic contact dermatitis from stainless steel, *Contact Dermatitis*, 31, 299–303, 1994.

Kanerva, L., Estlander, T., and Jolanki, R., Bank clerk's occupational allergic nickel and cobalt contact dermatitis from coins, *Contact Dermatitis*, 38, 217–218, 1998.

Kasting, G.B., Smith, R.L., and Cooper, E.R., Effect of lipid solubility and molecular size on percutaneous absorption, in *Skin Pharmacokinetics*, Shroot, B. and Schaefer, H., Eds., S. Karger, Basel, 1987, pp 138–153.

Kolpakov, F.I., Skin permeability to nickel compounds, *Ark. Patol.*, 25, 38–45, 1963.

Lidén, C., Menné, T., and Burrows, D., Nickel-containing alloys and platings and their ability to cause dermatitis, *Br. J. Dermatol.*, 134, 193–198, 1996.

Lidén, C. et al., Nickel release from tools on the Swedish market, *Contact Dermatitis*, 39, 127–131, 1998.

Lloyd, G.K., Dermal absorption and conjugation of nickel in relation to the induction of allergic contact dermatitis–preliminary results, in *International Conference on Nickel Toxicology 1980, Swansea, Wales,* Brown, S.S. and Sunderman, F.W., Eds., Academic Press, New York, 1980, pp. 145–148.

Maibach, H.I. and Feldman, R., Systemic absorption of pesticides through the skin of man, in *Occupational Exposure to Pesticides,* Federal Working Group on Pest Management, Washington, D.C., 1994, pp. 120–127.

Mali, J.W.H., Spruit, D., and Seutter, E., Chelation in human sweat, *Clin. Chim. Acta Int. Clin. Chem.*, 9, 187–190, 1964.

Malmqvist, K.G. et al., The use of PIXE in experimental studies of the physiology of human skin epidermis, *Biol. Trace Element Res.*, 12, 297–308, 1987.

Menczel, E. et al., Skin binding during percutaneous penetration, in *Percutaneous Absorption. Mechanisms, Methodology, Drug Delivery*, Bronaugh, R.I. and Maibach, H.I., Eds., Marcel Dekker, New York, 1985, pp. 43–56.

Menné, T. et al., Patch test reactivity to nickel alloys, *Contact Dermatitis*, 16, 255–259, 1987.

Nørgaard, O., Investigations with radioactive Ni[57] into the resorption of nickel through the skin in normal and in nickel-hypersensitive persons, *Acta Derm. Venereol.*, 35, 111–117, 1955.

Nørgaard, O., Investigations with radioactive nickel, cobalt and sodium on the resorption through the skin in rabbits, guinea-pigs and man, *Acta Derm. Venereol.*, 37, 440–445, 1957.

Odintsova, N.A., Permeability of the epidermis for lead acetate according to fluorescence and electron-microscopic studies, *Vestn. Dermatol. Venerol.*, 19–24, 1975.

Pinkus, H., Examination of the epidermis by the strip method of removing horny layers. I. Observation on thickness of the horny layer, and on mitotic activity after stripping, *J. Investigative Dermatol.*, 16, 383–386, 1951.

Potts, R.O. and Guy, R.H., Predicting skin permeability, *Pharm. Res.*, 9, 663–669, 1992.

Potts, R.O., Guy, R.H., and Francoeur, M.L., Routes of ionic permeability through mammalian skin, *Solid State Ionics*, 53–56, 165–169, 1992.

Potts, R.O. and Guy, R.H., A predicitve algorithm for skin permeability: the effects of molecular size and hydrogen bond activity, *Pharm. Res.*, 12, 1628–1633, 1995.

Preininger, T., Überempfindlichkeit gegen Nickelgeld, *Dermatol. Wochenschr.*, 99, 1082–1084, 1934.

Ridout, G.R. et al., The effects of zwitterionic surfactants on skin barrier function, *Fundam. Appl. Toxicol.*, 16, 41–50, 1991.

Rothman, S., Überempfindlichkeit gegen Hartgeld, *Dermatol. Wochenschr.*, 90, 98–99, 1930.

Rougier, A. et al., Regional variation in percutaneous absorption in man: measurement by the stripping method, *Arch. Dermatol. Res.*, 278, 465–469, 1986.

Samitz, M.H. and Katz, S.A., Nickel — epidermal interactions: diffusion and binding, *Environ. Res.*, 11, 34–39, 1976.

Santucci, B. et al., Nickel dermatitis from cheap earrings, *Contact Dermatitis*, 21, 245–248, 1989.

Santucci, B. et al., The influence exerted by cutaneous ligands in subjects reacting to nickel sulfate alone and in those reacting to more transition metals, *Exp. Dermatol.*, 7, 162–167, 1998.

Scheuplein, R.J., Mechanism of percutaneous absorption. I. Routes of penetration and the influence of solubility, *J. Investigative Dermatol.*, 45, 334, 1965.

Scheuplein, R.J. and Blank, I.H., Molecular structure and diffusional processes across intact skin, *Report to the U.S. Army Chemical R&D Laboratories*, Edgewood Arsenal, MD, 1967.

Scheuplein, R.J. and Blank, I.H., Permeability of the skin, *Physiol. Rev.*, 51, 707–747, 1971.

Schwindt, D.A., Wilhelm, K.P., and Maibach, H.I., Water diffusion characteristics of human *stratum corneum* at different anatomical sites *in vivo*, *J. Investigative Dermatol.*, 111, 385–389, 1998.

Spruit, D., Mali, J.W.H., and De Groot, N., The interaction of nickel ions with human cadaverous dermis. Electric potential, absorption, swelling, *J. Investigative Dermatol.*, 44, 103–106, 1965.

Tanojo, H., Nickel dermatitis from cheap earrings; new design of a flow-through diffusion cell for studying in vitro permeation across biological membranes, *J. Controlled Release*, 45, 41–47, 1997.

Tanojo, H. et al., In vitro permeation of nickel salts through human stratum corneum, *Acta Derm. Venereol. (Suppl.)*, 212, 19–23, 2001.

Templeton, D.M., Xu, S.X., and Stuhne-Sekalec, L., Isotope-specific analysis of Ni by ICP-MS: applications of stable isotope tracers to biokinetic studies, *Sci. Total Environ.*, 148, 253–262, 1994.

Tiemessen, H.L.G.M. et al., A two-chambered diffusion cell with improved flow-through characteristics for studying the drug permeability of biological membranes, *Acta Pharmacol. Technol.*, 34, 99–101, 1988.

Wahlberg, J.E. and Skog, E., Percutanous absorption of mercuric chloride in guinea-pigs. Effect of potassium iodide and the pretreatment of the skin with irritant concentrations of mercury, *Acta Derm. Venereol.*, 42, 418–425, 1962.

Wahlberg, J.E. and Skog, E., The percutaneous absorption of sodium chromate (^{51}Cr) in the guinea pig, *Acta Derm. Venereol.*, 43, 102–108, 1963.

Wahlberg, J.E., "Disappearance measurements," a method for studying percutaneous absorption of isotope-labelled compounds emitting gamma-rays, *Acta Derm. Venereol.*, 45, 397–414, 1965a.

Wahlberg, J.E., Percutaneous absorption of sodium chromate, (^{51}Cr), cobaltous(^{58}Co), and mercuric(^{203}Hg) chlorides through excised human and guinea pig skin, *Acta Derm. Venereol.*, 45, 415–426, 1965b.

Wahlberg, J.E., Percutaneous absorption of trivalent and hexavalent chromium, *Arch. Dermatol.*, 92, 315–318, 1965c.

Wahlberg, J.E., Percutaneous absorption from chromium (^{51}Cr) solutions of different pH, 1.4–12.8, *Dermatologica*, 137, 17–25, 1968a.

Wahlberg, J.E., Percutaneous absorption of radioactive strontium chloride Sr 89 (^{89}SrCl$_2$). A comparison with 11 other metal compounds, *Arch. Dermatol.*, 97, 336–339, 1968b.

Wahlberg, J.E., Transepidermal or transfollicular absorption? *Acta Derm. Venereol.*, 48, 336–344, 1968c.

Wahlberg, J.E., Percutaneous absorption of trivalent and hexavalent chromium (^{51}Cr) through excised human and guinea pig skin, *Dermatologica*, 141, 288–296, 1970.

Wahlberg, J.E., Nickel: the search for alternative, optimal and non-irritant patch test preparations. Assessment based on laser Doppler flowmetry, *Skin Res. Technol.*, 2, 136–141, 1996.

Wells, G.C., Effects of nickel on the skin, *Br. J. Dermatol.*, 68, 237–242, 1956.

6 Diagnostic Testing for Nickel Allergic Hypersensitivity: Patch Testing versus Lymphocyte Transformation Test

Jurij J. Hostýnek, Katherine E. Reagan, and Howard I. Maibach

CONTENTS

Abstract 167
6.1   Introduction 168
6.2   Patch Testing 168
     6.2.1   General Comments 168
          6.2.1.1   Nickel Compounds 169
          6.2.1.2   Test Vehicle 169
          6.2.1.3   Test Concentration 169
          6.2.1.4   Test Site 171
          6.2.1.5   False-Positive and False-Negative Reactions 172
     6.2.2   Discussion of the Patch Test 173
6.3   The Lymphocyte Transformation Test (LTT) 174
     6.3.1   Methodology 174
     6.3.2   Review of Mechanism of LTT 174
     6.3.3   Discussion of the LTT 177
6.4   Summary 179
Abbreviations 179
References 180

ABSTRACT

This review evaluates the lymphocyte transformation test (LTT) as an *in vitro* alternative to traditional patch testing. Patch-test results require knowledge, practice, and experience for correct biological and clinical interpretation, and in spite of long-term use, the method is fraught with technical and interpretative limitations. Nickel in particular is an allergen eliciting false-positive reactions in patch testing due to the irritancy of test materials; it is sometimes difficult to distinguish an irritant reaction from a true allergic response, and patients may need to be tested more than once. Also, false-negative reactions can occur due to varying sensitivity of the patient. It therefore appears reasonable to search for a more objective, *in vitro* alternative; the LTT appears one procedure that gives relatively reliable results. Still, at this point this method can be used only in association with patch testing, and it has often given results inconsistent with the patch test.

6.1 INTRODUCTION

In vivo patch testing in the clinical setting is a commonly used diagnostic test to ascertain sensitization of the organism, or to assess the skin-sensitization potential of chemicals. Such sensitization is a two-stage process involving induction and elicitation. Induction occurs upon first-time exposure of the skin to an environmental agent and is characterized by the formation of immune memory cells (T cells). These antigen-sensitized T cells can recognize the specific agent upon repeated exposure. The second, or elicitation phase, follows at a distance in time (delayed by 1 to 6 or 7 days) when the skin is reexposed to the original agent, causing a reaction by memory T cells to the antigen, which results in an eczematous skin reaction.

Nickel is an allergen that on skin patch testing can elicit false-positive as well as false-negative reactions; correct application and evaluation of patch tests requires skill and experience. For optimal diagnosis, patch testing should be done with materials supplied by commercial sources, and in combination with a thorough evaluation of a patient's history of allergy and morphology (Ale and Maibach, 1995).

The lymphocyte transformation test (LTT) is one of several *in vitro* diagnostic tests under development for the investigation of allergic conditions in general and of nickel allergy, capable of distinguishing nickel-sensitive individuals from controls, and is ideally used in association with patch testing.

Hypersensitivity may be accompanied by antigen-specific circulating T-lymphocytes in the blood, as is the case for nickel allergic hypersensitivity (NAH). These cells (lymphocytes) can be reactivated (transformed) by the antigen *in vitro* in peripheral blood lymphocyte cultures. The LTT reaction usually takes one to several days to develop. The technical procedure is of importance, and because of the generally low sensitivity of the LTT, the value of a positive LTT could be estimated as higher than a negative outcome of that test.

6.2 PATCH TESTING

6.2.1 GENERAL COMMENTS

Patch testing is the standard procedure to establish the presence of allergy by provoking an elicitation reaction; it consists of the application to the skin of a certain amount of the suspected allergen placed on adhesive tape, in a suitable concentration and a suitable vehicle. Penetration through the stratum corneum (SC) is promoted by airtight occlusion. The test unit is left on for at least 24 h, as seen in about one third of studies, but because many test substances are slow to diffuse through the SC and reactions accordingly develop with substantial delays, patches are usually removed only after 2 days (in about 2 out of 3 studies) in order to promote penetration.

Usual application and occlusion time for NAH testing is 48 h. Although more practical, the routinely used 24 h occlusion in patch testing has proven to lead to 20% false-negative readings, due to the low penetration rate of nickel salts in general, and nickel sulfate in particular (Mali et al., 1964; McDonagh et al., 1992; Nielsen and Menné, 1993; Ale, Laugier, and Maibach, 1996).

Verification of NAH in practice typically involves skin exposure to 184 mg Ni/cm^2 over 2 to 4 days in a patch test with 5% $NiSO_4$ in petrolatum. These experimental conditions reflect the results of the investigations conducted toward optimal NAH diagnosis, as itemized in the following.

6.2.1.1 Nickel Compounds

The pronounced irritancy of nickel salts (nickel sulfate, nickel nitrate, nickel chloride) is one difficulty encountered in the appropriate performance of NAH diagnostic patch testing (Wahlberg, 1996). For that reason, the role of the counterion on the irritation potential of nickel salts under simulated patch test conditions has been investigated in human skin *in vivo*, whereby irritation potential was considered the expression of skin permeability (Fullerton et al., 1986; Samitz and Katz, 1976; Wahlberg, 1990). The irritation potential of the salts was determined by application under occlusion on healthy volunteers and evaluation of irritancy by objective measurement with the laser Doppler technique. Comparison of equimolal concentrations in the range of 0.01 to 0.38 m showed a clear dose-response relationship, whereby the chloride and the nitrate were more irritating than the sulfate; 0.30 m nickel chloride and nickel nitrate caused erythema, while lower concentrations (0.01 to 0.10m) did not affect skin blood flow (Wahlberg, 1996).

6.2.1.2 Test Vehicle

Petrolatum is generally the vehicle of choice for nickel sulfate, although uniform distribution of the crystalline salt is problematic and poor penetration from petrolatum make that formulation less than ideal (Fischer and Maibach, 1984a).

Nevertheless, nickel patch test materials are preferably formulated in petrolatum due to their lesser irritancy to the skin in that base, and convenience in storing and dosing. Nickel salts are also used in an aqueous medium; such an alternate patch test system is the T.R.U.E. TEST®, using nickel sulfate in a hydoxypropylcellulose gel (Andersen et al., 1993).

6.2.1.3 Test Concentration

Suppliers of ready-to-use standard patch test allergens traditionally present concentrations as a percentage, but such designation is ambiguous as it is not clear if this means weight/weight, volume/volume, volume/weight, or weight/volume. Relevant is the number of moles applied; e.g., the concentration of nickel ions is 20.9% in nickel sulfate (hexahydrate), compared to 24.7% in the chloride (hexahydrate). It is essential that in studies comparing different salts the same molality is used.

No definite value can be assigned to the threshold inducing sensitization, nor to a concentration which will elicit reaction in those already sensitized, as observed in numerous investigations reviewed here. This due to considerable individual variation in susceptibility, which also depends on gender and which also changes with age (Nethercott et al., 1994).

Several investigations have attempted a definition of threshold values using serial dilutions of nickel, only to find that some patients react to relatively high concentrations, while others react even to surprisingly small amounts (Allenby and Basketter, 1993; Emmett et al., 1988; Al-Tawil et al., 1985). Different response values determined in those studies underscore the individual variation in susceptibility to sensitization and in reactivity. In a study conducted by Magnusson and Hersle (1965) to determine the highest concentration which would not elicit sensitivity reactions to nickel, the one which still resulted in positive patch test reactions to $NiSO_4$ in 10% of highly nickel sensitized individuals, at 48 h, under occlusion and on normal forearm skin compromised by pretreatment with SDS, was 0.5 ppm (3 out of 12). Also, there was a pronounced difference in reactivities depending on test site (Magnusson and Hersle 1965).

Nickel sulfate at 0.039% in water was the lowest concentration eliciting positive patch test reactions in 5 of 53 eczema patients with NAH (9.4%), when they were tested with the nickel salt in either water or petrolatum (Wahlberg and Skog, 1971).

Three hundred and thirty-two patients with previously diagnosed contact allergy to nickel or a history suggestive of nickel allergy were tested with serial dilutions of nickel sulfate (exposure 24 to 48 h, reading at 72 h or later). Nickel sulfate 0.0005% patch tests were negative in all patients; at 0.001% patch tests were positive in 4 patients (1.2%); at 0.005% positive in 5 patients (1.5%); at 0.01% positive in 19 patients (5.7%) (Uter et al., 1995).

The effect of repeated exposure of the hands to low nickel concentrations over 2 weeks was evaluated by patch testing post exposure in a study of 17 nickel-sensitive volunteers, to simulate occupational exposure. Nickel chloride at 0.02% was positive in 4 patients (23.5%); at 0.01% positive in 4 patients (23.5%); at 0.001% positive in 1 patient (5.8%) (Nielsen et al., 1999).

Elicitation reactions to nickel on contact with irritated skin were investigated in a hand-immersion experiment with nickel-sensitive volunteers. Upon exposure twice daily for 23 days to a surfactant solution, 12 of 20 individuals tested showed positive reactions to 10 ppm aq. nickel sulfate (60%), 6 of 12 to 5 ppm (50%), 3 of 20 to 1 ppm (15%), and 2 of 20 to 0.5 ppm (10%). Difference in test site also determined a difference in reactivity (Allenby and Basketter, 1993). In a similar study, no reaction was seen upon repeated open nickel sulfate application at 1 ppm for 23 days on the skin of 4 sensitized volunteers following irritant application of SDS (Allenby and Basketter, 1994).

In a single open application on the forearm of nickel-sensitive individuals with and without addition of SDS, of 51 subjects none reacted to a concentration of 100 ppm nickel chloride or lower (range of 0.1 to 4000 ppm), an indication that in that cohort the elicitation threshold lay above that level (Menné and Calvin, 1993).

Twenty-five nickel-sensitive patients were patch tested by application of a dilution series of nickel sulfate (Allenby and Goodwin, 1983). In 9 patients (36%) 112 ppm nickel (0.05% $NiSO_4$) caused reactions, 1.12 ppm in one of the patients tested (4%).

The thresholds of sensitivity in individuals with positive reactions to nickel was determined in a serial dilution test with nickel sulfate in petrolatum. Four individuals reacted to 390 ppm, six to 190 ppm, and one to 100 ppm (Rystedt and Fischer, 1983).

Handley, Todd, and Dolan (1996) noted how allergic patch test reactions are remarkably long-lasting in nickel-sensitized individuals. A median duration of response to nickel sulfate was 9 days, and 15% of responses extended to 17 days or longer. Nickel quantification in involved versus noninvolved tissue showed no significant qualitative or quantitative differences in the immunocytochemistry of the tissues, however (difference in surface receptors on activated T-lymphocytes or Langerhans cells). This was seen as an indication that the elevated, local nickel concentration occurring at the challenge sites does not play a significant role in the time course of the immune reaction.

Patch tests under occlusion using nickel sulfate in a hydroxypropylcellulose gel (T.R.U.E. TEST) were conducted by Andersen et al. (1993) on the back of 72 test subjects who were confirmed as NAH positive, and left for 48 h; reaction was read at 96 h. They established the dose–response relationship for nickel sulfate hexahydrate patch-test response over a dose range of 0.01 to 300 $\mu g/cm^2$. The results showed that 38 subjects (52.7%, the largest group of responders) reacted to 3 to 0.3 μg Ni/cm^2 (threshold value). A number of subjects also reacted to lower concentrations, however (three doubtful at 0.03 $\mu g/cm^2$, two positive, 4.2%, at 0.1 $\mu g/cm^2$). This wide range in response indicates the individual variation that prevails in susceptibility to sensitization and in reactivity.

Problems in appropriate dosing due to such individual variability may be compounded by fluctuations in test allergen concentration of commercial materials, adding to the uncertainty of diagnostic test validity. Recent investigation of five currently marketed standard patch test materials from Sweden, Germany, and Japan demonstrated that since earlier, similar studies (Fischer and Maibach, 1984b) suppliers have markedly reduced the variance in test concentrations (Nakada et al., 1998).

From a literature survey Menné (1994) concluded that elicitation of nickel dermatitis is unlikely for concentrations <0.1 to 1 $\mu g/cm^2$ with occluded exposure, and 15 $\mu g/cm^2$ when nonoccluded. Highly sensitized individuals might react to 0.5 ppm nickel (0.0075 $\mu g/cm^2$) under occlusion when exposing inflamed skin.

6.2.1.4 Test Site

Studies have been conducted associating patch test responses or skin permeability with anatomical site, pointing to regional variation in SC thickness and thereby reactivity within the same specimen (Magnusson and Hersle 1965; Rougier et al., 1986; Williams, Cornwell, and Barry, 1992; van der Valk and Maibach, 1989; Basketter and Allenby, 1990). For nickel in particular, notably lesser reactivity of the skin on the back was noted on occluded exposure to nickel sulfate, as compared to the forearm (Basketter and Allenby, 1990). False-negative test results can be obtained when testing on the lower back or on the volar forearm (Magnusson and Hersle, 1965). Nevertheless, traditionally the preferred site for patch testing is the upper back, while the intrascapular area and the outer aspect of the upper arm are also acceptable (Belsito, 1989).

Grading of patch test reactions in accordance with the International Contact Dermatitis Research Group follows degree of skin involvement:

No visible reaction	Negative	Score 1
Erythema	Doubtful	Score 2
Erythema/infiltration	Weak	Score 3
Erythema/infiltration/papules	Strong	Score 4
Erythema/infiltration/papules/vesicles	Extreme	Score 5

6.2.1.5 False-Positive and False-Negative Reactions

Cutaneous patch testing for nickel sensitivity has a limited reliability, as a clear distinction on morphologic grounds cannot be made between moderate irritation and an allergic reaction to nickel compounds (Nielsen et al., 1999). Clinical experience also suggests the existence of different degrees of sensitivity among patients allergic to the same chemical. Several authors proposed a quantitative concept of "strong" versus "normal" or "weak" contact allergy. According to this concept the skin reactions to different concentrations of a chemical correlate with the grade of the previous sensitization, rendering an individual more (or less) likely to respond to skin contact with a given quantity of allergen (Hindsén et al., 1997; Meneghini and Angelini, 1979).

The most common cause for false-positive diagnosis is the irritant effect of the patch test concentration used, as testing is performed at levels close to the irritating dose; also uneven distribution of the salt (usually nickel sulfate crystals) in the vehicle (usually petrolatum) may cause foci of high concentration under the patch (Wahlberg, 1996; Fullerton et al., 1986; Samitz and Katz, 1976). Intradermal testing has been proposed as an alternative, bypassing the SC barrier (Meneghini and Angelini, 1979; Herbst et al., 1993).

Occurrence of active sensitization of a naive organism induced by patch testing with nickel salts has been investigated as a risk factor by Agrup and by Meneghini, found to be of minor import. By definition, active sensitization is a flare-up at 10 to 20 days after a negative patch test reaction, and a positive reaction after 2 to 4 days at retesting. The authors found that the risk of such induction by nickel was minor when compared to the overall benefits of that diagnostic procedure. Of 379 hand eczema patients retested with 11 substances applied earlier, 73 (19%) had become positive, but only 2 (0.5%) to nickel (Agrup, 1968). Re-patch testing of 208 patients with the standard series (31 substances) showed that 25% had developed new sensitivities, but only two of them to nickel (<1%) (Meneghini and Angelini, 1977). Active sensitization is uncommon, but a typical complication of patch testing. For nickel in particular, however, the benefits of patch testing outweigh such risks. Reproducibility of the test is not 100%, and positive retest outcome does not automatically indicate active sensitization. Test outcome has to be put in context with the individuals who were negative on retesting.

A potential cause of false-positive, clinically nonrelevant reactions on patch testing is hyperreactive skin, also known as the Excited Skin Syndrome or "angry back" (Mitchell and Maibach, 1997; Mitchell, 1975). This condition can result from multiple inflammatory skin conditions or from strong positive patch-test reactions magnifying adjacent patch-test responses (Cronin, 1975). Such untoward reaction was investigated by specifically testing reactivity of nickel-sensitive individuals to a dilution series of nickel sulfate (Fischer and Maibach, 1984b). Multiple applications and strong reactions to high concentrations did not statistically magnify the response to adjacent lower concentrations of the compound.

False-negative results may occur due to actual allergen concentrations which fall short of label concentration (Fischer and Maibach, 1984b) or the extremely long induction or lag times, demonstrated in skin penetration experiments with nickel salts (Wahlberg, 1996; Fullerton et al., 1986; Samitz and Katz, 1976). In practice, also 2.5% nickel sulfate is used in the U.S., Sweden, and Japan instead of 5% (Nakada et al., 1998), but, as Cronin (1975) pointed out, up to 20% of true nickel sensitivities can thereby be missed. Cases with a clinical history of nickel sensitivity have occasionally shown negative test results also when patch tested with the standard 5% (0.19 M) nickel sulfate in petrolatum, possibly due to the considerable lag time involved in the salt's penetration through the SC and the likelihood of depot formation there (Samitz and Katz, 1976; Mali et al., 1964; Cotton, 1964; Spruit et al., 1965; Fullerton et al., 1988; Santucci et al., 1998; Seidenari et al., 1996a). Upon pretreatment of nickel test areas with SDS, however, such asymptomatic sensitivity will nevertheless become manifest, the inflammatory reaction elicited by the pretreatment facilitating the penetration of the immunogen (Seidenari et al., 1996b).

6.2.2 Discussion of the Patch Test

The "gold" standard test for ACD remains to be the patch test, in spite of its limitations (false negatives and positives). As noted by Ale and Maibach (1995), because of these limitations a semiquantitative analysis of the results provides a more facile and robust clinical interpretation. Hence, we review this bioassay in context of an operational definition, as described by Marrakchi and Maibach (1944).

Appropriate diagnosis of ACD is based on two essential criteria: (1) the presence of contact allergy should be firmly established, and (2) the clinical relevance should be demonstrated. Certain guidelines may be helpful in satisfying these prerequisites.

- To eliminate uncertainty in the case of ambivalent test reactions, retesting can confirm or deny the presence of hypersensitivity. If the initial positive reaction is not reproducible on retesting, allergy may be excluded; reactivity may have subsided, or the initial reaction may have been a false positive due to Excited Skin Syndrome (Mitchell and Maibach, 1997; Mitchell, 1975). In repeating the patch test, a dose-response assessment (serial dilution) may lead to the appropriate assessment, and also potentially to definition of a threshold sensitivity.
- Assessment of clinical relevance is based on a stepwise elucidation of factors. The patient is queried as to history of exposure to the putative

sensitizer (occupational/nonoccupational; dose; frequency; site; skin area affected; severity). A use test, such as a Provocation Use Test or the Repeated Insult Patch Test, may then be performed.

6.3 THE LYMPHOCYTE TRANSFORMATION TEST (LTT)

6.3.1 METHODOLOGY

Mononuclear cells are isolated from heparinized peripheral blood by Ficoll-isoplaque centrifugation prior to or 2 to 3 weeks after skin testing, and are cryopreserved (Nowell, 1960). The cells are cultured in RPMI 1640 supplemented with 4-(2-hydroxyethyl)-1-piperazineethanesulfonic acid (HEPES) buffer, antibiotics, and either 20% inactivated pooled human serum or 20% inactivated autologous serum. Nickel sulfate hexahydrate is used as antigen in the cultures in final concentrations of 0, 7, 14, 40, and 80 μM. At day six radiolabelled thymidine uptake is measured using liquid scintillation counting. Nickel-specific stimulation is expressed as:

$$\text{Stimulation index (SI)} =$$
$$\text{mean CPM w. nickel sulfate/mean cpm w/o nickel sulfate (Nowell, 1960).}$$

6.3.2 REVIEW OF MECHANISM OF LTT

Antigens possess the capability of transforming lymphocytes, enlarging and transforming them into blast cells, a process that can be assessed morphologically using various techniques to stain for RNA, DNA, and nucleoli (Mills, 1966). Since uptake of radiolabeled thymidine by lymphocyte nucleic acids in culture also correlates well with transformation, it led to its use as a method of assessment of such transformation.

Lymphocyte transformation can be specific for the antigen to which the organism has become sensitized, and often correlates with delayed hypersensitivity (Aspegren and Rorsman, 1962). By adding antigen to a sample from an NAH individual, transformation is likely to be increased over that of a non-NAH person's sample.

Aspegren and Rorsman (1962), following the report by Nowell (1960), investigated the ability of nickel to transform lymphocytes from Ni-allergic subjects. At high nickel concentrations they found suppression of mitosis, while at lower concentrations they failed to demonstrate any differences in transformations compared to controls. Pappas, Orfanos, and Bertram (1970) also found nonspecific transformation in response to nickel acetate, similar to previous reports of the nonspecific mitogenic effects of mercury salts (Schopf, Schultz, and Isensee, 1969). In contrast, Macleod, Hutchinson, and Raffle (1970) found no significant thymidine uptake in controls, but significant uptake occurred in lymphocyte cultures from 7 of 12 nickel-sensitive patients (58%). Using nickel sulfate and nickel acetate as antigens, Gimenez-Camarasa et al. (1975) reported specific transformation in nickel-sensitive patients, with neither salt acting in a nonspecific capacity. There have been reports of similar findings (Millikan, Conway, and Foote, 1973; Kim and Schopf, 1976). In addition to demonstrating transformation in response to nickel challenge of lymphocytes from Ni-allergic subjects, several authors found a weak, nonspecific mitogenic effect in control patients, taken as an indication that mechanisms other than those mediated by lymphocytes may be operating under patch test conditions (Svejgaard et al., 1978; Silvennoinen-Kassinen, 1981; Nordlind, 1984a; Nordlind, 1984b; Al-Tawil et al., 1981). Furthermore, cord blood lymphocytes showed the capacity to transform lymphocytes following incubation with nickel, a trend becoming more pronounced at higher nickel concentrations (Al-Tawil et al., 1985; Hutchinson et al., 1971).

Comparison of results obtained by the various investigators using the LTT as an *in vitro* means of assessing hypersensitivity to a particular contact allergen such as nickel has proven difficult due to numerous technical difficulties encountered in the test and the many different techniques used (Macleod, Hutchinson, and Raffle, 1982). Results from *in vitro* testing often are inconsistent with clinical observations and *in vivo* sensitization data (patch test data). Some of the procedural alternatives pursued in the endeavor to establish optimal conditions for the LTT are described in the following.

Methods of white cell (lymphocyte) separation vary among authors, even though the techniques used may affect the overall levels of transformation. These methods include gravity sedimentation, with or without dextran, and density sedimentation. Gravity sedimentation results in less pure lymphocyte cultures, but may lead to higher transformational values following stimulation with nickel (Elves, 1976) and phytohaemagglutinin (Gimenez-Camarasa et al., 1975).

The LTT has been used to study metal sensitivity in patients receiving total joint replacements (Gilboa et al., 1988): significant levels of lymphocyte transformation were observed in samples obtained from patients with positive patch tests for nickel, while none of the samples from nonsensitized (naive) subjects showed significantly increased lymphocyte transformation. In the case of patch test negatives among recipients of total joint prosthesis, however, an elevated transformation index was found in 7 out of 15.

The LTT using nickel sulfate in various concentrations was performed in a study involving 8 patients with contact dermatitis and positive nickel patch test, 7 patients with CD due to other factors and a negative nickel patch test, and 9 other subjects, 7 of whom suffered from other dermatological disorders (Silvennoinen-Kassinen, 1981). While all except 1 of the nickel allergics showed significant response to nickel in the LTT, at least 3 individuals with a negative patch test responded positively in the LTT. As reported by others (Pappas et al., 1970), this is also taken as an indication that nickel sulfate may have nonspecific mitogenic properties causing lymphocyte transformation.

In the attempt to improve the LTT in diagnosing NAH, Nordlind (1984a, 1984b) compared cell subpopulation separation techniques in the *in vitro* study of 9 patients with NAH and nine control subjects. The highest lymphocyte thymidine uptake was found in Percoll-separated cells, with less uptake in those separated using Ficoll-Paque and the lowest in gravity-sedimented lymphocytes. According to the results, the LTT was not improved if the cells were separated into different subpopulations on the basis of density.

A more significant difference in thymidine uptake between NAH and control subjects was obtained with unseparated cells (Silvennoinen-Kassinen, 1981). The value of the LTT for diagnosis was limited by a high percentage of positives in healthy controls. Also, in a substantial number of patch test negative individuals, circulating nickel-sensitive lymphocytes were seen to proliferate on contact with nickel, yet are not able to mount a clinically manifest allergic reaction.

Dual parameter analysis, however, combining LTT and the macrophage migration inhibition test (MMIT), allows a reliable diagnosis in most cases (Nowell, 1960). Correlation between skin test and *in vitro* reactivity for individuals with matching *in vitro* results (both tests positive or negative) was 60% of total. In individuals with discordant *in vitro* data (40%), skin testing still appears crucial for NAH diagnosis (Nowell, 1960).

Forty-three patients with NAH participated in a study attempting to correlate *in vivo* and *in vitro* response (Al-Tawil et al., 1985). The results showed a weak correlation of 0.42 and 0.46 between the two diagnostic approaches (patch testing and LTT) when tested for linear and logarithmic correlation, respectively. The authors surmise that this may be attributable to individual factors, such as the degree of substance diffusivity through the SC and epidermis ($NiSO_4$ applied in water).

Limited agreement was found in the quantitative comparisons of the patch test and lymphocyte responses (LTT) in a cohort of 30 cashiers tested (Gilboa, Al-Tawil, and Marcusson, 1988): only 3 *in vitro* positives (42%) were seen out of 7 *in vivo* positive subjects, indicating that subjects with positive cutaneous response outnumber those with positive *in vitro* responses.

In a study comparing nickel sulfate versus chloride for sensitization potential in the guinea pig maximization test, the stimulation indices in the LTT for the animals exposed to the two salts were nearly identical, in contrast to skin patch test results, where for the sulfate the responses were significantly different between exposed and control groups. Thereby use of the skin test appears preferable in sensitization experiments in the guinea pig (Dorn, Warner, and Ahmed, 1988).

Performance of the LTT was validated in distinguishing between 66 NAH subjects and 43 nonsensitive controls. In 6 and 7-day assays using 5 µg/ml nickel sulfate, 61 out of 66 (92%) of those sensitized to nickel had positive stimulation indices, the remaining 5 giving false-negative readings. There were no false positives among the controls (Everness et al., 1990).

Toward optimizing the diagnostic value of the LTT in identifying NAH, Räsänen and Tuomi (1992) compared outcome of the proliferation test performed over a range of nickel sulfate concentrations in cultures with results obtained from patch testing 21 nickel-allergic subjects versus 23 controls. Patch test results were verified by intradermal testing, and in 2 nickel-sensitive cashiers the cause of eczema was confirmed by coin provocation. Optimized at <10 µg/ml nickel sulfate hexahydrate and incubation times of 6 to 7 days, the provocation test differentiated between allergic patients and controls in 86% of cases. Nickel sulfate concentrations greater than 10 µg/ml appeared to cause nonspecific lymphocyte stimulation, resulting in false-positive results.

Elaborating on their earlier observation that T cells from most subjects with no history of allergy and negative to patch testing with nickel sulfate can be reactive to nickel, Lisby et al. (1999a; 1999b) investigated which particular cell population is responsible for such nickel-mediated activation in nonallergic individuals. When peripheral blood mononuclear cells from nonallergic subjects were separated into macrophages and nonadherent, HLA-DR-depleted T cells, only monocytes and macrophages led to T-cell proliferation upon preincubation with nickel sulfate, and not the T cells. Further, nickel sulfate-induced proliferation could be blocked by antibodies to major histocompatibility complex class II (HLA-DR) molecules. The result points to nickel-inducible T cell activation occurring in nonallergic individuals. Nickel has been shown to bind directly to the HLA-class II antigens. Therefore it is not surprising that blocking of HLA-DR molecules results in reduced or absent proliferation (Sinigaglia et al., 1985). In the effort to identify an early-warning test in nonsymptomatic persons, Lisby et al. (1999b) investigated the background for nickel reactivity of T cells capable of recognizing nickel-modified peptides in the peripheral blood of 18 apparently nonsensitized subjects on exposure to nickel sulfate. They found Ni-specific activation and proliferation of peripheral blood mononuclear cells in 16 of the 18 naive individuals (89%). Also cytokine release of nickel-inducible cells was investigated in allergics and nonallergics upon exposure to the antigen. T cells from both groups released interferon-γ but no interleukin-4. This is taken as an indication of equivalent function of T cells in both NAH and nonallergic individuals.

MELISA (memory lymphocyte immuno-stimulation assay), a lymphoproliferative assay, had been suggested by Stejskal et al. as a valuable instrument for the diagnosis of metal allergy (Stejskal et al., 1994). It is a modification of the LTT, specifically adapted to the study of lymphocyte reactivity to metals. Defibrinated blood is used in place of heparin, and monocyte and macrophage content is reduced by plastic adherence before analyzing for DNA synthesis, with the proviso that an increase in DNA synthesis be accompanied by the presence of lymphoblasts. Using the patch test as reference, sensitivity and specificity of the LTT and the MELISA were calculated, based on reactions from 34 patients with various metal contact allergies (Cederbrant et al., 1997). Neither sensitivity nor specificity was seen to differ significantly between the two *in vitro* test methods for the three metals gold, palladium, and nickel (se = 82%; sp = 17%). In both tests specificity was found to be unacceptably low for all three metals.

6.3.3 DISCUSSION OF THE LTT

While there is universal agreement among investigators that in the case of nickel the concentration used to stimulate lymphocytes *in vitro* is critical, for the LTT the optimum stimulatory concentration varies from laboratory to laboratory. Too high a concentration causes toxic and nonspecific mitogenic effects, while too low a concentration fails to exhibit any mitogenic effects. Amounts of nickel as mitogen vary from 23,770 µg with positive results, down to 0.01 µg with negative results (Kim and Schopf, 1976). Certain authors (Millikan et al., 1973) suggest testing at more than one concentration because of "high dilution responders" and "low-dilution responders" among patients.

Nickel sulfate is the most commonly used source of nickel and corresponds with that used in patch testing, but nickel acetate and chloride are also reported. Radiolabeled thymidine uptake, besides being the most widely used method of assessing lymphocyte transformation, is not standardized. Different radiolabeled isotopes may be added to cell culture from 1 to 24 h prior to assessment of uptake. Duration of cell culture varies from 3 to 7 days, with maximum response usually reported from 5 to 7 days. Following culture, the preparation of cells prior to measurement of thymidine uptake also varies.

The timing of the LTT in relation to patch testing might be important. Powell (1975) noted increased transformation following epicutaneous challenge of human volunteers with experimentally induced contact allergy to dinitrochlorobenzene. This problem was considered by Veien et al. (1979) in the context of NAH. They found no difference in transformation before and after epicutaneous challenge, although they did report increased transformation following oral challenge.

Again taking nickel as one of the most frequently investigated allergens, in spite of the inability to compare results between different laboratories, several investigators report significant differences between lymphocyte transformation in nickel-sensitive patients and controls (Svejgaard et al., 1978). Unfortunately, however, there is often a degree of overlap between affected subjects and controls, which makes it unreliable to diagnose nickel allergy on the basis of the LTT alone. Significantly, the test was reported as positive in an NAH patient whose patch testing had reverted to negative (Svejgaard et al., 1978). Recent papers clearly demonstrate that *in vitro* reactivity to nickel in apparently nonallergic individuals is mediated by Ni-specific T cells. Data by Borg et al. (2000) and Cavani et al. (1998; 2001) indicate that regulatory T cells are a factor in attenuating or limiting the severity and duration of hypersensitivity reactions in the skin. Ultimately clinical expression of disease is brought to an end, avoiding excessive tissue damage. Thus status allergicus may resolve in time, but antigen-specific T cells persist in the tissue, leading to *in vitro* reactivity observed in the LTT..

It would be premature to draw the conclusion that *in vitro* testing may, in certain circumstances, be more sensitive than testing *in vivo*, or even propose that the LTT replace *in vivo* testing.

While lymphocyte transformation has been investigated and used over the past 30 years, no attempt at interlaboratory validation of the assay has yet been attempted, nor have double-blind tests been conducted so far. No agreement exists on the question of which nickel salt to use and what the optimal concentration for antigenic challenge would be.

Thus, some of the questions that still await resolution are:

- Optimal dose of the allergen
- Optimal number of cells
- Optimal culture conditions
- Separation of cell types

In spite of extensive efforts expended, the test method still remains under investigation. We now still await new insights as to how the LTT is to be conducted optimally. Although the system is still under development in 2002, it has the potential to become an effective *in vitro* approach for investigating hypersensitivity.

The LTT is one of several *in vitro* tests available for the investigation of nickel allergy, capable of distinguishing nickel-sensitive individuals from controls. Results of most studies, however, show an overlap between nickel-allergic and non–nickel allergic subjects, possibly due to a nonspecific, concentration-dependent mitogenic

TABLE 6.1
Performance of the Lymphocyte Transformation Test in the Diagnosis of Nickel Allergy

Reference	Nickel antigen	Concentration (µg/ml)	Patients (Sensitivity)	Controls (Specificity)
Kalimo et al. (1989)	Sulfate	0.78–50	5 (100)	N/A
Everness et al. (1990)	Sulfate	5	66 (92)	43 (100)
Räsänen et al. (1992)	Sulfate	<10	21 (86)	23 (91)
Cederbrant et al. (1997)	Chloride	2.5–10	31 (82)	N/A (17)

Note: N/A = not available.

effect by nickel. The comparison of data from different investigations remains difficult due to variations in LTT methodology between laboratories, since the method has not been standardized. An *in vitro* technique must be simple, quick, and reproducible. The LTT execution is still too cumbersome to appear adaptable to routine use and is practicable only on a research basis.

The more relevant references published since the compilation presented in a review by von Blomberg et al. (1987) are summarized in Table 6.1.

6.4 SUMMARY

A direct comparison between the LTT and patch test remains qualitative, rather than quantitative. Both assays have limitations (false positives and false negatives) and quantitative aspects that are nonlinear. This lack of current comparability leads us to refer to a clinical interpretation as defined operationally (Marrakchi and Maibach, 1944).

Standardizing the *in vitro* assay has tested two generations of bench workers; unfortunately, the assay remains tedious, tricky, and time consuming (as compared to a patch test). Thus, after decades of research we still lack double validation assays.

Taken together, the current value of the patch test resides in a century of experience in performing and interpretation, while the LTT unfortunately remains a specialized *in vitro* research tool. We hope that this overview stimulates further simplification and clinical validation of the LTT.

ABBREVIATIONS

aq. aqueous
ACD allergic contact dermatitis
SC stratum corneum
SDS sodium dodecyl sulfate
ICDRG International Contact Dermatitis Research Group
LTT lymphocyte transformation test
NAH nickel allergic hypersensitivity

REFERENCES

Agrup, G., Sensitization induced by patch testing, *Br. J. Dermatol.*, 80, 632–634, 1968.

Alder, J.F. et al., Depth concentration profiles obtained by carbon furnace atomic absorption spectrometry for nickel and aluminium in human skin, *J. Anal. At. Spectrom.*, 1, 365–367, 1986.

Ale, S.I. and Maibach, H.I., Clinical relevance in allergic contact dermatitis, *Dermatosen*, 43, 119–121, 1995.

Ale, S.I., Laugier, J.P., and Maibach, H.I., Spacial variability of basal skin chromametry on the ventral forearm of healthy volunteers, *Arch. Dermatol. Res.*, 288, 774–777, 1996.

Allenby, C.F. and Goodwin, B.F., Influence of detergent washing powders on minimal eliciting patch test concentrations of nickel and chromium, *Contact Dermatitis*, 9, 491–499, 1983.

Allenby, C.F. and Basketter, D.A., An arm immersion model of compromised skin (II). Influence on minimal eliciting patch test concentrations of nickel, *Contact Dermatitis*, 28, 129–133, 1993.

Allenby, C.F. and Basketter, D.A., The effect of repeated open exposure to low levels of nickel on compromised hand skin of nickel allergic subjects, *Contact Dermatitis*, 30, 135–138, 1994.

Al-Tawil, N.G., Marcusson, J.A., and Möller, E., Lymphocyte transformation test in patients with nickel sensitivity: an aid to diagnosis, *Acta Derm. Venereol. (Stockh.)*, 61, 511–515, 1981.

Al-Tawil, N.G. et al., Correlation between quantitative in vivo and in vitro responses in nickel-allergic patients, *Acta Derm. Venereol. (Stockh.)*, 65, 385–389, 1985.

Andersen, K.E. et al., Dose-response testing with nickel sulphate using TRUE test in nickel-sensitive individuals, *Br. J. Dermatol.*, 129, 50–56, 1993.

Aspegren, N. and Rorsman, H., Short-term culture of leucocytes in nickel hypersensitivity, *Acta Derm. Venereol. (Stockh.)*, 42, 412–417, 1962.

Basketter, D. and Allenby, F., A model to simulate the effect of detergent on skin and evaluate any resulting effect on contact allergic reactions, *Contact Dermatitis*, 23, 291, 1990.

Belsito, D.V., The immunologic basis of patch testing, *J. Am. Acad. Dermatol.*, 21, 822–829, 1989.

Borg, L. et al., Nickel-induced cytokine production from mononuclear cells in nickel-sensitive individuals and controls. Cytokine profiles in nickel-sensitive individuals with nickel allergy-related hand eczema before and after nickel challenge, *Arch. Dermatol. Res.*, 292, 285–291, 2000.

Cavani, A. et al., Patients with allergic contact dermatitis to nickel and nonallergic individuals display different nickel-specific T cell responses. Evidence for the presence of effector CD8+ and regulatory CD4+ T cells, *J. Invest. Dermatol.*, 111, 621–628, 1998.

Cavani, A. et al., Effector and regulatory T cells in allergic contact dermatitis, *Trends Immunol.*, 22, 118–120, 2001.

Cederbrant, K. et al., In vitro lymphocyte proliferation as compared to patch test using gold, palladium and nickel, *Int. Arch. Allergy Immunol.*, 112, 212–217, 1997.

Cotton, D.W.K., Studies on the binding of protein by nickel, *Br. J. Dermatol.*, 76, 99–109, 1964.

Cronin. E., Patch testing with nickel, *Contact Dermatitis*, 1, 56, 1975.

Dorn, C.R., Warner, R.D., and Ahmed, W., Comparison fo $NiSO_4$ and $NiCl_2$ as sensitizers in the guinea pig, *Int. Arch. Allergy Immunol.*, 85, 332–336, 1988.

Elves, M.W., Transformation in the presence of metals of lymphocytes from patients with total joint prostheses, *J. Pathol.*, 122, 35–41, 1976.

Emmett, E.A. et al., Allergic contact dermatitis to nickel: bioavailability from consumer products and provocation thershold, *J. Am. Acad. Dermatol.*, 19, 314–322, 1988.

Everness, K.M. et al., The discrimination between nickel-sensitive and non-nickel-sensitive subjects by an in vitro lymphocyte transformation test, *Br. J. Dermatol.*, 122, 293–298, 1990.

Fischer, T. and Maibach, H., Finn chamber patch test technique, *Contact Dermatitis*, 11, 137–140, 1984a.

Fischer, T. and Maibach, H., Amount of nickel applied with a standard patch test, *Contact Dermatitis*, 11, 285–287, 1984b.

Fullerton, A. et al., Permeation of nickel salts through human skin in vitro, *Contact Dermatitis*, 15, 173–177, 1986.

Fullerton, A., Andersen, J.R., and Hoelgaard, A., Permeation of nickel through human skin in vitro — effect of vehicles, *Br. J. Dermatol.*, 118, 509–516, 1988.

Gilboa, R., Al-Tawil, N.G., and Marcusson, J.A., Metal allergy in cashiers, *Acta Derm. Venereol. (Stockh.)*, 68, 317–324, 1988.

Gimenez-Camarasa, J.M. et al., Lymphocyte transformation test in allergic contact nickel dermatitis, *Br. J. Dermatol.*, 92, 9–15, 1975.

Handley, J., Todd, D., and Dolan, O., Long-lasting allergic patch test reactions to nickel sulfate: analysis by nickel quantification and immunochemistry, *Contact Dermatitis*, 34(2), 101–105, 1996.

Herbst, R., Lauerma, A., and Maibach, H.I., Intradermal testing in the diagnosis of allergic contact deermatitis — a reappraisal, *Contact Dermatitis*, 29(1), 1–5, 1993.

Hindsén, M., Bruze, M., and Christensen, O.B., The significance of previous allergic contact dermatitis for elicitation of delayed hypersensitivity to nickel, *Contact Dermatitis*, 37, 101–106, 1997.

Hutchinson, F., Macleod, T.M., and Raffle, E.J., Lymphocyte transformation, *Br. J. Dermatol.*, 85, 300–301, 1971.

Hutchinson, F., Raffle, E.J., and Macleod, T.M., The specificity of lymphocyte transformation in vitro by nickel salts in nickel sensitive patients, *J. Invest. Dermatol.*, 58, 362–365, 1972.

Kalimo, K. et al., PUVA treatment of nickel contact dermatitis: effect on dermatitis, patch test sensitivity, and lymphocyte transformation reactivity, *Photodermatology*, 6, 16–19, 1989.

Kim, C.W. and Schopf, E., A comparative study of nickel hypersensitivity by the lymphocyte transformation test in atopic and non-atopic dermatitis, *Arch. Dermatol. Res.*, 257, 57–65, 1976.

Lisby, S. et al., Nickel-induced proliferation of both memory and naive T cells in patch test-negative individuals, *Clin. Exp. Immunol.*, 117, 217–222, 1999a.

Lisby, S. et al., Nickel-induced activation of T cells in individuals with negative patch test to nickel sulfate, *Arch. Dermatol. Res.*, 291, 247–252, 1999b.

Macleod, T.M., Hutchinson, F., and Raffle, E.J., The uptake of labelled thymidine by leucocytes of nickel sensitive patients, *Br. J. Dermatol.*, 82, 487–492, 1970.

Macleod, T.M., Hutchinson, F., and Raffle, E.J., In vitro studies on blastogenic lymphokine activity in nickel allergy, *Acta Derm. Venereol. (Stockh.)*, 62, 249–250, 1982.

Magnusson, B. and Hersle, K., Patch test methods. II. Regional variation of patch test responses, *Acta. Derm. Venereol. (Stockh.)*, 45, 257–260, 1965.

Mali, J.W.H. et al., Quantitative aspects of chromium sensitization, *Acta Derm. Venereol. (Stockh.)*, 44, 44–48, 1964.

Marrakchi, S. and Maibach, H.I., What is occupational contact dermatitis? An operational definition, *Occup. Derm.*, 12, 477–484, 1944.

McDonagh, A.J.G. et al., Nickel sensitivity: the influence of ear piercing and atopy, *Br. J. Dermatol.*, 126, 16–18, 1992.

Meneghini, B. and Angelini, G., Behaviour of contact allergy and new sensitivities on subsequent patch tests, *Contact Dermatitis*, 3, 138–142, 1977.

Meneghini, C. and Angelini, G., Intradermal test in contact allergy to metals, *Acta Derm. Venereol. (Stockh.)*, 85 (Suppl.), 123–124, 1979.

Menné, T. and Calvin, G., Concentration threshold of non-occluded nickel exposure in nickel-sensitive individuals and controls with and without surfactant, *Contact Dermatitis*, 29, 180–184, 1993.

Menné, T., Quantitative aspects of nickel dermatitis. Sensitization and eliciting threshold concentrations, *Sci. Total Environ.*, 148, 275–281, 1994.

Millikan, L.E., Conway, F., and Foote, J.E., In vitro studies of contact hypersensitivity: lymphocyte transformation in nickel sensitivity, *J. Invest. Dermatol.*, 60, 88–90, 1973.

Mills, J.A., The immunologic significance of antigen induced lymphocyte transformation in vitro, *J. Immunol.*, 97, 239–247, 1966.

Mitchell, J. and Maibach, H.I., Managing the excited skin syndrome: patch testing hyperirritable skin, *Contact Dermatitis*, 37, 193–199, 1997.

Mitchell, J.C., The angry back syndrome: eczema creates eczema, *Contact Dermatitis*, 1, 193–194, 1975.

Nakada, T., Hostýnek, J.J., and Maibach, H.I., Nickel content of standard patch test materials, *Contact Dermatitis*, 39, 68–70, 1998.

Nethercott, J.R. et al., Multivariate analysis of the effect of selected factors on the elicitation of patch test response to 28 common environmental contactants in North America, *Am. J. Contact Dermatitis*, 5, 13–18, 1994.

Nielsen, N.H. and Menné, T., Nickel sensitization and ear piercing in an unselected Danish population, *Contact Dermatitis* 29, 16–21, 1993.

Nielsen, N.H. et al., Effects of repeated skin exposure to low nickel concentrations: a model for allergic contact dermatitis to nickel on the hands, *Br. J. Dermatol.*, 141, 676–682, 1999.

Nordlind, K., Lymphocyte transformation test in diagnosis of nickel allergy, *Int. Arch. Allergy Appl. Immun.*, 73, 151–154, 1984a.

Nordlind, K., Further studies on the lymphocyte transformation test in diagnosis of nickel allergy, *Int. Arch. Allergy Appl. Immun.*, 75, 333–336, 1984b.

Nowell, P.C., Phytohemagglutinin, an initiator of mitosis in cultures of normal human lucocytes, *Cancer Res.*, 20, 462–466, 1960.

Pappas, A., Orfanos, C.E., and Bertram, R., Non-specific lymphocyte transformation in vitro by nickel acetate. A possible source of errors in lymphocyte transformation test (LTT), *J. Invest. Dermatol.*, 55, 198–200, 1970.

Powell, J.A., Whalen, J.J., and Levis, W.R., Studies on the contact sensitization of man with simple chemicals. IV. Timing of skin reactivity, lymphokine production and blastogenesis following rechallenge with DNCB using an automated microassay, *J. Invest. Dermatol.*, 64, 447–451, 1975.

Räsänen, L. and Tuomi, M., Diagnostic value of the lymphocyte proliferation test in nickel contact allergy and provocation in occupational coin dermatitis, *Contact Dermatitis*, 27, 250–254, 1992.

Rougier, A. et al., Regional variation in percutaneous absorption in man: measurement by the stripping method, *Arch. Dermatol. Res.*, 278, 465–469, 1986.

Rystedt, I. and Fischer, T., Relationship between nickel and cobalt sensitization in hard metal workers, *Contact Dermatitis*, 9, 195–200, 1983.

Samitz, M.H. and Katz, S.A., Nickel - epidermal interactions: diffusion and binding, *Environ. Res.*, 11, 34–39, 1976.

Santucci, B. et al., The influence exerted by cutaneous ligands in subjects reacting to nickel sulfate alone and in those reacting to more transition metals, *Exp. Dermatol.*, 7, 162–167, 1998.

Schopf, E., Schultz, K.H., and Gromm, M., Transformation and mitosis lymphocytes in vitro by mercury II-chloride, *Naturwissenschaften*, 5, 568–569, 1967.

Schopf, E., Schultz, K.H., and Isensee, I., Investigation of the LTT in mercury allergy. Non-specific transformation due to mercury compounds, *Arch. Klin. Exp. Dermatol.*, 234, 420–433, 1969.

Seidenari, S. et al., Comparison of 2 different methods for enhancing the reaction to nickel sulfate patch tests in negative reactors, *Contact Dermatitis*, 35, 308, 1996a.

Seidenari, S., Motolese, A., and Belletti, B., Pretreatment of nickel test areas with sodium lauryl sulfate detects nickel sensitivity in subjects reacting negatively to routinely performed patch tests, *Contact Dermatitis*, 34, 88–92, 1996b.

Silvennoinen-Kassinen, S., The specificity of a nickel sulphate reaction in vitro: a familial study and a study of chromium-allergic subjects, *Scand. J. Immunol.*, 13, 231–235, 1981.

Sinigaglia, F.J. et al., Isolation and characterization of Ni-specific T cell clones from patients with Ni contact dermatitis, *Immunology*, 135, 3929–3932, 1985.

Spruit, D., Mali, J.W.H., and De Groot, N., The interaction of nickel ions with human cadaverous dermis. Electric potential, absorption, swelling, *J. Invest. Dermatol.*, 44(2), 103–106, 1965.

Stejskal, V.D.M. et al., MELISA-an in vitro tool for the study of metal allergy, *Toxicol. In Vitro*, 8, 991–1000, 1994.

Svejgaard, E. et al., Lymphocyte transformation induced by nickel sulfate: an in vitro study of subjects with and without a positive nickel patch test, *Acta Derm. Venereol. (Stockh.)*, 58, 245–250, 1978.

Uter, W. et al., Patch test results with serial dilution of nickel sulfate (with and without detergent), palladium chloride, and nickel and palladium metal plates, *Contact Dermatitis*, 32, 135–142, 1995.

van der Burg, C.K.H. et al., Hand eczema in hairdressers and nurses: a prospective study, *Contact Dermatitis*, 14, 275–279, 1986.

van der Valk, P.G.M. and Maibach, H.I., Potential for irritation increases from the wrist to the antecubital fossa, *Br. J. Dermatol.*, 121, 709–712, 1989.

Veien, N.K., Svejgaard, E., and Menné, T., In vitro lymphocyte transformation to nickel: a study of nickel-sensitive patients before and after epicutaneous and oral challenge with nickel, *Acta Derm. Venereol. (Stockh.)*, 59, 447–451, 1979.

von Blomberg-van der Flier, M. et al., In vitro studies in nickel allergy: diagnostic value of a dual parameter analysis, *J. Invest. Dermatol.*, 88, 362–368, 1987.

Wahlberg, J.E. and Skog, E., Nickel allergy and atopy (threshold of nickel sensitivity and immunoglobulin E determinators), *Br. J. Dermatol.*, 85, 97–104, 1971.

Wahlberg, J.E., Nickel chloride or nickel sulfate? Irritation from patch-test preparations as assessed by laser doppler flowmetry, *Dermatol. Clin.*, 8, 41–44, 1990.

Wahlberg, J.E., Nickel: the search for alternative, optimal and non-irritant patch test preparations. Assessment based on laser Doppler flowmetry, *Skin Res. Technol.*, 2, 136–141, 1996.

Wells, G.C., Effects of nickel on the skin, *Br. J. Dermatol.*, 68, 237–242, 1956.

Williams, A.C., Cornwell, P.A., and Barry, B.W., On the Gaussian distribution of human skin permeabilities, *Int. J. Pharm.*, 86, 69–77, 1992.

7 Orally Induced Tolerance to Nickel: The Role of Oral Exposure (Orthodontic Devices) in Preventing Sensitization

Jurij J. Hostýnek, Katherine E. Reagan, and Howard I. Maibach

CONTENTS

Abstract 185
7.1 Background 186
7.2 Molecular Basis of Antigen-Specific Tolerance Induction 187
7.3 Experimental Hyposensitization on the T Cell Level 188
7.4 Experimental Hyposensitization in Animals 189
7.5 Hyposensitization in Humans 189
7.6 Clinical Observation of Nickel Tolerance Induced
     by Orthodontic Devices 190
7.7 Nickel Released from Orthodontic Devices *in Vitro* and *in Vivo* 192
7.8 Summary 195
7.9 Conclusions 196
7.10 Acknowledgment 197
References 197

ABSTRACT

A number of observations made in animals first, and then in humans, led to the hypothesis that systemic delayed hypersensitivity reactions can be suppressed following prior oral exposure to haptens under certain specific conditions, i.e., if low-level, prolonged antigenic contacts occurred during childhood and adolescence of immunologically naive individuals (Chase–Sulzberger phenomenon) (Chase, 1946). Since the late 1980s, dermatologists and immunologists have endeavored to confirm such a correlation, in particular since the prevalence of nickel allergic hypersensitivity (NAH) was seen to increase steadily in the young population, a phenomenon attributed to the pervasive practice of skin perforation with base metal objects for the sake of embellishment. Potential relationships between NAH, hyposensitization, and the induction of tolerance through oral intake are reviewed. Part of the discussion is the importance of priming the naive organism through oral exposure to nickel contained in orthodontic devices, as becomes evident from epidemiological studies, and the mechanism regulating the induction of tolerance on the T-cell level. Data available on the release of nickel from dental materials in the actual oral environment or *in vitro* are presented.

7.1 BACKGROUND

Sensitization to nickel is the most common cause of allergic contact sensitization (Menné et al., 1989). It is not limited to occupational exposure, and is more prevalent in the general population (Johansen et al., 2000). This is attributed to the release of the metal from objects of everyday use, such as jewelry and clothing fasteners, that on direct and prolonged contact with the skin may release traces of divalent nickel ion due to oxidation by skin exudates. The resulting low molecular mass species of the metal then can penetrate the stratum corneum (Hostýnek et al., 2001), and through complex formation the metal ion becomes attached to specific proteins (Griem et al., 1998). This forms the antigen that leads to allergic contact sensitization, the most common response in the human immune system. Immune reactions to nickel are not limited to this type IV, T-cell-mediated or delayed hypersensitivity, but include also the type I, B-cell-mediated or immediate reactivity (Hostýnek, 1997). Recent population studies from industrialized countries show that 8 to 15% of females and 2 to 5% of males are hypersensitive to nickel. An Italian multicenter study demonstrated an increase in NAH among dermatology patients nonoccupationally and occupationally: a prevalence of 38.5% overall in 1988, with 45.5% and 18.2%, respectively. This compares with the 1984 data of 26.2% overall, with 32.8% and 13%, respectively (Gola et al., 1992). Recent data gathered in Denmark suggest that, while that trend continues directionally, the nickel regulation promulgated in the European Union (EU, 1994) has had the desired effect of reversing the trend among the young, the age group at greatest risk (Johansen et al., 2000; Veien et al., 2001).

In all surveys so far NAH is most prevalent in females, believed to be due to the frequency and patterns of hapten exposure, rather than to a difference between females and males in predisposition to develop NAH.

Through the introduction of nickel in orthodontic devices, another potential type of exposure to nickel was added. Nickel in dental materials is subject to corrosion in the oral environment, putting dental patients at risk of developing allergic contact stomatitis, gingivitis, or cheilitis (confirmed histologically), conditions that disappeared following removal of the devices (Romaguera et al., 1989; Temesvári and Racz, 1988; van Loon et al., 1984; Veien et al., 1994). Also cases of generalized, systemic NAH without oral involvement were recorded following application of orthodontic devices not associated with dental appliances (Trombelli et al., 1992; Wilson and Gould, 1989). Chronic urticaria and eczema (type I allergy) have been observed in dental patients, attributed to oral exposure to nickel in orthodontic appliances (España et al., 1989; Bezzon, 1993).

Epidemiological survey shows that the prevalence of NAH among students, faculty, and employees of a medical center is significantly higher than is seen among the average dermatological patients: in an analytical study of 403 cases, 31.9% of the women and 20.7% of the men showed positive reactions to patch tests with $NiSO_4$ (Blanco-Dalmau et al., 1984).

A new phenomenon has been noted, however, that has the potential to counteract the potential untoward effects of nickel exposure and that, if applied prophylactically and in a timely fashion, may reverse the trend (Table 7.2). Observations first made with nickel exposure in animal experiments (Vreeburg et al., 1984) and correlations obtained from studies of human cohorts (van der Burg et al., 1986) led to the hypothesis that nickel hypersensitivity reactions may be prevented by prior oral exposure to the hapten, generally known as the Chase-Sulzberger phenomenon, if long-term, low-level antigenic contact occurred in the naive organism. Suppression of NAH reaction can be achieved in sensitized individuals (Sjövall et al., 1987). Since the late 1980s, then, dermatologists and immunologists focused on obtaining corroborating evidence of such correlation, motivated particularly by a steady increase in the prevalence of NAH in the young, attributed to the growing practice of skin perforation with objects releasing nickel.

A number of studies that followed van der Burg's serendipitous observation of induced nickel tolerance in humans has repeatedly confirmed occurrence of the phenomenon in humans (Kerosuo et al., 1996; Todd and Burrows, 1989; van Hoogstraten et al., 1989, 1991a, 1991b), as well as in animals (van Hoogstraten et al., 1992, 1993).

7.2 MOLECULAR BASIS OF ANTIGEN-SPECIFIC TOLERANCE INDUCTION

Induction of tolerance has been investigated for several antigens by Tomasi (1980). Oral tolerance of either humoral (type I) or cellular (type IV) immunity is defined as antigen-specific immunologic unresponsiveness after gastrointestinal (GI) exposure to the antigen prior to systemic immunization. It reflects the ability of the intestinal immune system to down-regulate local and systemic hypersensitivity reactions, a highly complex phenomenon that may involve a wide range of regulatory mechanisms, depending on the nature of the antigen used. As first observed in animals by Mowat, the tolerogenic effect of oral exposure to diverse types of antigen seems to affect all aspects of the systemic immune response that have been studied: IgM, IgG, and IgE antibody response, as well as the cell-mediated immunity, measured by lymphocyte proliferation *in vitro* or delayed-type hypersensitivity *in vivo* (Mowat, 1987). Although there is some evidence obtained by Challacombe and Tomasi (1980) that production of IgA may inhibit intestinal uptake of immunogenic protein, there is no direct evidence that this prevents hypersensitivity *in vivo*.

From observations made in rodents, it appears established that adverse reactions to xenobiotics are initiated and maintained by T cells (Goldman et al., 1991). In a study conducted in humans it was determined that antigen feeding of keyhole limpet hemocyanin induces systemic tolerance of the T-cell compartment, resulting in a markedly diminished delayed (type IV) skin test (peripheral) reactivity to this substance (Husby et al., 1994). While the B cell system can also be tolerized by antigen feeding, it requires larger doses (Challacombe and Tomasi, 1980). Two subpopulations of T helper cells Th1 and Th2 promote different forms of hypersensitivity. Activation of Th1 cells results in the secretion of soluble cytokines that promote the cell-mediated response; activation of Th2 cells results in the induction of antibody-mediated, immediate-type hypersensitivity. As broadly defined by Ishii et al. (1993), Polak et al. (1975), and Vreeburg et al. (1984), oral tolerance is the inhibition by antigen-specific T suppressor cells of Th1 responses in the periphery, identical to the phenomenon of antibody (IgG)-mediated suppression of the immune response. Local immune response in the gut-associated lymphoid tissue (GALT) of the GI tract, a well-developed immune network developed to protect the host, is the first line of defense against ingested allergens. The primary areas where specific immune responses are generated in the GALT are the villi and Peyer's patches. Such a response is the induction of regulatory T cells that then migrate to the systemic immune system and secrete suppressive cytokines following antigen-specific triggering. This is described by Chen et al. (1994) as one among the primary mechanisms by which oral antigen suppresses systemic immunity. Antigens that are able to penetrate this first line of defense gain access to the systemic site, where a down-regulated systemic response constitutes a second, specific defense against antigens. This reaction is activated by suppressor factors and a suppressor cell population. Certain antigens appear to be tolerogenic through their ability to induce antigen-specific suppressor T cells that are activated by intestinally processed tolerogen in the mucosa, Peyer's patches, or in systemic lymphoid tissues. It has been hypothesized by Challacombe and Tomasi (1980) that T suppressor cells generated in Peyer's patch migrate from there to mesenteric lymph node and the spleen, inhibiting the systemic immune response.

An alternative explanation for reduced clinical symptoms of hypersensitivity is the gradual decrease and finally disappearance in GI absorption due to the phenomenon termed immune exclusion; e.g., antibodies formed locally in the intestinal tract serve to limit the absorption of antigen (Walker and Isselbacher, 1977). The specific mechanism for induction of tolerance to nickel is not known, but may be one of those mentioned above.

7.3 EXPERIMENTAL HYPOSENSITIZATION ON THE T CELL LEVEL

Hyposensitization has been achieved by Boerrigter and Scheper (1987) to both immediate and delayed hypersensitivity reactions, to systemic as well as contact allergens. Skin exposure of guinea pigs to contact-sensitizing agents induced both systemic and local unresponsiveness for a certain period. Oral, epicutaneous, subcutaneous, and intramuscular exposure of allergen were shown to diminish or eliminate the allergic reaction in experimental animals and NAH subjects (Bagot et al., 1995; Christensen, 1990; Jordan and King, 1979; Panzani et al., 1995; Santucci et al., 1988; Sjövall and Christensen, 1990; Sjövall et al., 1987). Also UV exposure is known to have significant down-regulatory effects on T cell–mediated responses to contact allergens (Cooper et al., 1992; Prens et al., 1987).

While oral tolerance of both humoral and cellular immunity has been demonstrated by Husby et al. (1994) in rodents by feeding protein antigen, orally induced tolerance in humans using a similar procedure induced only systemic T-cell tolerance, and resulted in B-cell priming using keyhole limpet hemocyanin.

Hyposensitization has also been observed by Troost et al. (1995) following UVB irradiation, which has a marked effect on patch test responses to nickel; a considerable clinical improvement in the hypersensitivity state can be achieved by UVB pretreatment, although hyposensitization did not induce significant changes in the immunological findings in patients with NAH.

7.4 EXPERIMENTAL HYPOSENSITIZATION IN ANIMALS

Various mechanisms are operative in the induction of immunological tolerance by antigens, and the existence of one single mechanism that could account for the complex events involved in hyposensitization is highly improbable. Since the observation by Mowat (1987) regarding the physiological ability of the intestinal immune system to down-regulate local and systemic hypersensitivity reactions to most soluble antigens, oral administration of a variety of T-dependent antigens, nickel salts among them, has been reported to cause antigen-specific immune suppression of peripheral response in animals. In a number of experiments on mice and guinea pigs, persistent immune tolerance to nickel was induced by oral dosing with nickel prior to cutaneous exposure (Ishii et al., 1993; van Hoogstraten et al., 1992; Vreeburg et al., 1984). It was observed that intragastric priming with nickel sulfate prior to sensitization successfully reduced the cutaneous delayed-type hypersensitivity response to cutaneous application of the same antigen in mice in a dose-dependent manner, as measured by ear swelling (van Hoogstraten et al., 1993).

In this context it is interesting to note that attempts at sensitization of mice or guinea pigs to nickel apparently met with difficulties (Cornacoff et al., 1984; Möller, 1984; Vreeburg et al., 1992; Vreeburg et al., 1984). At the time such results were seen as a confirmation of the finding that nickel is not a potent sensitizer (Wahlberg, 1989). The apparent failure to sensitize the mice in that experiment can now be attributed to the fact that the animals had been raised and maintained in nickel-releasing metal cages, an environment that practically had led to oral induction of tolerance through long-term licking of the cage wire. However, van Hoogstraten noted in the guinea pig that nonsensitizing epicutaneous skin contact with antigen prevents subsequent induction of oral tolerance (van Hoogstraten et al., 1994).

7.5 HYPOSENSITIZATION IN HUMANS

It has been shown that significant down-regulation of patients with NAH can be achieved by keeping them on a controlled nickel diet. In a study involving 24 patients with nickel allergy, nickel sulfate was administered p.o. at differing doses and rates. Hyposensitization was achieved differentially by Sjövall et al. (1987) over 6 weeks at 5.0 mg Ni/day, measured as patch test reaction, demonstrating that such an effect depends on the size of the dose administered at specific intervals, rather than the total amount of allergen given.

Another approach has also been taken by Santucci et al. (1988) to achieve such an effect in humans, by a scheduled, gradual increase in oral exposure. Twenty-five NAH female patients were given a large amount of nickel as the sulfate (10 mg) p.o. in a single dose. Following a rest period of 15 days, 17 patients were given gradually increasing amounts of the allergen for 3 months (month 1 = 0.67 mg Ni/day, month 2 = 1.34 mg Ni/day, month 3 = 2.24 mg Ni/day). The study showed that the dose–response is not uniform, i.e., the organism is not able to cope with a sudden substantial challenge, but does adapt to a gradual increase. The majority of those tested with a single dose reacted with a generalized flare-up. The same patients, on a continuous and gradually increasing dose, experienced no worsening of symptoms. The authors hypothesized that the effect may be due to intestinal adaptivity, rather than to immunological tolerance, i.e., hyposensitization. They invoke as analogy the oral tolerance observed to other metals, such as arsenic, presumably leading to adaptive impermeability of intestinal cells upon sustained exposure.

More recently, in a cohort of 51 patients with preexisting allergy to nickel (of both type I and type IV), extended hyposensitization to the allergen could be induced by Panzani et al. (1995) in a majority of cases presenting with ACD, generalized urticaria, angioedema, or generalized erythema following oral exposure to 0.1ng $NiSO_4$/day for 3 years. This result is put in doubt, however, in contrast with animal findings, where attempts to induce antigen-specific hyposensitization have failed in case of previous contact with the sensitizer, even on chronic exposure to nonsensitizing levels of antigen (van Hoogstraten et al., 1994).

7.6 CLINICAL OBSERVATION OF NICKEL TOLERANCE INDUCED BY ORTHODONTIC DEVICES

Induction and elicitation reactions to nickel are seen in consequence of various types of systemic exposure: oral (España et al., 1989; Romaguera et al., 1989; Bezzon, 1993; Kerosuo et al., 1996), GI (Menné and Thorboe, 1976; Cronin et al., 1980), respiratory (Shirakawa et al., 1987; Shirakawa et al., 1992; Novey et al., 1983), parenteral, or iatrogenic (Stoddard, 1960; Menné, 1983; Sunderman, 1983; Grandjean, 1989). Conversely, there is increasing evidence that low-level, long-time oral or cutaneous exposure to nickel can have a desensitizing effect in nickel-sensitized individuals, or can induce tolerance in nickel-sensitized individuals (Bagot et al., 1995; Christensen, 1990; Mitchell and Shibata, 1969; Morris, 1998; Sjövall and Christensen, 1990; van Hoogstraten et al., 1992).

This conclusion is reached from a number of *post faestum* observations that also unintentional, long-term oral exposure to low levels to nickel substantially reduces the prevalence of hypersensitivity upon later challenge (van der Burg et al., 1986). This observation motivated closer scrutiny of early exposure history to nickel in humans. In the anamnesis of the growing numbers of dermatology patients with

NAH and also of large cohorts of adolescents without symptoms of allergy, particular attention now focuses on the fact of preexposure to orthodontic appliances as a potential tolerizing factor.

In a prospective study of 303 hairdressers and nurses, an effect contrary to sensitization was noted for the first time if oral exposure to nickel occurred in the form of orthodontic treatment at an early time in life, mainly prior to ear piercing. Female nurses in particular who had worn a dental prosthesis in childhood had a markedly lower incidence of NAH than those without orthodontic treatment (P < 0.05) (van der Burg et al., 1986):

No. with prosthesis: 74	Ni positive: 4 (5.4%)
No. without prosthesis: 114	Ni positive: 21 (18.4%)

Since van der Burg (1986) happened to notice a significant decrease in the prevalence of NAH among patients who had early orthodontic treatment, i.e., prior to having their ears pierced, several other European dermatologists pursued that clue further and repeatedly confirmed the tolerizing effect of slow oral release of nickel invariably occurring from dental prostheses (Kerosuo et al., 1996; Peltonen and Terho, 1989; Todd and Burrows, 1989).

A European multicenter study of 485 males and 1252 females showed that orthodontic treatment did not contribute to NAH. Preliminary results showed that early orthodontic treatment among those with pierced ears significantly reduced the incidence of sensitization (P < 0.05) (van Hoogstraten et al., 1989):

No. with prosthesis: 86	Ni positive: 24 (27.9%)
No. without prosthesis: 431	Ni positive: 168 (39%)

Final results of this international retrospective study were obtained from 2176 patients, in seven western European clinics, who were queried by questionnaire. Occurrence of NAH was correlated with early oral exposure to nickel-releasing appliances, in function of age and gender. When the wearing of dental braces preceded ear piercing, NAH in female patients was seen in 25.0 versus 39.3% in those previously unexposed to dental braces (P < 0.006). Among males the difference was 7.7 versus 22.5%, but the difference was not significant. Specifically, in the Netherlands this difference was 15.6 versus 37.5% (P < 0.025) and in Denmark 21.7 versus 38.0% for female and male patients, respectively (P < 0.05) (van Hoogstraten et al., 1991a) (Table 7.1).

In another study, relationships between development of NAH and previous ear piercing or orthodontic treatment with nickel-containing appliances were studied in 294 patients by Todd and Burrows (1989). Seventy-seven (31.2%) patients with pierced ears were allergic to nickel compared with only 3 (6.4%) patients without pierced ears, representing a significant difference. When orthodontic treatment followed ear piercing the frequency of NAH was 36%, compared with 25% when orthodontic treatment preceded ear piercing. These results confirm the correlation between ear piercing and the frequency of NAH, although statistically significant in female patients only. This also supports the view that oral exposure to nickel at an

TABLE 7.1
Tolerogenic Effect of Oral Exposure to Nickel in Function of Age (van Hoogstraten et al., 1991a)

Age	Dental Prosthesis	Sample	Patch Test Positives	% Patch Test Positive
10–14	Yes	45	11	24.4
	No	200	76	38.0
15–20	Yes	140	46	32.9
	No	56	14	25.0
21–25	Yes	15	2	13.3
	No	31	8	25.8
26–30	Yes	5	1	20.0
	No	17	6	35.3

early age, such as wearing a dental metal prosthesis, may induce a state of cutaneous tolerance to nickel allergy also (Table 7.2).

A study of 700 Finnish adolescents from 14 to 18 years of age showed: (a) orthodontic treatment did not increase the prevalence of NAH; and (b) orthodontic treatment with fixed appliances preceding ear piercing prevented NAH altogether. Appliances like quadhelix or headgear, with a smaller surface area than fixed appliances, did not show a significant reduction in NAH rate, possibly an indication that nickel release did not reach the apparent threshold limit necessary to induce tolerance. In that cohort, 35% who had their ears pierced prior to orthodontic treatment were found to be sensitized to nickel (Kerosuo et al., 1996).

7.7 NICKEL RELEASED FROM ORTHODONTIC DEVICES *IN VITRO* AND *IN VIVO*

The release of nickel from orthodontic devices such as crowns, bands, brackets, wire retainers, and bridgework in the oral cavity is due to electrochemical corrosion

TABLE 7.2
Effect of Timing of Oral Exposure versus Ear Piercing on Tolerance to Nickel (Todd and Burrows, 1989)

Status	Sample Size	M (%)	F (%)	Total (%) Sensitized Individuals
Pierced	247	2 (33)	75 (31)	77 (31)
Not pierced	47	2 (10)	1 (4)	3 (6)
Brace	6			1 (17)
No brace, not pierced	185			55 (30)
Brace before piercing	36			9 (25)
Brace after piercing	26			13 (36)

occurring in microenvironments of varying composition (Bumgardner and Lucas, 1994; Bumgardner and Lucas, 1995; Gjerdet et al., 1991; Grimsdottir et al., 1992; Kerosuo et al., 1995; Park and Shearer, 1983). The oral cavity in particular provides exceptional conditions for this process, due to a combination of endogenous and exogenous factors. The products of corrosion may then be taken up either through the oral mucosa directly, or by the soft tissues of the GI tract. Transported by blood throughout the organism, they can elicit an allergic reaction in specific target organs such as the skin or, conversely, induce tolerance to the hapten if nickel release occurs in the developmental stage of the immunologically naive organism (van Hoogstraten et al., 1991a).

Immersed in a 0.05% sodium chloride solution, a level typical for saliva, at 37°C such appliances released an average of 40 μg Ni per day, corrosion products with cumulative values of 125 μg ± 22 over 12 days. This appears as a minor factor in relation to an average dietary nickel intake of 300 to 500 μg per day (Park and Shearer, 1983).

Nickel release from orthodontic appliances (face-bows, brackets, molar bands, and arch wires) was also investigated in 0.9% sodium chloride over a period of 14 days by Grimsdottir et al. (1992a). The largest amounts of nickel and chromium were leached out from the face-bows (0.5 to 10.4 μg Ni) and the least from the arch wires (0 to 0.1 μg).These release levels appeared to bear no relation to the metal composition of the appliances themselves, but rather to the amount of silver solder used in their manufacture (the highest levels used in face bows), which appears to facilitate the release of nickel (Berge et al., 1982). The authors found that nickel levels released were not proportional to the nickel content of the alloys. While a single metal undergoes dissolution in function of its position on the electromotive scale, other metals present in an alloy have a bearing on metal corrosion and release, depending on the electromotive gradients in the local galvanic elements created ("pile phenomenon").

Cavelier et al. (1985) investigated nickel release from clothing objects and the tolerance of NAH patients for such objects and for nickel-plated metal discs. They concluded that good tolerance can only be observed if use of nickel is avoided altogether. They also disqualify the DMG spot test as indicator of tolerable nickel release because of its limited sensitivity (DMG pos. = 10 ppm), potentially yielding false negative results (van Ketel and Liem, 1981; Wall, 1992).

The surface compositions of four commercially available nickel–chromium dental alloys, Neptune™, Rexalloy™, Regalloy T™, and Vera Bond™, were compared as to corrosion behavior in the oral environment and correlated to the alloys' ability for protective surface oxide formation (and reforming following surface damage). Also the role of beryllium, added to alloys for improved castability, was investigated for its role in the corrosion rate of dental restorative materials. The alloys were chosen to be representative of alloys with acceptable and unacceptable chromium levels, with and without Be additions. In this investigation, Neptune had the best corrosion characteristics of the nickel–chromium dental casting alloys evaluated, forming a homogenous oxide surface responsible for the alloy's corrosion resistance, which also easily reformed when damaged. Neptune was followed by Rexalloy, Regalloy T, and Vera Bond. The results also showed that the presence of beryllium led to inferior corrosion resistance by interfering with the formation of homogenous surface oxides (Bumgardner and Lucas, 1993).

Bumgardner and Lucas (1994) evaluated corrosion and surface properties of those four nickel–chromium dental-casting alloys using electrochemical corrosion testing and Auger electron microscopy under cell culture conditions after cold solution sterilization of test samples. The results of the surface and corrosion analyses were correlated to cytotoxicity to assess the biocompatibility of the materials. As in the previous study, the surface and electrochemical corrosion analyses demonstrated that the alloys without beryllium were more resistant to accelerated corrosion processes as compared to the beryllium-containing alloys. Although the corrosion products released from the alloys tested failed to alter the cellular morphology and viability of human gingival fibroblasts, they did cause reductions in cellular proliferation.

Release of metal ions from the four commercial nickel–chrome dental-casting alloys was further investigated by Bumgardner and Lucas (1995) in incremental three-dimensional cell-culture tests. Metal ion release was correlated to changes in cellular morphology, viability, and proliferation. Morphology or viability were not affected by the alloys' corrosion products, but cellular proliferation did decrease. Analysis of nickel levels showed that of the alloys tested, Neptune released the statistically lowest amount of nickel, and also caused the smallest decrease in cellular proliferation. Pure nickel samples released greater than 324 ppm nickel over the 24 to 72 h tests. These levels are 1000 times greater than those determined from the commercial alloys. All alloys released statistically increasing amounts of nickel ions at successive test intervals. Based on this and the previous studies (Bumgardner and Lucas, 1993; Bumgardner and Lucas, 1994) the authors express concern over corrosion resistance and the biocompatibility of certain dental alloys, due to a perceived potential for accelerated corrosion and the exposure of local and systemic tissues to elevated levels of corrosion products. They conclude, however, that nickel-based dental-casting alloys containing sufficient chromium (16 to 27%) to create a homogenous surface oxide layer are most desirable for corrosion stability of dental appliances.

Release of nickel from different types of simulated orthodontic appliances was determined *in vitro* by immersion in a simulated oral medium under both static and dynamic conditions by Kerosuo et al. (1995). Five identical samples, each consisting of a fixed appliance, a headgear, and a quad-helix equivalent to one half of a dental appliance were immersed in 0.9% sodium chloride for 2 h, 24 h, and 7 days. A control appliance was subjected to dynamic test conditions in a specially built "oral simulator" under similar test conditions. A significant release of nickel was detected from the quad-helix during the first 2 h in static conditions, whereas during the following two periods significantly less nickel was released from the quad helix than from the other appliances. The fixed appliance with simulated function showed a significantly higher cumulative release of nickel than the similar appliance in static conditions, 44.2 versus 17.1 μg. The results indicate certain differences in the amount and pattern of nickel release from different stainless-steel orthodontic appliances *in vivo*. The release rate of nickel from fixed appliances under dynamic conditions was found to be accelerated compared with nickel released under static conditions.

Intraoral corrosion and release of nickel was recorded in a study of 34 patients outfitted with orthodontic appliances by Gjerdet et al. (1991). The levels of nickel in the saliva of 6 of the patients sampled within hours of placement of the appliances in the mouth was significantly elevated versus levels detected for the average of 34 patients prior to treatment (median of 67.6 ng/ml versus 8.2 ng/ml; $p < 0.05$; range of 0.0 to 104 ng/ml). These levels decreased again dramatically in the 3 weeks posttreatment, to 7.8 ng/ml in three individuals tested, values not significantly different from those seen prior to treatment.

Edie et al. (1981) compared the corrosion effect occurring under clinical conditions on examples of Nitinol™ wire with that on stainless steel wire by electron microprobe. Formation of a passive oxide layer in the aqueous environment appears to equally prevent corrosion on either materials.

Nickel and chromium concentrations were investigated in saliva of patients with different types of fixed appliances by Kerosuo et al. (1997) to document any differences in metal corrosivity occurring in the oral cavity, when compared with data generated under artificial *in vitro* conditions. For clinical analysis purposes, saliva samples were collected from orthodontic patients (1) before insertion of the appliance, (2) 1 to 2 days after, (3) 1 week after, and (4) 1 month after insertion of the appliance. No significant differences were found between the no-appliance saliva samples and those from the same patients after insertion of the appliances. The results suggest that fixed orthodontic appliances do not significantly affect nickel and chromium concentrations in saliva during the first month of exposure.

Changes in blood nickel concentrations were analyzed by Bishara et al. (1993) in a study to determine whether orthodontic patients ($n = 31$) accumulate measurable amounts of the metal during the initial course of orthodontic therapy. Blood samples were collected at three different time periods: before the placement of orthodontic appliances, 2 months after their placement, and 4 to 5 months after their placement. Biodegradation of orthodontic appliances in patients with fully banded and bonded orthodontic appliances, or appliances made of alloys containing nickel–titanium, did not lead to either a significant or consistent increase of nickel blood levels during the first four to five months of orthodontic therapy.

Release of metal ions from oral implants with superstructures of different metals and alloys used in clinical dentistry over time was determined by Cortada et al. (1997) in an artificial saliva environment at 37°C. Using Inductively Coupled Plasma Mass Spectrometry as the analytical technique, a high level of ion release was noted when a titanium oral implant was coupled with a chromium–nickel alloy. Chromium, nickel, and molybdenum levels reached 50 ng/ml over 15 days when the titanium implant was coupled with different metals, while the titanium implant coupled with a titanium superstructure presented a low level of <8 to 12 ng/ml titanium ion release during the 560-h test.

7.8 SUMMARY

According to current knowledge on induction of oral tolerance and hyposensitization to nickel, the following effects could be achieved, depending on exposure:

- Oral exposure: Tolerance obtained in animal and man. Desensitization in animal and man may be only temporary.
- Epicutaneous exposure: Temporary desensitization, observed in animals only.

Experimental evidence for induction of oral tolerance in general, as it has previously been observed in rodents, has recently been obtained in man also, where it seems to target cellular immunity in particular (Husby et al., 1994). Epidemiological studies in man show that long-term, low-level ingestion of nickel as it is released from dental materials appears to significantly impart tolerance in both males and females, as long as the target organism is naive to the antigen. A number of studies documenting human immunotolerance to nickel involve cohorts of school-age children and young adults. Consistently, contact with nickel through ear piercing at an early age showed increased prevalence of NAH, while a lower prevalence was observed among those who previously were subjects of orthodontic treatment involving nickel-releasing appliances. Such tolerogenic effect appears to be permanent. Conversely, a number of studies show an increase in NAH incidence when fitting of dental braces followed piercing of the ear lobes. A salient fact remains that the immunological status of the individual determines the result of exposure to allergen.

Truly permanent desensitization in the previously sensitized organism, as was described in one study, could not be definitely confirmed due to contrary experimental evidence obtained in other investigations. Most likely, then, with the evidence on hand, antigen-specific hyposensitization by oral administration in case of contact allergy is indeed possible, but appears to be a temporary effect only.

7.9 CONCLUSIONS

The animal studies are readily interpreted in that all necessary controls are included. The human studies, however, lack a matched control group. An optimized nonirritating patch-test concentration for nickel is still not available.

Testing for metal release should be conducted in a relevant medium for dental appliances (0.05% saline).

Some practical implications can be perceived in this overview:

In theory, it might be feasible to use oral dosing, such as with capsules, to prevent sensitization in the naive. A precedent was set by Epstein et al. (1974; 1982) in the attempt to desensitize to toxicodendron.

Limiting factors are:

- The relative novelty of the concept
- Toxicity of the nickel salt chosen
- Immunologic properties of the salt chosen

It is not obvious that orthodontic devices will be a long-term solution. Nevertheless, slow-release devices attached to teeth or the mucosa might provide a practical prophylactic method. Suggested is a cohort study involving children before they have been exposed to both orthodontic treatment and ear piercing. Quantification of exposure to nickel ion released from orthodontic devices should be conducted. It is important to note that epidemiological studies often overstate the real incidence due to the occurrence of significant false positives. Furthermore, patch-test positivity is often equated to clinical disease. In epidemiological studies, serial dilution data are lacking that could define the level of sensitivity (Andersen et al., 1993).

7.10 ACKNOWLEDGMENT

We gratefully acknowledge the financial support by the Nickel Producers Environmental Research Association (NiPERA) toward this review project.

REFERENCES

Andersen, K.E. et al., Dose-response testing with nickel sulphate using TRUE test in nickel-sensitive individuals, *Br. J. Dermatol.,* 129, 50–56, 1993.

Bagot, M. et al., Oral desensitization in nickel allergy induces a decrease in nickel-specific T-cells, *Eur. J. Dermatol.,* 5, 614–617, 1995.

Berge, M., Gjerdet, N.R., and Erichsen, E.S., Corrosion of silver soldered orthodontic archwires, *Acta Odontol. Scand.*, 40, 75–79, 1982.

Bezzon, O.L., Allergic sensitivity to several base metals: a clinical report, *J. Prosthetic Dentistry,* 69, 243–244, 1993.

Bishara, S.E., Barrett, R.D., and Moustafa, I.S., Biodegradation of orthodontic appliances. Part II. Changes in the blood level of nickel, *Am. J. Orthodont. Dentofacial Orthop.*, 103, 280–285, 1993.

Blanco-Dalmau, L., Carrasquillo-Alberty, H., and Silva-Parra, J., A study of nickel allergy, *J. Prosthet. Dent.*, 52, 116–119, 1984.

Boerrigter, G.H. and Scheper, R.J., Local and systemic desensitization induced by repeated epicutaneous hapten application, *J. Invest. Dermatol.*, 88, 3–7, 1987.

Bumgardner, J.D. and Lucas, L.C., Surface analysis of nickel–chromium dental alloys, *Dental Materials,* 9, 252–259, 1993.

Bumgardner, J.D. and Lucas, L.C., Corrosion and cell culture evaluations of nickel-chromium dental castings, *J. Appl. Biomat.*, 5, 203–213, 1994.

Bumgardner, J.D. and Lucas, L.C., Cellular response to metallic ions released from nickel-chromium dental alloys, *J. Dent. Res.*, 74, 1521–1527, 1995.

Cavelier, C., Foussereau, J., and Massin, M., Nickel allergy: analysis of metal clothing objects and patch testing to metal samples, *Contact Dermatitis*, 12, 65–75, 1985.

Challacombe, S.J. and Tomasi, T.B., Systemic tolerance and secretory immunity after oral immunization, *J. Exp. Med.*, 12, 1459–1472, 1980.

Chase, M.W., Inhibition of experimental drug allergy by prior feeding of the sensitizing agent, *Proc. Soc. Exp. Biol. Med.*, 61, 257–259, 1946.

Chen, Y. et al., Regulatory T cell clones induced by oral tolerance: suppression of autoimmune encephalomyelitis, *Science,* 265, 1237–1240, 1994.

Christensen, O.B., Nickel dermatitis — an update, *Dermatol. Clin.*, 8, 37–40, 1990.

Cooper, K.D., Oberhelman, L., and Hamilton, T.A., UV exposure reduces immunization rates and promotes tolerance to epicutaneous antigens in humans: relationship to dose, CD1a-DR+ epidermal macrophage induction, and Langerhans cell depletion, *Proc. Nat. Acad. Sci. USA,* 89, 8497–8501, 1992.

Cornacoff, J.B., House, R.V., and Dean, J.H., Comparison of a radioisotopic incorporation method and the mouse ear swelling test MEST for contact sensitivity to weak sensitizers, *Fund. Appl. Toxicol.*, 10, 40–44, 1984.

Cortada, M. et al., Metallic ion release in artificial saliva of titanium oral implants coupled with different metal superstructures, *Bio-Med. Mat. Eng.*, 7, 213–220, 1997.

Cronin, E., Di Michiel, A.D., and Brow, S.S., Oral challenge in nickel-sensitive women with hand eczema, in *International Conference on Nickel Toxicology, 1980, Swansea, Wales*, Brown, S.S. and Suderman, F.W., Eds., Academic Press, New York, 1980, pp. 150–152.

Edie, J.W., Andreasen, G.F., and Zaytoun, M.P., Surface corrosion of nitinol and stainless steel under clinical conditions, *Angle Orthodontry*, 51, 319–324, 1981.

Epstein, W.L., Baer, H., and Dawson, C.R., Poison oak hyposensitization: evaluation of purified urushiol, *Arch. Dermatol.*, 109, 356–360, 1974.

Epstein, W.L., Byers, V.S., and Frankart, W., Induction of antigen specific hyposensitization to poison oak in sensitized adults, *Arch. Dermatol.*, 118, 630–633, 1982.

España, A. et al., Chronic urticaria after implantation of 2 nickel-containing dental prosthesis in a nickel-allergic patient, *Contact Dermatitis*, 21, 204–206, 1989.

EU, Nickel, *Official Journal of the European Communities*, 22.7.94, 1–2, 1994.

Gjerdet, N.R. et al., Nickel and iron in saliva of patients with fixed orthodontic appliances, *Acta Odontol. Scand.*, 49, 73–78, 1991.

Gola, M. et al., GIRDCA Data Bank for Occupational and Environmental Contact Dermatitis (1984 to 1988), *Am. J. Contact Dermat.*, 3, 179–188, 1992.

Goldman, M., Druet, P., and Gleichmann, E., Th2 cells in systemic autoimmunity: insights from allogeneic diseases and chemically-induced autoimmunity, *Immunology Today*, 12, 223–227, 1991.

Grandjean, P., Nielsen, G.D., and Andersen, O., Human nickel exposure and chemobiokinetics, in *Nickel and the Skin: Immunology and Toxicology*, Maibach, H.I. and Menné, T., Eds., CRC Press, Boca Raton, FL, 1989, pp. 9–34.

Griem, P. et al., Allergic and autoimmune reactions to xenobiotics: how do they arise?, *J. Immunol.*, 150, 1191–1204, 1998.

Grimsdottir, M.R., Gjerdet, N.R., and Hensten-Pettersen, A., Composition and in vitro corrosion of orthodontic appliances, *Am. J. Orthodont. Dentofal. Orthoped.*, 101, 525–532, 1992.

Hostýnek, J.J., Metals, in *Contact Urticaria Syndrome*, Amin, S., Lahti, A., and Maibach, H.I., Eds., CRC Press, Boca Raton, FL, 1997, pp. 189–211.

Hostýnek, J.J. et al., Human stratum corneum adsorption of nickel salts: investigation of depth profiles by tape stripping in vivo, *Acta Derm. Venereol. (Suppl.)*, 212, 11–18, 2001.

Husby, S. et al., Oral tolerance in humans. T-cell but not B-cell tolerance after antigen feeding, *J. Immunol.*, 152, 4663–1970, 1994.

Ishii, N. et al., Nickel sulfate-specific suppressor T cells induced by nickel sulfate in drinking water, *J. Dermatol. Sci.*, 6, 159–164, 1993.

Johansen, J. et al., Changes in the pattern of sensitization to common contact allergens in Denmark between 1985–86 and 1997–98, with a special view to the effect of preventive strategies, *Br. J. Dermatol.*, 142, 490–495, 2000.

Jordan, W.P. and King, S.E., Nickel feeding in nickel-sensitive patients with hand eczema, *J. Am. Acad. Dermatol.*, 1, 506–508, 1979.

Kerosuo, H., Moe, G., and Kleven, E., In vitro release of nickel and chromium from different types of simulated orthodontic appliances, *Angle Orthodontist*, 65, 111–116, 1995.

Kerosuo, H. et al., Nickel allergy in adolescents in relation to orthodontic treatment and piercing of ears, *Am. J. Orthod. Dentofac. Orthoped.*, 109, 148–154, 1996.

Kerosuo, H., Moe, G., and Hensten-Pettersen, A., Salivary nickel and chromium in subjects with different types of fixed orthodontic appliances, *Am. J. Orthod. Dentofac. Orthoped.*, 111, 595–598, 1997.

Menné, T. and Thorboe, A., Nickel dermatitis — nickel excretion, *Contact Dermatitis*, 2, 353–354, 1976.

Menné, T., Reactions to systemic exposure to contact allergens, in *Dermatotoxicology*, Marzulli, F.N. and Maibach, H.I., Eds., Hemisphere, Washington, 1983, pp. 483–499.

Menné, T., Christophersen, J., and Green, A., Epidemiology of nickel dermatitis, in *Nickel and the Skin: Immunology and Toxicology*, Maibach, H.I. and Menné, T., Eds., CRC Press, Boca Raton, FL, 1989, pp 109–115.

Mitchell, J.C. and Shibata, S., Immunologic activity of some substances derived from lichenized fungi, *J. Invest. Derm.*, 52, 517–520, 1969.

Möller, H., Attempts to induce contact allergy to nickel in the mouse, *Contact Dermatitis*, 10, 65–68, 1984.

Morris, D.L., Intradermal testing and sublingual desensitization for nickel, *Cutis*, 61, 129–132, 1998.

Mowat, A.M., The regulation of immune responses to dietary protein antigens, *Immunology Today*, 8, 93–96, 1987.

Novey, H.S., Habib, M., and Wells I.D., Asthma and IgE antibodies induced by chromium and nickel salts, *J. Allergy Clin. Immunol.*, 72, 407–412, 1983.

Panzani, R.C. et al., Oral hyposensitization to nickel allergy: preliminary clinical results, *Int. Arch. Allerg. Immunol.*, 107, 251–254, 1995.

Park, H.Y. and Shearer, T.R., In vitro release of nickel and chromium from simulated orthodontic appliances, *Am. J. Orthodont.*, 84, 156–159, 1983.

Peltonen, L. and Terho, P., Nickel sensitivity in schoolchildren in Finland, in *Current Topics in Contact Dermatitis*, Frosch, P.J. et al., Eds., Springer-Verlag, Heidelberg, 1989, pp. 184–187.

Polak, L., Geleick, H., and Turk, J.L., Reversal by cyclophosphatide of tolerance in contact sensitization, *Immunology*, 28, 939–943, 1975.

Prens, E.P., Benne, K., and van Joost, T., UVB treatment induces decreased patch test responses and in vitro lymphocyte proliferation to nickel sulphate in nickel allergic patients, in *Human Exposure to Ultraviolet Radiation: Risks and Regulation*, Passchier, W.F. and Bosnjakovic, B.F.M., Eds., Elsevier, Amsterdam, 1987, pp. 117–120.

Romaguera, C., Vilaplana, J., and Grimalt, F., Contact stomatitis from a dental prosthesis, *Contact Dermatitis*, 21, 204, 1989.

Santucci, B. et al., Nickel sensitivity: effects of prolonged oral intake of the element, *Contact Dermatitis*, 19, 202–205, 1988.

Shirakawa, T. et al., Positive bronchoprovocation with cobalt and nickel in hard metal asthma, *Am. Rev. Resp. Dis.*, 135, 233–236, 1987.

Shirakawa, T. et al., Hard metal asthma: cross immunological and respiratory reactivity between cobalt and nickel?, *Thorax*, 45, 267–271, 1990.

Sinigaglia, F., The molecular basis of metal recognition by T cells, *J. Invest. Dermatol.*, 102, 398–401, 1994.

Sjövall, P., Christensen, O.B., and Möller, H., Oral hyposensitization in nickel allergy, *J. Am. Acad. Dermatol.*, 17, 774–778, 1987.

Sjövall, P. and Christensen, O.B., Oral hyposensitization in allergic contact dermatitis, *Sem. Dermatol.*, 9, 206–209, 1990.

Staerkjaer, L. and Menné, T., Nickel allergy and orthodontic treatment, *Eur. J. Orthodont.*, 12, 284–289, 1990.

Stoddard, J.D., Nickel sensitivity as a cause of infusion reactions, *Lancet*, 2, 741–742, 1960.

Sunderman, F.W., Potential toxicity from nickel contamination of intravenous fluids, *Ann. Clin. Lab. Sci.*, 13, 1–4, 1983.

Temesvári, E. and Racz, I., Nickel sensitivity from dental prosthesis, *Contact Dermatitis*, 18, 50–51, 1988.

Todd, D.J. and Burrows, D., Nickel allergy in relationship to previous oral and cutaneous nickel contact, *Ulster Med. J.*, 58, 168–171, 1989.

Tomasi, T.B., Oral tolerance, *Transplantation*, 29, 353–356, 1980.

Trombelli, L. et al., Systemic contact dermatitis from an orthodontic appliance, *Contact Dermatitis*, 27, 259–260, 1992.

Troost, R.J.J. et al., Hyposensitization in nickel allergic contact dermatitis: clinical and immunologic monitoring, *J. Am. Acad. Dermatol.*, 32, 576–583, 1995.

van der Burg, C.K.H. et al., Hand eczema in hairdressers and nurses: a prospective study, *Contact Dermatitis*, 14, 275–279, 1986.

van Hoogstraten, I.M.W. et al., Preliminary results of a multicenter study on the incidence of nickel allergy in relationship to previous oral and cutaneous contacts, in *Current Topics in Contact Dermatitis*, Frosch, P.J. et al., Eds., Springer-Verlag, Heidelberg, 1989, pp. 178–183.

van Hoogstraten, I.M.W. et al., Reduced fequency of nickel allergy upon oral nickel contact at an early age, *Clin. Exp. Immunol.*, 85, 441–445, 1991a.

van Hoogstraten, I.M.W. et al., Effects of oral exposure to nickel or chromium on cutaneous sensitization, in *Metabolic Disorders and Nutrition Correlated with Skin*, Vermeer, B.J. et al., Eds., S. Karger, Basel, 1991b, pp. 237–241.

van Hoogstraten, I.M.W. et al., Persistent immune tolerance to nickel and chromium by oral administration prior to cutaneous sensitization, *J. Invest. Dermatol.*, 99, 608–616, 1992.

van Hoogstraten, I.M.W. et al., Oral induction of tolerance to nickel sensitization in mice, *J. Invest. Dermatol.*, 101, 26–31, 1993.

van Hoogstraten, I.M.W. et al., Non-sensitizing epicutaneous skin test prevent subsequent induction of immune tolerance, *J. Invest. Dermatol.*, 102, 80–83, 1994.

van Ketel, W.G. and Liem, D.H., Eyelid dermatitis from nickel contaminated cosmetics, *Contact Dermatitis*, 7, 217, 1981.

van Loon, L.A.J. et al., Contact stomatitis and dermatitis to nickel and palladium, *Contact Dermatitis*, 11, 294–297, 1984.

Veien, N.K. et al., Stomatitis or systemically-induced contact dermatitis from metal wire in orthodontic materials, *Contact Dermatitis*, 30, 210–213, 1994.

Veien, N.K., Hattel, T., and Laurberg, G., Reduced nickel sensitivity in young Danish women following regulation of nickel exposure, *Contact Dermatitis*, 45, 104–106, 2001.

Vreeburg, K.J.J. et al., Induction of immunological tolerance by oral administration of nickel and chromium, *J. Dent. Res.*, 63, 124–128, 1984.

Vreeburg, K.J.J. et al., Successful induction of allergic contact dermatitis to mercury and chromium in mice, *Int. Arch. Allergy Appl. Immunol.*, 96, 179–183, 1992.

Wahlberg, J.E., Nickel: animal sensitization assays, in *Nickel and the Skin: Immunology and Toxicology*, Maibach, H.I. and Menné, T., Eds., CRC Press, Boca Raton, FL, 1989, pp. 65–73.

Walker, W.A. and Isselbacher, K.J., Intestinal antibodies, *New Engl. J. Med.*, 297, 767–773, 1977.

Wall, L.M., Spot tests and chemical analysis for allergen evaluation, in *Textbook of Contact Dermatitis*, Rycroft, R.J.G. et al., Eds., Springer-Verlag, Heidelberg, 1992, pp. 277–285.

Wilson, A.G. and Gould, D.J., Nickel dermatitis from a dental prosthesis without buccal involvement, *Contact Dermatitis*, 21, 53, 1989.

8 Biochemical Aspects of Nickel Hypersensitivity: Factors Determining Allergenic Action

Baldassarré Santucci, Emanuela Camera, and Mauro Picardo

CONTENTS

8.1 Introduction 201
8.2 Biological Properties of Nickel Ions *In Vivo* and *In Vitro* 203
8.3 Genetic Predisposition 204
8.4 Geometry of the Complexes 206
8.5 Oxidation States 207
8.6 Complexing with Proteins 208
8.7 Metal–Metal Interactions 211
References 213

8.1 INTRODUCTION

Over the last century, the wide use of heavy metals has increased both environmental pollution and the number of harmful effects for human beings (Manaham, 1994).

Direct contact with transition metals such as nickel, cobalt, chromate, palladium, platinum, gold, mercury, etc. frequently occurs in either domestic or industrial settings, and is difficult for everyone to avoid. Since the skin is one of the largest organs that function as structural interface between body and its environment, it becomes one of the main targets of the action of metals.

Several biological effects (immunogenic, toxic, carcinogenic, etc.) often caused by the intervention of the same factors may develop after single or repeated exposure to these metals (Guy et al., 1999). The nature of these effects and some of the mechanistic details at play are partly known.

Since all these metals are small, low molecular weight, highly reactive elements, they can enter into the body easily. Once penetrated, depending upon their half-lives, they may settle for variable times in biologic environments, acting along different pathways and to different degrees.

A general property of these metals in biological systems is their ability to react with several extracellular (i.e., enzymes etc.) or cellular (i.e., DNA etc.) targets, modifying, often not in a reversible way, their ability to perform previous functions (Jones, 1995). The appearance of the effects is mostly conditioned upon exposure, physicochemical properties of the metals, and individual reactivity that makes some people more susceptible than others.

The amounts in solutions and the chemical forms of the metals (anionic, cationic, or neutral) allow covalent or noncovalent binding with membrane proteins (the preferred targets of the action of the metals) and different effects on the cellular structures and functions.

While some of these metals are known to be essential nutrients, others are toxic for organ systems. Moreover, the effects they cause depend either on the intensity of the exposure or on their biologic requirement. Likely, moderate exposure to metals which have unknown function in cells is enough to cause toxic effects, whereas exposure to metals which are essential for normal cellular functions and/or partici-pate in biochemical processes leads to toxic effects only when it exceeds certain levels (Lansdown, 1995).

From a chemical point of view, transition metals have either electrovalences (that is, the number of negative charges carried by the anions) or coordination numbers (that is, the number of anions or neutral molecules that is associated with the cation). One of the main characteristics they show is that they all have partly filled d shells. d orbitals project well out of the periphery of the atom and ions and the occupying electrons are strongly influenced and, in turn, influence very significantly the surroundings of the ions (Cotton and Wilkinson, 1988). This means that the behavior of these metals in biological systems can be conditioned upon arrangement of the electrons filling the orbitals of the outer-most shells.

Transition metals act like Lewis acids. Their general trend is to accept lone pairs from organic or inorganic moieties (ligands), giving rise to a multiplicity of com-pounds called *coordination compounds* or *complexes*, which play a biological role. Chemical properties and role of the complexes depend upon important factors such as atomic radius, redox potential of the elements, coordination number, the possi-bility to form sandwich complexes, solubility in biological fluids, and competition for reactive sites of proteins. The large variability of the disposable ligands in biological environments makes it difficult to understand the site of action for metals or the pathways followed in causing harmful effects. Despite the complexity of the subject (readers may find further details in more specialized books (see, for example, Goyer and Cherian, 1995; Guy et al., 1999; Nieboer and Nriagu, 1992; Siegel, 1988), some key points appear sufficiently clarified.

The distribution, absorption, disposition, retention, and excretion of these metals are regulated by concentrations and affinities of extracellular and intracellular ligands (Dawson and Ballatori, 1995).

Metals do not necessarily display a high ligand specificity (Dawson and Balla-tori, 1995). While some metals such as mercury are almost invariably associated with one type of chemical group, i.e., sulphydryl groups, others like nickel are able to bind several ligands (Andrews et al., 1988).

Nature and accessibility of the disposable ligands may exert a protective effect against the toxic metals. Likely, the skin, similar to other organs of the body and thanks to its collocation, has developed defensive systems that keep metals away from critical targets or limit their toxic effects. Although the nature of these defensive mechanisms is still poorly understood, it is conceivable to think that the availability of the cutaneous ligands regulates both the activity of metals and their removal from the organ. Therefore, the inherited variability of the ligands could lead to the formation of complexes with different physicochemical properties that are capable of promoting not only their interaction with targets, but also their elimination.

8.2 BIOLOGICAL PROPERTIES OF NICKEL IONS
IN VIVO AND *IN VITRO*

A large part of harmful health effects develops following exposure to several nickel compounds in occupational or domestic environments. Nickel and nickel compounds are capable of inducing toxic effects that vary from organ to organ and depend upon the physical and chemical characteristics of the forms, concentration, length and route of exposure, distribution in the tissues, and individual sensitivity. When contacting the skin, nickel may cause irritation, eczema, or allergic contact dermatitis (Barceloux, 1999; Savolainen, 1996; Sunderman, 1992; Toxicology Update, 1997). However, the main hazard posed by the soluble nickel compounds is the development of allergic contact dermatitis.

Nickel is the 24th most abundant element in the earth's crust. Its whole-body load is comparable to that of trace elements such as manganese, cobalt, and molybdenum, which are involved in enzymatic or coenzymatic activities (IARC, 1984; Mracussen, 1960). In humans, nickel's essential status remains to be established (Nielsen and Sandstead, 1974). The presence of the ion in several important catalyst enzymes such as urease, methylcoenzyme M reductase, hydrogenase, and carbon monoxide dehydrogenase seems to suggest that trace levels of the metal are necessary for several biological processes (Hausinger, 1992; Thauer, 2001).

Experimentally, nickel has been considered only a moderate sensitizer in humans and animals (Guy et al., 1999), even though contact allergy is the most common form of cell-mediated contact hypersensitivity in the industrialized parts of the world. The dermatitis has emerged, over the last decades, into a significant and continuously expanding social problem with economic effects on workers' compensation and disability. At least 10% of the women, 20% of young women, and 1 to 2% of the men are allergic to nickel and the frequency of this type of dermatitis continues to spread nationwide (Menné et al., 1982; Nielsen and Menné, 1992; Peltonen, 1979). Prolonged contacts are generally required to induce sensitization in unsensitized people, whereas minute amounts of nickel are sufficient to elicit the clinical manifestations once sensitization has been acquired. A large interpersonal variability, either in acquiring hypersensitivity or in inducing the dermatitis in already sensitized subjects, has been observed (Gawkrodger, 1996).

At least three main factors concur in causing the high incidence of nickel dermatitis:

1. About 40% of the nickel produced is used in the manufacture of steel and other alloys that are widely used in domestic objects and especially in jewelry (Toxicology Update, 1997). Therefore, daily contacts often depending on fashion are extremely frequent.
2. Even if in everyday use the majority of the objects are not made of pure nickel but are electroplated with nickel, they are intended to come into direct and occluded contact with the skin (Basketter et al., 1993; Flint, 1998; Lidén, 1992; Lidén et al., 1996). Although the level of absorption through the skin is, in theory, lower than that from inhalation or ingestion, the intimate contact of metal objects with the skin, together with concurring factors, facilitates the formation and the penetration of nickel ions, favoring the onset of contact dermatitis.

These contributing factors include shape and mode of use of the objects, duration of exposure, extension of exposed area, trauma, maceration, temperature and humidity, pH, etc. Nickel reacts slowly with sweat, but prolonged skin contacts with nickel-containing objects favor the development of an electrochemical reaction between metal objects and sweat, leading to the formation of different amounts of Ni(II) ions, the most responsible of toxic action. The rate of formation of these divalent ions — more than the absolute nickel concentration of the objects contacting the skin — is a critical factor in inducing contact dermatitis (Flint, 1998).

3. Nickel is a transition metal with a peculiar coordination and redox chemistry. It easily forms several coordination structures and its reactions are strictly controlled by the quality and quantity of ligands in the environment (Kasprzack, 1995).

The penetration of nickel through the skin is a prerequisite for the development of dermatitis. In general, the solubility of the compounds conditions the absorption, distribution, and elimination of the metal in biological systems (Barceloux, 1999). Highly soluble nickel salts (sulfate, chloride, acetate, etc.) have a half-life of about 1 day, whereas poor soluble compounds (oxides, sulfides, etc.) have half-lives estimated to up to 3 years and may undergo phagocytosis by various cell types (Savolainen, 1996).

The adsorbed nickel may be partly retained at the site of application, and a delayed elimination facilitates the uptake of the metal which occurs in keratinocytes more than in fibroblasts (Lacy et al., 1996).

8.3 GENETIC PREDISPOSITION

For several years it has been established that both exposure and individual genetic susceptibility play a determinant role in inducing allergic contact dermatitis to nickel compounds. Several studies have attempted to evaluate the role of the genetic factors. Most of the studies performed on guinea pigs lead to the conclusion that the mode of inheritance is autosomal and irregularly dominant (Baer, 1995). By contrast, studies of the mode of inheritance in humans do not allow us to confirm these statements and additional work must be carried out before a firm conclusion can be reached.

In humans, the influence of genetic factors has been evaluated by epidemiological, family, and twin studies. Fleming et al. (1999) used patch tests and questionnaires to study patients with allergic contact dermatitis to nickel and their relatives. They reported that the latter group was at high risk of developing nickel dermatitis.

Genetic predisposition to nickel allergy has been evaluated in a study including 115 twin pairs (Hange, 1981). The partners with suspected nickel allergy were further investigated with clinical examination and patch testing. The concordance rates of nickel allergy were higher in a statistically significant way in monozygotic than in dizygotic twins. In a Danish study only twin partners with a history of dermatitis in relation to direct contact with cheap metals showed positive patch test responses to nickel (Menné and Holm, 1983).

Since HLA antigen expression is necessary for the development of ACD, numerous studies using both serological methods and genomic typing have been performed to evaluate whether the tendency to develop nickel sensitivity was associated with alleles of the HLA class II region. Some authors reported that the antigens HLA-B7, B21, B12, BW22, B35, B40, DR4, and DRw6 were increased (Baer, 1995; Fleming et al., 1999; Mozzanica et al., 1990; Olerup and Emtestam, 1988), whereas others concluded that the distribution of several HLA class II alleles was similar in both nickel-sensitive and nickel-nonsensitive subjects (Emtestam, 1992).

The majority of the authors conclude that the tendency to develop metal sensitivity is not associated with alleles of the HLA class II (Emtestam et al., 1993; Ikaheimo et al., 1993; Karvonen et al., 1984).

Isolated studies concerning HLA class III polymorphisms in nickel-sensitive subjects put in evidence a statistically significant high frequency of the subtype BF FB (Orecchia et al., 1992). The authors suggested that this polymorphic serum protein might be involved in the pathogenesis of the disease. Recently, a study was undertaken to see whether the genes TAP1 and TAP2, whose alleles control the immune response to peptides, were involved in the susceptibility to nickel allergy (Silvernnoinen-Kassinen et al., 1997). Two populations of 55 nickel-sensitive subjects and 54 nonsensitive subjects were TAP1 and TAP2 typed by amplification refractory mutation system-polymerase chain reaction. While the allele and phenotypic frequencies of TAP2B were significantly increased, the allele frequency of TAP2C was decreased in nickel-sensitive subjects. The conclusion drawn by the authors was that TAP2B increases the risk for nickel allergy with a considerably high etiological factor.

In conclusion, even if some people with genetic background are more frequently sensitized than others to nickel, it is likely that the elevated number of subjects affected by nickel sensitization mostly depends on the degree of the exposure.

8.4 GEOMETRY OF THE COMPLEXES

Recognized by the Swedish chemist Cronsted in 1754 and isolated as a pure metal by Berthier in 1820, nickel belongs to the first transition series group VIIIB of the periodic table and has partly filled three-dimensional shells either in the ground state of the atom or in one or more of its chemically important ions (Cotton and Wilkinson, 1988). The outer electron configurations of Ni(0), Ni(II), and Ni(III) are $3d^8 4s^2$, $3d^8$, and $3d^7$, respectively (Figure 8.1). The electronic structure, together with the natural tendency of the element to achieve a more stable coordination sphere, makes all the nickel ions capable of binding several ions or molecules containing unshared pairs of electrons. Donating bonds (dative or coordinate bonds) to the metal ions can be formed by several ions or molecules that share electron pairs with the element. Nickel may combine with oxygen, nitrogen, and sulfur-containing ligands and donors from rows IV, V, VI, and VII of the periodic table (Coogan et al., 1989).

The coordinated groups around the cation tend to achieve different geometrical arrangements which are of great biological importance. For example, a ternary complex is necessary for L-histidine in removing nickel from the protein albumin (Coogan et al., 1989). The octahedral complexes formed by nickel and other divalent cations may explain some ionic interactions occurring between nickel and divalent essential cations (Andrews et al., 1988). Nickel has several coordination numbers and geometries, and in forming complexes it may engage a number of orbitals varying from 3 to 6 due to the large capability of the orbital hybridization (Cotton and Wilkinson, 1988) (Figure 8.2).

Ni(I) tends to be tetrahedral, whereas Ni(II) has oxidation numbers of 4, 5, and 6 and forms several types of complexes with unpaired or paired electrons. In the tetra-coordinate form, the prevalent complexes are tetrahedral and square planar polyhedral; in the five-coordinate form, the prevalent complexes are square pyramidal and trigonal bipyramidal. Last, in the six-coordinate form, the prevalent complex is distorted octahedral.

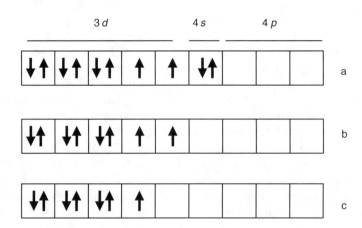

FIGURE 8.1 Outer electronic configuration of (a) Ni(0); (b) Ni(II); (c) Ni(III).

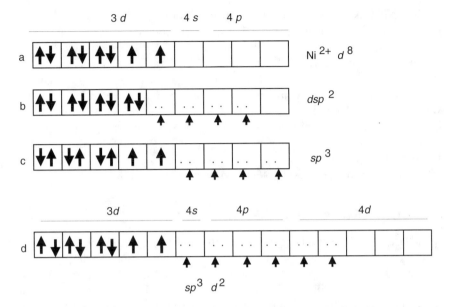

FIGURE 8.2 (a) Nickel hybridization; (b) diamagnetic square complex; (c) paramagnetic tetrahedral complex; (d) paramagnetic octahedral complex.

Ni(III) is 5–6-coordinated and may form trigonal, bypyramidal, or distorted octahedral configurations.

In solutions, nickel generally forms several complexes with different stability. In fact, the bonds which hold the coordinated groups together have different strengths that vary depending on the nature of the ligands, the pH, and the ionic strength of the immediate environment. Moreover, equilibria of nickel complexes with different geometrical arrangements undergoing rapid interconversion between them are frequently found in solution (Boyle and Robinson, 1988). All the soluble nickel complexes can be rapidly translocated in biological systems and the nickel movement between different compartments needs a ligand exchange (Coogan et al., 1989).

8.5 OXIDATION STATES

The nickel oxidation states vary from -1 to $+4$. In biological systems the soluble Ni(II), classically considered responsible for the induction of contact allergy, is the one most frequently found. It exists either in particulate form or as a coordination complex with water alone — as a green hexaquinonickel (II) ion ($[Ni(H_2O)_6]^{2+}$) — or with water and other ligands (Coogan et al., 1989). The electrochemical reaction between metal objects and sweat leads to the formation of different amounts of Ni(II) ions *in vivo*. In Ni-enzymes the oxidation state of nickel is II in active dehydrogenase, hydrogenase, and urease, whereas it is I in active methyl-coenzyme M reductase (Thauer, 2001).

Ni(III) can derive from electrochemical oxidation of Ni(II) complexes in aqueous solutions. Protein-Ni(III) complexes play a predominant role in enzymology (Andrews, 1988).

The Ni(II)/Ni(III) redox couple is active in biological systems because in aqueous solutions electrochemical oxidation of Ni(II) complexes can produce Ni(III) species (Cross et al., 1985). The likelihood that nickel can undergo redox cycling between Ni(II) and Ni(III) implies a geometrical reorganization and may play a role in its toxicity (Cross et al., 1985; Nieboer et al., 1984).

Ni(III) and Ni(IV) are considered strong oxidizing agents with low stability in water (Cotton and Wilkinson, 1988). However, as stated below, Artik et al. (1999) observed that when administering nickel in the presence of hydrogen peroxide they were able to induce contact hypersensitivity (Artik et al., 1999). In their opinion Ni(III) and Ni(IV) generated from Ni(II) by reactive oxygen species released during inflammation were able, besides Ni(II), to sensitize naive T cells.

8.6 COMPLEXING WITH PROTEINS

In the last three decades a large number of studies have enhanced our understanding of the complex interactions between nickel compounds and the host's immune response. However, our knowledge of the circumstances under which nickel antigen(s) are formed is still incomplete. It has been generally assumed that the small-sized nickel hapten has to conjugate with cellular or matrix proteins of the skin to be recognized as a full antigen (Lepoittevin and Berl, 1998).

Although nickel and cobalt are chelated by histidine residues to form protein complexes (Romagnoli and Sinigaglia, 1991), the nature and the importance of the carrier protein(s) in allergic contact dermatitis still remain speculative (Büdinger and Hertl, 2000; Chu et al., 1989). In theory, nickel is able to form complexes either with single amino acids or with di-, tri-, and higher peptides including proteins. Furthermore, nickel ions display a propensity to reaction with patterns varying from organ to organ, with a large variety of nucleophilic ligands such as carboxyl, hydroxyl, amino, sulfydryl groups, imidazole ring, etc. (Boyle and Robinson, 1988; Coogan et al., 1989).

The stability constant of the complex formed with nickel has been established for several amino acids. According to the defined values, nickel is able to form complexes preferentially with L-cysteine (pKa1 = 8.7) followed by L-histidine (pKa1 = 8.66) and L-aspartate (pKa1 = 7.15). The remaining amino acids show comparably lower values of the stability constant of their complex with nickel. L-Lysine is considered to form the less stable complex (Andrews et al., 1988).

In neutral solutions, nickel is capable of binding sulfur and nitrogen in cysteine and histidine residues, respectively, and, less frequently, amino and tryptophane's indole groups (Boyle and Robinson, 1988; Coogan et al., 1989).

Under physiological conditions, Ni(II) is transported throughout the body bound to proteins and amino acids. In plasma, nickel is mostly bound to high molecular mass proteins such as albumin and to a low molecular mass component forming Ni(II)–amino-acid complexes. The affinity of albumin for nickel is low, the complex is reasonably unstable, and albumin does not seem to be a significant carrier in producing an antigen (Ciccarelli and Wetterhahan, 1984; Nieboer et al., 1992; Sunderman, 1977).

In human and bovine serum albumin, the imidazole groups are considered to be the primary nickel-binding sites. Free L-histidine shows greater affinity for nickel than albumin and forms strong complexes with Ni(II) that, due to their molecular weight, are able to cross biological membranes (Glennon and Sarkar, 1982; Rao, 1962; Sarkar, 1983).

In order to understand the role played by low-molecular-mass constituents of human blood in binding Ni(II), Lucassen and Sarkar (1979), testing a series of 22 amino acids, found that at physiological pH, L-histidine was the prevalent Ni(II) binding amino acid. An active role for histidine motifs in the incorporation of nickel in hydrogenase and urease has been reported (Coogan et al., 1989; Hausinger, 1992). In addition, hystidine has a potential as an efficient, nontoxic, nickel chelator. Rostenberg and Perkins (1951) first discovered that nickel chelation could prevent the symptoms of nickel allergic contact dermatitis. Other investigators have demonstrated the effect *in vivo* using a variety of organic ligands (Healy et al., 1998; Gawkrodger et al., 1995). Fullerton et al. (1988) tested the ability of three metal chelating agents (ethylenediamine tetracetic acid disodium salt, L-histidine and D-penicillamine) in removing nickel from its binding sites in the epidermis; L-histidine was effective only at high concentrations. Nearly all of these studies used patch testing and demonstrated that a positive reaction to nickel was avoided by application of a ligand-based preparation.

The role played by the cutaneous amino acids in allergic contact dermatitis is difficult to assess. The exact distribution of the nickel between the various amino acids is unknown. In theory, all the nucleophilic amino acids included in peptidil chains or free are competitors for nickel binding. They may react either by their side chains or by both their amino and carboxylic termini (Romagnoli and Sinigaglia, 1991).

Samitz and Katz (1976), performing binding experiments using epidermis powder and inactivating functional groups through methylation, reached the conclusion that the carboxyl groups of amino acids were involved in the binding of nickel to a greater extent than amino groups.

It is likely that exposure to nickel ions gives rise to a continuous reformation of networks of bonds between nickel and amino-acid ligands. The nature of these interactions varies, depending upon the abundance of the ligands, the values of the binding constants of Ni ions for the different amino acids, and last, upon the concentration of the metal. Consequently, complexes with various proteins showing different immunogenic properties are conceivably formed (Chu et al., 1989). They are processed in different ways and target different biomolecules.

T-lymphocyte response to an antigen is governed by the chemical properties of that antigen (Kalish, 1995; Allen, 1987), and the percentage of responders varies, depending on the chemistry of the contacting agent (Basketter et al., 1995). In allergic contact dermatitis to nickel, the specific T-cell response is often induced by a trimolecular complex formed by MHC II molecules, peptide, and T-cell receptor (Büdinger and Hertl, 2000). However, in some cases, nickel may interact either directly with some T cells in the absence of antigen-presenting cells or with MHC class II molecules (Pellettier and Druet, 1995; Sinigaglia et al., 1985).

In patients suffering from nickel contact dermatitis, a broad repertoire of the T-cell clones has been isolated from both peripheral blood and lesional tissue biopsies (Kapsemberg et al., 1987). The presence of different clones in the same subject probably indicates recognition of different nickel complexes (Büdinger and Hertl, 2000; Chu et al., 1989; Pellettier and Druet, 1995). Moreover, the susceptibility of certain subjects to the toxic effects of the metal may be dependent on both the individual immune response and the nature of constitutive ligands, which varies among individuals.

Like other transition metals nickel is capable of inducing proinflammatory actions and, depending on the applied concentrations, cytotoxic effects in cultured human keratinocytes. To date, we do not know if these effects are able to elicit an immune system intervention, at least in some individuals.

Studies conducted in rats demonstrated the connection between lipoperoxidation, cytokine production, and hepatoxicity after exposure to acute $NiCl_2$ poisoning (Chen et al., 1998). Accordingly, elevated levels of malonyldialdehyde in serum were associated with interleukin-1 (IL-1), tumor necrosis factor-alpha (TNF-α), and transforming growth factor-beta (TGF-β) expression (Goebler et al., 1993).

Nickel salts applied to the skin of nonsensitized individuals can induce an inflammatory reaction and, in sensitive subjects, induces keratinocytes to express immune-associated surface antigens such as human leukocyte antigen-DR (HLA-DR) and intracellular adhesion molecule-1 (ICAM-1) at levels comparable with interferon-gamma (IFN-γ), suggestive of a participation of these cells to the sensitization process by facilitating the binding and recruitment of T lymphocytes and monocytes through the leukocyte function antigen (LFA-1) (Garioch et al., 1991; Vejlsgard et al., 1989).

Even though some authors report that the up-regulation of ICAM-1 in response to $NiSO_4$ is relatively modest in comparison to that obtained with IFN-γ, they reported that this relatively slight induction of ICAM-1 expression was enough to ensure T-cell binding to keratinocytes (Little et al., 1998).

Nickel ions, at subtoxic concentrations, are also able to activate keratinocytes into producing IL-1α, IL-1β, and IL-1RA, whose increments take place in this order: IL-1RA > IL-1α > IL-1β. Moreover, up-regulation of TNF-α mRNA ultimately inducing ICAM-1 expression by indirect mechanisms has been shown (Goebler et al., 1993; Guèniche et al., 1994; Picardo et al., 1990).

The mechanism involved in the stimulation process remains to be determined, but some findings suggest that nickel could activate the lipoxygenase pathway, favoring the generation of lipoperoxides, ultimately altering the cell membranes (Friedman et al., 1993; Goebler et al., 1993, 1994; Guèniche et al., 1994; Lange-Wantizin et al., 1988; Picardo et al., 1990; Sterry et al., 1991; Trenam et al., 1992).

Activation of the peroxidative process associated with nickel ions could have a role in the inflammatory reaction obtained even in nonsensitized subjects (Wells, 1956).

Recent studies have compared the effect of various sensitizing agents in cultured normal human keratinocytes and transformed human keratinocyte HaCaT cell lines and in conditions favoring either cell proliferation or differentiation. In the proliferative HaCaT cell line, following 24-h exposure, nickel produced a concentration-dependent up-regulation of ICAM-1 expression without reducing cell viability. In normal human keratinocytes, $NiSO_4$ induced ICAM-1 expression to a significantly greater extent in proliferative cells than in differentiated cells. Interestingly, among the nickel-containing compounds tested, $NiSO_4$, $NiCl_2$, NiCitrate, and $Ni(His)_2$ complex, the latter was the less effective in the up-regulation of ICAM-1 expression (Wagner et al., 1997).

Nickel ions are also able to induce the expression of the adhesion molecules ICAM-1, VCAM-1, and E-selectin in other cell types such as human cultured endothelial cells in relation to the hapten capacity to activate nuclear factor-kappaB (NF-κB) (Wagner et al., 1997). Furthermore, a dose-dependency induction of mRNA production and protein secretion of the NF-κB-controlled proinflammatory cytokines IL-6 and IL-8 in endothelial cells stimulated with $NiCl_2$ was found (Wagner et al., 1997). Another transcription factor, AP-1, was also increased in human umbilical vein endothelial cells stimulated by $NiCl_2$ (Wagner et al., 1997).

Thus, pathomechanisms leading to contact hypersensitivity to $NiCl_2$ appear to involve direct effects on other immunocompetent cells such as keratinocytes and endothelium cells, besides Ag-specific Langherans- and T-cell-dependent events (Wagner et al., 1997).

The release of reactive oxygen species, such as hydrogen peroxide and hypochlorite produced by phagocytes during the inflammatory process, may play a role in the sensitizing potential of Ni(II), which, in this condition, can be oxidized to the higher oxidation states Ni(III) and Ni(IV), species associated with a pronounced chemical reactivity. Co-administration of irritants with Ni(II) or administration of nickel at higher oxidation states induces contact hypersensitivity to Ni(II) in mice when Ni(II) given alone was ineffective in T-cell priming (Artik et al., 1999).

8.7   METAL–METAL INTERACTIONS

The toxicity of nickel may be associated with its ability to bind several biomolecules at sites that are normally occupied by other essential divalent metals, thereby replacing the latter. Since conformation and physiological functions of these molecules depend on the bound ion, replacement alters their structure causing different harmful effects (Wagner et al., 1997).

In experimental systems, the toxic and carcinogenic effects of nickel can be significantly inhibited to a different degree by the concurrent administration of some metals such as Mn, Mg, Zn, Fe, or Ca. The inhibiting effects depend on the choice of metal, its chemical form and dose, and, in most cases, the mode of administration. In addition, minimum effective time and elevated concentrations are necessary for divalent cations to interact at the biological level (Kasprzack and Rodriguez, 1992).

While some divalent cations such as Mg, Mn, and Fe exert predominantly localized effects, Zn seems to exert a systemic inhibitory effect on the response to nickel, suggesting that another mechanism may act during the zinc–nickel interaction at the sites of biomolecules (Kasprzack, 1992).

The exact sites and mechanisms by which essential metals inhibit the nickel action are not completely understood. For example, it is not known whether their capability to replace nickel depends on the level reached at intracellular or extracellular sites.

In some cases, interactions are facilitated by their biochemical similarities. Nickel and magnesium cations have almost identical crystal ionic radii, form octahedral complexes, and show similar quantitative affinities for ligands like oxygen or nitrogen (Coogan et al., 1989). In addition, Zn and Ni are borderline elements that can form complexes of comparable stabilities. Divalent metals, however, may act through different mechanisms, blocking the immunosuppressive effects exerted by nickel on macrophages, T cells, and NK cells. Furthermore, they either inhibit the nickel transport at cell membranes (e.g., magnesium) or interact at binding sites of extracellular and intracellular molecules (e.g., enzymes and nucleic acids).

The question may arise whether these metal–metal interactions also occur in nickel allergic contact dermatitis.

When patch tested to aqueous solutions containing nickel sulfate 2.9% (0.1 M) mixed to equimolar amounts of sulfates of Mg, Zn, and Cu, patients sensitive to nickel sulfate 5% petrolatum (pet.) showed a variable significant modification of their positive patch tests read at 48 h (Santucci et al., 1993). Magnesium was the strongest inhibitor. To answer the question of whether the inhibiting effect was due to the magnesium itself or to the counter-ions sulfate and chloride in nickel allergic reactions, nickel sulfate-sensitive patients were initially patch tested with aqueous solutions containing nickel sulfate mixed with magnesium sulfate at different concentrations. The results showed that when the applied concentrations of magnesium sulfate were increased, the percentage of patients with reduced or suppressed nickel reactions increased proportionally. In contrast, when testing patients sensitive to nickel chloride with aqueous solutions containing nickel chloride mixed with higher concentrations of magnesium chloride, by increasing the amount of magnesium chloride, both number and intensity of the positive patch test reactions to nickel chloride increased (Santucci et al., 1995).

Later, the influence exerted in patch test reactions by both the counter-ions sulfate and chloride was evaluated by testing nickel-sensitive patients with solutions containing nickel sulfate mixed with magnesium chloride or with sodium chloride, and nickel chloride mixed with magnesium sulfate or with sodium sulfate. The different effects observed stressed the role exerted either by the cation or by its counter-ions. A possible explanation was that the two counter-ions favored the formation of different nickel complexes (Santucci et al., 1995).

Further experiments showed that in human beings, a part of nickel sulfate patch test positive reactions was abolished by the simultaneous administration of higher doses of sulfates of other divalent ions such as Zn, Mg, and Mn. In contrast, sulfates of Cu and Cd exerted synergistic effects (Santucci et al., 1996). Conversely, it was impossible to inhibit the patch test positive reactions to nickel chloride with chlorides of Zn, Mg, and Mn (Santucci et al., 1998). The conclusions we drew were that the two chemical forms of nickel probably caused allergic reactions through the formation of complexes with different ligands that hit different targets.

The influence exerted by cutaneous ligands was emphasized when the patch test reactions to some aqueous nickel salts (sulfate, chloride, nitrate, and acetate) at different concentrations (47 and 12 µg, respectively) were compared in two groups of subjects reacting to nickel sulfate alone and to nickel sulfate and other transition metals. Patch tests results were that subjects belonging to the latter group showed a higher percentage of strong positive responses to the four salts tested. When considering the QS–AR (Quantitative Structure–Activity Relationship) model, either the low concentrations tested or the consequent minimal differences in the rate of nickel penetration through the skin could not explain the difference in the sensitizing properties of the four nickel salts in the two groups tested. It was likely that in individuals reacting to more than one metal, these differences could be explained by a more uniform availability of cutaneous ligands conditioning the formation of complexes more immunogenic (Santucci et al., 1999).

The systemic effects exerted by zinc were evaluated in a group of nickel-sensitive patients with different patterns of contact dermatitis and variable degrees of itching. In all subjects, the positive reactions to 0.1 M nickel sulfate were inhibited by 0.3 M zinc sulfate. Orally administered zinc sulfate at doses of 300 mg/day for 30 days improved the clinical manifestations, mostly itching, and abolished or reduced the majority of patch test reactions (Hoogenraad, 1995). These results confirmed the preliminary observations of improvement of cases of nickel dermatitis following oral administration of $ZnSO_4$ for a short period of treatment (Hoogenraad, 1995; Weissmann and Mennè, 1989).

Although the possible mechanism of action of $ZnSO_4$ remains to be clarified, part of the ionic interactions between nickel and other divalent cations, described in several biological models, seems to occur even in allergic contact dermatitis. We do not know if these interactions occur during the antigen formation phase or successively. However, although we need to improve our knowledge of the mechanism of nickel sensitization, this different approach may suggest that the treatment of nickel dermatitis may be carried out not only by modulating the immune response, but also by preventing the antigen formation.

REFERENCES

Allen, P.A., Antigen processing at molecular level, *Immunol. Today*, 8, 270, 1987.

Andrews, R.K. et al., Nickel in proteins and enzymes, in *Metal Ions in Biological Systems, Vol. 23. Nickel and Its Role in Biology*, Siegel, H., Ed., Marcel Dekker, New York, 1988, p. 165.

Artik, S. et al., Nickel allergy in mice: enhanced sensitization capacity of nickel at higher oxidation states, *J. Dermatol.*, 1143, 1999.

Baer, R.L., The pathogenesis of allergic contact hypersensitivity, in *Fisher's Contact Dermatitis*, 4th ed., Rietscel, R.L. and Fowler, J.F., Eds., Williams & Wilkins, Baltimore, 1995, p. 1.

Barceloux, D.G., Nickel, *Clin. Toxicol.*, 37(2), 239, 1999.

Basketter, D.A. et al., Nickel, cobalt and chromium in consumer products: a role in allergic contact dermatitis? *Contact Dermatitis*, 28(1), 15, 1993.

Basketter, D. et al., The chemistry of contact allergy: why is a molecule allergenic? *Contact Dermatitis*, 32, 65, 1995.

Bergstresser, P.R., Contact dermatitis. Old problems and new techniques, *Arch. Derm.*, 25, 276, 1989.

Boyle, R.W. and Robinson, H.A., Nickel in natural environment, in *Metal Ions in Biological Systems. Vol. 23. Nickel and Its Role in Biology*, Siegel, H., Ed., Marcel Dekker, New York, 1988, p. 165.

Büdinger, L. and Hertl, M., Immunologic mechanisms in hypersensitivity reaction to metal ions: an overview, *Allergy*, 55, 108, 2000.

Burrows, D. et al., Metals, in *Occupational Skin Disease*, 3rd ed., Adams, R.M., Ed., W.B. Saunders, Philadelphia, 1999, p. 417.

Chen, C.Y. et al., Association between oxydative stress and cytokine production, in nickel-treated rats, *Arch. Biochem. Biophys.*, 356, 127, 1998.

Chu, T. et al., Allergic contact dermatitis: carrier proteins for nickel. Current topics, in *Contact Dermatitis*, Frosh, P.J., Dooms Gossens, A., Lachapelle, J.M., and Ryicroft, Springer-Verlag, Berlin, 1989.

Ciccarelli, R.B. and Wetterhahan, K.E., Molecular basis for the activity of nickel, in *Nickel in the Human Environment,* Sunderman, F.W. et al., Eds., IARC, Lyon, France, 1984.

Coogan, T.P. et al., Toxicity and carcinogenicity of nickel compounds, *CRC Crit. Rev. Toxicol.*, 19(4), 341, 1989.

Cotton, A.F. and Wilkinson, G., *Advanced Inorganic Chemistry,* 5th ed., John Wiley & Sons, New York, 1988.

Cross, J.E. et al., Critical review of the evidence for Ni(III) in animals and man, in *Progress in Nickel Toxicology*, Brown., S.S. et al., Eds., Blackwell Scientific, London, 1985.

Dawson, D.C. and Ballatori, N., Membrane transports as site of action and routes of entry for toxic metals, in *Toxicology of Metals: Biochemical Aspects,* Goyer, A. and Cherian, G., Eds., Springer-Verlag, Berlin, 1995, p. 52.

Emtestam, L., The human major histocompatibility complex, in nickel sensitivity, in *Nickel and Human Health: Current Perspectives*, Nieboer, E. and, Nriagu, J.O., Eds., John Wiley & Sons, New York, 1992.

Emtestam, L. et al., HLA-DR,-DQ and DP alleles in nickel, chromium, and cobalt sensitive individuals: genomic analysis based on restriction fragment length polymorphism, *J. Invest. Derm.*, March, 100(3), 271, 1993.

Fleming, C.J. et al., The genetics of allergic contact hypersensitivity to nickel, *Contact Dermatitis,* 41, 251, 1999.

Flint, G.N., A metallurgical approach to metal contact dermatitis, *Contact Dermatitis,* 39(5), 213, 1998.

Friedman, P.S. et al., Early time course of recruitment of immune surveillance in human skin after chemical provocation, *Clin. Exp. Immunol.*, 91, 351, 1993.

Fullerton, A. and Hoelgaard, A., Binding of nickel to human epidermis in vitro, *Br. J. Dermatol.*, November, 119(5), 675, 1988.

Garioch, J.J. et al., Keratinocytes expression of intercellular adhesion molecule–1 (ICAM-1) correlated with infiltration of lymphocyte function associated antigen 1 (LFA-1) positive cells in evolving allergic contact dermatitis reaction, *Hystopathology*, 19, 351, 1991.

Gawkrodger, D.J. et al., The prevention of nickel contact dermatitis. A review of the use of binding agents and barrier creams, *Contact Dermatitis*, 32, 257, 1995.

Gawkrodger, D.J., Nickel dermatitis: how much nickel is safe?, *Contact Dermatitis*, 35(5), 267, 1996.

Glennon, J.D. and Sarkar, B., Nickel II transport in human blood serum, *Biochem. J.*, 203, 15, 1982.

Goebler, M. et al., Nickel chloride and cobalt chloride, two common contact sensitizer, directly induce expression of intracellular adhesion molecule 1 (ICAM-1), vascular cell adhesion molecule 1 (VCAM), and endothelial leukocyte adhesion molecule 1 (ELAM-1) by endothelial cells, *J. Invest. Dermatol.*, 100, 759, 1993.

Goyer, A. and Cherian, M.C., *Toxicology of Metals: Biochemical Aspects,* Springer-Verlag, Berlin, 1995, p. 52.

Guèniche, A. et al., Effect of various metals on intercellular adhesion molecule-1 expression and tumor necrosis factor alpha production by normal keratinocites, *Arch. Dermatol. Res.*, 286, 466, 1994.

Guy, R.H., Hostýnek, J.J., Hinz, R.S., and Lorence, C.R., Eds., *Metals and Skin. Topical Effects and Systemic Absorption,* Marcel Dekker, New York, 1999, p. 283.

Hange, M., The Danish Twin Register, in *Prospective Longitudinal Research. An Empirical Basis for the Primary Prevention of Psychosocial Disorders,* Mednick, S.A., Baert, A.L., and Bachmann, B.P., Eds., Oxford University Press, Oxford, 1981, p. 217.

Hausinger, R.O., Biological utilization of nickel, in *Nickel and Human Health: Current Perspectives,* Nieboer, E. and Nriagu, J.O., Eds., John Wiley & Sons, New York, 1992, p. 21.

Healy, J. et al., An in vitro study of the use of chelating agents in cleaning nickel-contaminated human skin: an alternative approach to preventing nickel allergic contact dermatitis, *Contact Dermatitis*, 39, 171, 1998.

Hoogenraad, T.U., Zinc therapy: advance in the treatment of Wilson's disease, in *Genetic Response to Metals,* Sarkar, B., Ed., Marcel Dekker, New York, 1995, p. 361.

IARC, Nickel in the human environment, in *IARC Scientific Publication No. 53,* Sunderman, F.W., Ed., IARC, Lyon, France, 1984.

Ikaheimo, I. et al., HLA-DQA1 and DQB1 loci in nickel allergy patients, *Int. Arch. Allergy Immunol.*, 100(3), 248, 1993.

Jones, M.M., Chemistry of chelation: chelating agents antagonists for toxic metals, in *Toxicology of Metals: Biochemical Aspects,* Goyer, A. and Cherian, G., Eds., Springer-Verlag, Berlin, 1995, p. 279.

Kalish, R.S., Antigen processing: the gateway to the immunoresponse, *J. Am. Acad. Derm.*, 4, 640, 1995.

Kapsemberg, M.L. et al., Nickel specific T lymphocyte clones derived from allergic contact dermatitis lesions in man: heterogeneity based on requirement of dendritic antigen presenting cell subset, *Eur. J. Immunol.*, 17, 861, 1987.

Karvonen, J. et al., HLA antigens in nickel allergy, *Ann. Clin. Res.*, 168(4), 211, 1984.

Kasprzack, K.S. and Rodriguez, R.E., Inhibitory effects of zinc, magnesium, and iron on nickel subsulfide carcinogenesis in rat skeletal muscle, in *Nickel and Human Health: Current Perspectives*, Nieboer, E. and Nriagu, J.O., Eds., John Wiley & Sons, New York, p. 1992.

Kasprzack, K.S., Animal studies: an overview, in *Nickel and Human Health: Current Perspectives,* Nieboer, E. and Nriagu, J.O., Eds., John Wiley & Sons, New York, 1992, p. 387.

Kasprzack, K.S., Oxidative mechanism of Ni (II) and Co(II) genotoxicity, in *Genetic Response to Metals,* Sarkar, B., Ed., Marcel Dekker, New York, 1995, p. 69.

Lacy, S.A. et al., Distribution of nickel and cobalt following dermal and systemic administration with in vitro and in vivo studies, *J. Biochem. Mat. Res.*, 32, 279, 1996.

Lange-Wantizin, G. et al., The role of intracellular adhesion molecules in inflammatory skin reactions, *Br. J. Dermatol.*, 119, 141, 1988.

Lansdown, A.B.G., Physiological and toxicological changes in the skin resulting from the action and interaction of metal ions, *Clin. Rev. Toxicol.,* 25(5), 397, 1995.

Lepoittevin, J.P. and Berl, V., Chemical basis, in *Allergic Contact Dermatitis. The Molecular Basis*, Lepoittevin, J.P., Basketter, D.A., Goossens, A., and Karlberg, A.T., Eds., Springer-Verlag, Berlin, 1998.

Lidén, C. et al., Nickel containing alloys and platings and their ability to cause dermatitis, *Br. J. Derm.*, 134, 193, 1996.

Lidén, C., Nickel in jewellery and associated products, *Contact Dermatitis*, 26, 2, 1992.

Little, M.C. et al., The participation of proliferative keratinocytes in the preimmune response to sensitizing agents, *Br. J. Dermatol.*, 138, 45, 1998.

Lucassen, M. and Sarkar, B., Ni(II)-binding constituents of human blood serum, *J. Toxicol. Environ. Health*, 5, 897, 1979.

Manaham, S.E., Fundamentals of chemistry, in *Environmental Chemistry*, 6th ed., Manhan, S.E., Ed., CRC Press, Boca Raton, FL, 1994, p. 741.

Mennè, T. and Holm, N.V., Nickel allergy in a female twin population, *Int. J. Derm.*, 22, 1983.

Menné, T. et al., Nickel allergy and hand dermatitis, in a stratified sample of Danish female population: an epidemiological study including a statistical appendix, *Acta Derm. Ven.*, 62, 35, 1982.

Mozzanica, N. et al., HLA-A,B,C and DR antigens in nickel contact sensitivity, *Br. J. Derm.*, March, 122(3), 309, 1990.

Mracussen, P.V., Ecological considerations on nickel dermatitis, *Br. Ind. Med. J.*, 17, 65, 1960.

Nieboer, E. et al., Characterization of the Ni(III)/Ni(II) redox couple for the NiI(II) complex of human serum albumin, *Ann. Clin. Lab. Sci.*, 409, 14, 1984.

Nieboer, E. and Nriagu, J., *Nickel and Human Health: Current Perspectives,* John Wiley & Sons, New York, 1992.

Nieboer, E. et al., Absorption, distribution, and excretion of nickel, in *Nickel and Human Health. Current Perspectives*, Nieboer, E. and Nriagu, J.O., Eds., John Wiley & Sons, New York, 1992, p. 49.

Nielsen, F.H. and Sandstead, H.H., Are nickel, vanadium, silicon, fluorine and tin essential for man? A review, *Am. J. Clin. Nutr.*, 27, 515, 1974.

Nielsen, N.H. and Mennè, T., Allergic contact sensitization in an unselected Danish population. The Glostrup Allergy Study, Denmark, *Acta Derm. Ven.*, 72, 456, 1992.

Olerup, O. and Emtestam, L., Allergic contact dermatitis to nickel is associated with a Taq1 HLA-DA alleles restriction fragment, *Immunogenetics*, 28(5), 310, 1988.

Orecchia, G. et al., Polymorphism of HLA class III genes in allergic contact dermatitis, *Dermatology*, 184(4), 254, 1992.

Pellettier, L. and Druet, P., Immunotoxicology of metals, in *Toxicology of Metals: Biochemical Aspects,* Goyer, A. and Cherian, G., Eds., Springer-Verlag, Berlin, 1995.

Peltonen, L., Nickel sensitivity in the general population, *Contact Dermatitis*, 5, 27, 1979.

Picardo, M. et al., Nickel-keratinocyte interaction: a possible role in sensitization, *Br. J. Dermatol.*, 122, 729, 1990.

Rao, M.S.N., A study of intersections of the Ni II with bovine serum albumin, *J. Am. Chem. Soc.*, 84, 1788, 1962.

Romagnoli, P. and Sinigaglia, F., Selective interaction of nickel with an MHC-bound peptide, *EMBO J.*, 10, 1303, 1991.

Rostenberg, A., Jr. and Perkins, A.J., Nickel and cobalt dermatitis, *J. Allergy*, 22, 466, 1951.

Samitz, M.H. and Katz, S.A., Nickel-epidermal interactions. Diffusion and binding, *Environ. Res.*, 11, 34, 1976.

Santucci, B. et al., Interaction of metals in nickel-sensitive patients, *Contact Dermatitis*, 29, 251, 1993.

Santucci, B. et al., Nickel/magnesium interactions in nickel-sensitive patients, *Contact Dermatitis*, 33(1), 20, 1995.

Santucci, B. et al., Interactions of sulfates of divalent metals in nickel sulfate sensitive patients, *Exp. Dermatol.*, 5, 79, 1996.

Santucci, B. et al., Nickel chloride/chlorides of divalent metal interactions in nickel chloride sensitive patients, *Exp. Dermatol.*, 5, 254, 1996.

Santucci, B. et al., The influence exerted by cutaneous ligands in subjects reacting to nickel sulfate alone and in those reacting to more transition metals, *Exp. Dermatol.*, 7, 162, 1998.

Santucci, B. et al., $ZnSO_4$ treatment of $NiSO_4$-positive patients, *Contact Dermatitis*, 40, 281, 1999.

Sarkar, B., Biological specificity of the transport process of copper and nickel, *Chem. Scr.*, 21, 103, 1983.

Savolainen, H., Biochemical and clinical aspects of nickel toxicity, *Rev. Environ. Health*, 11, 167, 1996.

Siegel, H., *Metal Ions in Biological Systems. Vol. 23. Nickel and Its Role in Biology*, Marcel Dekker, New York, 1988, p. 165.

Silvernnoinen-Kassinen, S. et al., TAP1 and TAP2 genes in nickel allergy, *Int. Arch. Allergy Immunol.*, September, 114(1), 94, 1997.

Sinigaglia, F. et al., Isolation and characterization of Ni-specific T cell clones from patients with Ni-contact dermatitis, *J. Immunol.*, 135, 3929, 1985.

Sterry, W. et al., Cell trafficing in positive and negative patch test reactions: stereotypic migration pathway, *J. Invest. Dermatol.*, 96, 459, 1991.

Sunderman, F.W., A review of the metabolism and toxicology of nickel, *Ann. Clin. Lab. Sci.*, 7, 377, 1977.

Sunderman, F.W., Hazards from exposure to nickel: a historical account, in *Nickel and Human Health: Current Perspectives*, Nieboer, E. and Nriagu, J.O., Eds., John Wiley & Sons, New York, 1992.

Thauer, R.K., Enzymology: nickel to the fore, *Science*, 293(5533), 1264, 2001.

Toxicology update, nickel and some nickel compounds, *J. Appl. Toxicol.*, 17(6), 425, 1997.

Trenam, C.W. et al., Skin inflammation reactive oxygen species and the role of iron, *J. Invest. Dermatol.*, 99, 675, 1992.

Vejlsgard, G.L. et al., Kinetics and characterization of intercellular adhesion molecule-1 (ICAM-1) expression on keratinocytes in various inflammatory skin lesions and malignant cutaneous lymphomas, *J. Am. Acad. Dermatol.*, 20, 782, 1989.

Wagner, M. et al., Heavy metal ion induction of adhesion molecules and cytokines in human endothelial cells: the role of NF-κB, Iκ-α and AP-1, *Pathobiology*, 65(5), 241, 1997.

Weissmann, K. and Mennè, T., Nickel allergy and drug interaction, in *Nickel and the Skin: Immunology and Toxicology*, Maibach, H.I. and Mennè, T., Eds., CRC Press, Boca Raton, FL, 1989, p. 179.

Wells, G.C., Effect of nickel on the skin, *Br. J. Dermatol.*, 68, 237, 1956.

9 Nickel Metal and Alloys

G. Norman Flint and C. Peter Cutler

CONTENTS

9.1   Introduction 219
    9.1.1   Nickel: Properties of the Element 220
    9.1.2   Pure Nickel...220
    9.1.3   Nickel-Containing Alloys...221
        9.1.3.1   Stainless Steels...222
        9.1.3.2   High Nickel Alloys 223
        9.1.3.3   Other Nickel-Containing Alloys....................................223
    9.1.4   Industrial Contact with Nickel-Containing Alloys.........................224
9.2   Reaction of Nickel and Its Alloys with Sweat...224
    9.2.1   Higher Oxidation States of Nickel 226
    9.2.2   Nickel in Powder Form...226
    9.2.3   Alloys 227
        9.2.3.1   Nickel–Copper Alloys 228
        9.2.3.2   Copper–Nickel–Zinc Alloys 228
        9.2.3.3   Coinage Alloys...229
        9.2.3.4   Alloys of Iron and Chromium with Nickel....................230
        9.2.3.5   Stainless Steels...230
        9.2.3.6   Nickel–Iron–Chromium and Nickel–Chromium Alloys..232
        9.2.3.7   Other Nickel Alloys...233
        9.2.3.8   Alloys of Noble Metals and Nickel 233
    9.2.4   Nickel Coatings...234
        9.2.4.1   Top-Coats on Nickel Substrates 235
        9.2.4.2   Tin–Nickel Coatings 236
        9.2.4.3   Chemically Reduced (Electroless) Nickel Coatings........236
9.3   Conclusions 237
9.4   Acknowledgment..237
References..237

9.1   INTRODUCTION

This first section describes nickel, its characteristics, and where it is used, both in its pure form and as alloys. The emphasis is on materials that can come into contact with skin. This introduction provides the background for the second section, which gives a detailed discussion of the corrosion resistance of these materials and how that influences their interaction with sweat.

9.1.1 NICKEL: PROPERTIES OF THE ELEMENT

Nickel is a metallic element, atomic number 28. Its position in the periodic table — in the first series of the transition elements — accounts for many of its key characteristics. Nickel:

- Has a high melting point of 1453°C
- Forms an adherent oxide film
- Has good resistance to corrosion, especially by alkalis
- Has a face-centred cubic crystal structure, which confers ductility
- Alloys readily, both as a solute and as a solvent
- Is ferromagnetic at room temperature
- Is readily deposited by electroplating
- Displays catalytic behavior

This combination of properties is unique among the elements and makes nickel one of the most versatile metals, accounting for the thousands of applications of nickel-containing materials in today's society.

9.1.2 PURE NICKEL

After extraction from its ores and refining, metallic nickel is produced in various forms to suit its further processing — ingot, cathode (an electrodeposited plate that is often cut into pieces about 25 mm square), pellets (typically 5 to 15 mm diameter) and powder of various morphologies. Ferro-nickel, which contains 25 to 50% nickel, is produced by some refining processes and is used for subsequent alloy manufacture. Refined compounds include the oxide, chloride, and sulphate, which are used as feedstock for plating and other chemical processes.

These forms of metallic nickel are raw materials for other industrial processes such as melting and plating, or for conversion to other forms and so would not normally come into direct contact with the skin, particularly as far as the general public is concerned. Conventional metal processing routes such as melting, casting, extrusion, forging, rolling, tube making and wire drawing can all be used to produce nickel bar, plate, sheet and wire for direct use in further manufacture of finished products.

Nickel sheet has been blanked and stamped into coins for over 100 years, an application that continues today. It is readily formed, welded and machined. Nickel sheet and strip is used in the chemical industry, particularly for vessels and pipework to handle alkaline liquids. In all these operations, skin contact will be minimal because workers involved in either fabrication or operation are likely to be wearing gloves for normal safety reasons.

Manufacturing processes for electrical and electronic components utilizing pure nickel — batteries, transducers, and valves (vacuum tubes) — are normally automated, and the nickel will be fully encapsulated, resulting in minimal skin contact.

Few solid nickel objects are in everyday use, apart from some coins. However, there are many applications of nickel plating. This can be produced either electrolytically or by chemical reduction to provide a variety of corrosion-resistant and wear-resistant properties, especially for industrial tools and engineering components. The ability to reproduce fine detail is utilized to make moulds by electroforming for compact discs and similar moulded plastic objects. Overplating nickel plating with chromium or other metals can be used to alter the appearance and properties — the familiar decorative chromium surface being the most common example, which is used for items such as consumer goods and architectural products.

Nickel powder is used to catalyze the fat-hydrogenation step in margarine manufacture, in conductive paint to provide electromagnetic interference screening for electronic systems, in battery manufacture, and for metal injection moulding of small nickel-containing alloy steel automotive and similar engineering components.

9.1.3 Nickel-Containing Alloys

Almost 90% of nickel use is in the form of alloys. Alloys can be either single phase, where one element is in solid solution in the other, or they may be multiphase, where the phases may be solid solutions, intermetallics, or compounds with minor elements. The exact microstructure determines the properties and behavior of the alloy: it may vary in scale from nanometres to millimetres, and can be changed by hot working, cold working, and heat treatment.

Generally, the physical, mechanical, and corrosion-resistant properties of alloys are quite different from those of the constituent elements, and they are rarely just a mixture of the individual properties of the elements. This is why alloys are so useful in practice. Once alloyed, the constituent elements cannot be separated again by simple physical means.

The individual elements must be mixed intimately to produce an alloy. This can be achieved by:

- Melting, which allows the elements to mix in the liquid phase
- Sintering of powders, which allows the constituents to interdiffuse
- Mechanical alloying (high energy ball-milling, which causes repeated cold welding and fracture of the powder particles) followed by sintering
- Co-deposition by electrolysis
- Co-deposition by vapor deposition

Sometimes an actual chemical reaction occurs between the elements of an alloy so that an intermetallic compound is formed: thus nickel and aluminium can form Ni_3Al, which is very important in strengthening the superalloys used in gas turbines. Compounds can also form with some of the minor elements present in alloys, leading for example to carbides, nitrides, and sulphides. These minor elements may be present either as deliberate alloying additions or as impurities and can have a strong influence on an alloy's corrosion resistance and mechanical properties.

9.1.3.1 Stainless Steels

One of the most striking examples of the way in which alloying can change the properties of a base metal is the addition of chromium to iron to form stainless steel. When the chromium content is above about 10.5%, a thin continuous oxide layer (based on chromium oxide, Cr_2O_3) forms very rapidly when fresh surfaces are exposed to air. This layer is tightly adherent and protects the surface from further oxidation without getting significantly thicker. If it is damaged, this "passive layer" will repair itself equally rapidly in air and it is responsible for the "stainless" characteristic of these alloys. The passive layer protects stainless steel from general, uniform corrosion during service without the need for any further protective coating. However, as discussed below, situations can arise when the passive film can be broken down, allowing localized corrosion of the under-lying metal, leading to the formation of pits or to corrosion in crevices, e.g., in flanged joints.

In addition to the essential chromium, stainless steels can also contain nickel, molybdenum, and other alloying elements to enhance their mechanical and corrosion-resistant properties. Metallurgically, stainless steels can be classified according to their microstructure — ferritic, martensitic, austenitic, duplex, and precipitation hardening. The austenitic grades are the most widely used and contain 8 to 25% nickel. However, some of the other grades can contain up to 6% nickel.

As a result of their corrosion resistance, availability, and fabricability, stainless steels are used for equipment that is required to have long life with little maintenance, does not contaminate the product stream, is hygienic, can be cleaned readily, can handle aggressive and hazardous chemicals, and maintains its appearance. This has led to the wide usage of stainless steels in:

- Food, beverage, and pharmaceutical manufacturing plants
- Commercial catering equipment
- Domestic kitchen equipment and tableware
- Oil and gas production and processing facilities
- Chemical plants
- Water and waste-water treatment plants
- Surgical implants
- Watch cases and straps
- Automotive trim and exhaust systems
- Railcars and bus bodies
- Building fixtures and architectural trim
- Street furniture
- Radioactive waste disposal containers
- Coinage

It is apparent that across this range of applications, skin contact will vary from transitory to prolonged.

9.1.3.2 High Nickel Alloys

Alloys based on nickel with additions of chromium, molybdenum, cobalt and other elements offer extreme resistance to corrosion in aggressive environments from ambient to high temperatures, as well as retaining high strength at high temperatures. Thus they are used for vital components and structures in chemical and petrochemical plants, power generation, and aircraft engines, as well as heating elements in furnaces and domestic appliances.

9.1.3.3 Other Nickel-Containing Alloys

Nickel improves the toughness of steels, so it is found in alloys for automotive gears and also in alloys to handle liquified natural gas (LNG), where the toughness of steel containing 9% nickel is maintained to cryogenic temperatures.

An alloy of iron with 36% nickel has almost zero coefficient of thermal expansion at ambient temperatures. This has led to its use for instruments where dimensional stability is important — and on a much larger scale to line cryogenic tanks to store LNG. However, the largest use today is for shadow masks in color-television tubes. The expansion coefficient can be controlled by adjusting the nickel content, so iron alloys containing 36 to 50% nickel can be made to match the expansion coefficients of glasses and ceramics, allowing them to be used for glass-to-metal seals and the lead frames for electronic integrated circuit packages. The same alloy range, and the 78% nickel iron alloy, also have valuable magnetic properties that are used in components and electromagnetic shielding in much of today's electronic equipment.

Copper and nickel, both face-centred cubic metals, are mutually soluble over the whole range of compositions of copper–nickel alloys. The combination of physical, mechanical, and chemical properties, coupled with the biofouling resistance of the high copper alloys, resulted in a long history of application of the copper–nickel alloys in seawater handling systems (e.g., for cooling and firefighting), desalination plants, engineering applications, and coinage. The addition of copper to nickel increases its nobility and generally improves its resistance to corrosion by acids and chloride solutions. Typical applications are shown in Table 9.1.

TABLE 9.1
Copper–Nickel Alloys and Their Applications

Alloy	% Nickel	Application
400	67	Chemical industry; seawater pumps and valves, heat exchangers
	45	Thermocouples, electrical resistors, and control instruments
Copper–nickel	30	Seawater heat exchangers, condenser tubes
Copper–nickel	25	Coinage alloy
Copper–nickel	10	Power plant and marine condenser tubes

Nickel silvers, in spite of their name, are alloys of copper with 10 to 30% nickel and zinc. While they have had some applications in architecture for handles, door knobs, handrails, etc., their most significant consumer use is jewelry, cutlery, and tableware, which is often plated with silver.

9.1.4 INDUSTRIAL CONTACT WITH NICKEL-CONTAINING ALLOYS

Manufacture and conversion to final products of all the nickel-containing alloys follows the normal metallurgical practices: intermediate products are either melted and cast; or melted, cast and wrought; or made from consolidated powders. Hot and cold working, welding, and machining may then be involved in final component fabrication. Manufacturing, environmental, health, and safety controls restrict the opportunities for direct skin contact throughout all these processes.

9.2 REACTION OF NICKEL AND ITS ALLOYS WITH SWEAT

The contact of nickel and certain of its alloys with skin is not a direct cause of allergic dermatitis. The soluble products resulting from the corrosion of the metal by sweat are the direct cause (Flint, 1998). Thus there is a fundamental difference between dermatitis due to metal contact from that due to contact with a soluble nickel compound. The former requires the elapse of a period of time for the concentration of soluble corrosion products to reach a critical dose per unit area of skin before dermatitis can occur.

A number of consequences of practical significance follow:

- Transient skin contact is rarely damaging.
- The rate of reaction of a nickel alloy with sweat may be too slow to generate a critical dose.
- The nature of the exposure may be such that corrosion products are washed or abraded away.
- The rate of reaction may differ markedly between persons as a result of differences in corrosivity of their sweat.

Corrosion is an electrochemical process involving movement of electrons (e^-) through the metal from anodic to cathodic areas and related movement of ions in the electrolyte. At metal potentials and pH values occurring in sweat, anodic reactions for nickel and alloys include:

$$Ni \rightarrow Ni^{++} + 2e^-$$

$$Cu \rightarrow Cu^{++} + 2e^-$$

$$Fe \rightarrow Fe^{++} + 2e^-$$

$$Cr \rightarrow Cr^{+++} + 3e^-$$

The ions so formed may be oxidized further if oxidizing agents more powerful than air become available.

The electrons generated are consumed at the cathode, most commonly by reaction with oxygen:

$$O_2 + 2H_2O + 4e^- \rightarrow 4(OH)^-$$

but in acid sweat, evolution of hydrogen is feasible:

$$2H_2O + 2e^- \rightarrow 2(OH)^- + H_2$$

Other possibilities are the reduction of ferric, cupric, or other high-valency ions. Thus, if corrosion products such as ferric or cupric ions are retained at the site of reaction, it is possible for them to accelerate the rate of corrosion.

The situation with respect to a patch test on a metal specimen is shown in Figure 9.1. Sweat acts as the electrolyte. The anodic area occurs in the oxygen-deficient region in the crevice where metal is in contact with the skin, since oxygen

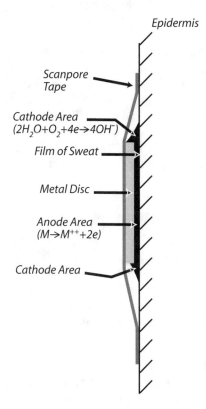

FIGURE 9.1 Corrosion of a metal or alloy at the region of skin contact in a patch test. The rate of production of metal ions is controlled primarily by the size of the cathode area and the electrical resistance of the sweat film.

in sweat derived from the epidermis or by diffusion from the atmosphere would soon be consumed. The cathodic area exists at the outer edges where sweat on the specimen is freely in contact with air.

The concentrations of nickel and other metal ions that develop in the area contacting the skin are governed by:

1. The rate of reaction of nickel metal or alloy, which in turn is controlled by their electrochemical characteristics, the extent of the area outside the crevice that is wetted by sweat, supply of oxygen or other reactant to that area, and the electrical resistance of the film of sweat.
2. The geometric configuration, which controls the diffusion of reactants, e.g., oxygen, to the reacting surfaces and of corrosion products away from reacting surfaces. (The reaction products may form insoluble compounds and although remaining on site may be present in an innocuous form.)
3. The supply of sweat and its composition.

The patch test represents a simple configuration that is generally undisturbed, usually for the 48 h test period. Acidity tends to develop in the creviced region due to hydrolysis of corrosion products, particularly if high valency ions such as Cr^{+++} are involved. In real life, articles in contact with the skin are often of complex shape and are not undisturbed, and the contact is rarely as tight or for as long a period as 48 h. Thus the patch test provides exposure conditions much more severe than those occurring in practice. Furthermore, the conditions developed in the patch test may differ substantially from those employed in tests in artificial sweat to determine release of nickel from articles intended to come into contact with the skin (CEN EN 1811:1998). Thus a discrepancy can occur in results from patch testing and those from nickel-release tests (see Figure 9.2) (Flint, 1998).

9.2.1 HIGHER OXIDATION STATES OF NICKEL

Trivalent and quadrivalent nickel ions are more powerful sensitizers than divalent nickel (Artik, et al., 1999). The nickel species produced by reaction with sweat on the skin is always the divalent form, but it is feasible for further oxidation to occur subsequently by reaction with reactive oxygen species such as peroxide or hypochlorite produced by phagocytes at inflamed areas. Thus nickel contact dermatitis develops more readily in irritated than in normal skin.

9.2.2 NICKEL IN POWDER FORM

Particular care has to be taken when handling nickel in powder form. Very fine powders, say less than 50 μm diameter, tend to cling to the skin and be difficult to dislodge. Since the surface area of fine particles can be very large, even a relatively short exposure may be enough to generate sufficient nickel ions to cause dermatitis in a sensitized person.

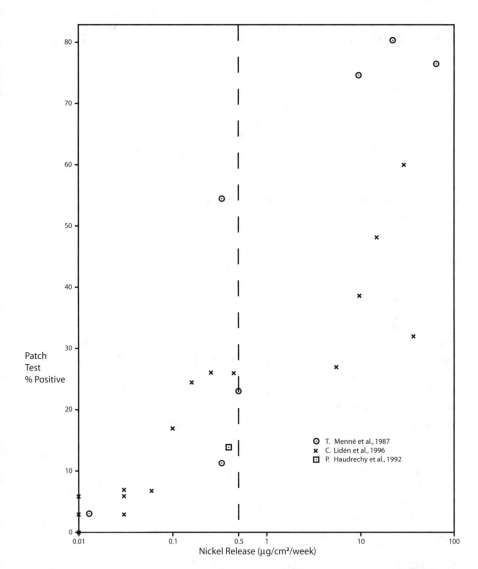

FIGURE 9.2 Discrepancies in the correlation between patch test positive results and nickel release tests. The dotted line shows the maximum release value of 0.5 μg/cm²/week specified in Directive 94/27/EC for articles in direct and prolonged contact with the skin.

9.2.3 ALLOYS

As outlined above, numerous alloys of nickel with other metals are known and have industrial applications. Those that the public is most likely to have contact with are iron–chromium–nickel (stainless steels), copper–zinc–nickel (nickel silver), copper–nickel (coinage alloys), and gold–copper–nickel (white gold).

The rates of reaction of nickel alloys exposed to sweat may differ markedly from those of nickel and the alloying metals when in the unalloyed state, particularly if chromium, aluminium, or titanium is present in sufficient quantity to provide surface oxide films that prevent corrosion. The most common example of such an alloy is stainless steel.

When the content of nickel in an alloy that does react with sweat is low, the rate of formation of nickel ions may be insufficient to allow a concentration to be achieved that will initiate an allergic response. However, if the duration of exposure is long and the area of such an alloy exposed to the skin is large, a low content of nickel in the alloy could suffice to elicit a response, especially in a hypersensitive person. Thus it is not possible to define a lower limit for the content of nickel in the alloy below which there would be no possibility of eliciting contact dermatitis. The European Union classifies an alloy as a skin sensitizer if it contains more than 1% of nickel. However, that classification is aimed primarily at the ability to induce sensitization and not to its elicitation in an already sensitized person. In practice, alloys containing less than 3% nickel are unlikely to arouse an allergic reaction, even in sensitized persons, especially if the duration of exposure is short (Menné et al., 1987; Lidén, Menné, and Burrows, 1996).

9.2.3.1 Nickel–Copper Alloys

The alloys of nickel and copper are widely used in the chemical, oil, marine, and power industries. Despite their nobility and their good resistance to seawater corrosion, their behavior in sweat and patch tests is sometimes inferior to that of wrought nickel. The rate of attack of metals in sweat is greater than that in seawater as a result of the high degree of aeration, the lower pH value, and higher temperature. A more significant feature for the nickel–copper alloys, however, is the concentration of copper corrosion products that can develop in the sweat. The presence of cupric ions facilitates corrosion by providing an alternative cathodic reaction — the reduction of cupric ions to the cuprous state — thus increasing the rate of release of nickel.

The nickel–copper alloys used in engineering are rarely handled by the public, but two groups that are in constant everyday use are the copper–nickel–zinc alloys (nickel silvers) and the coinage alloys.

9.2.3.2 Copper–Nickel–Zinc Alloys

The addition of nickel in amounts greater than 12% to copper–zinc alloys whitens the alloy and eliminates the yellow color of brass — hence the derivation of the term "nickel silver" for such alloys. The nickel addition also improves strength, resistance to corrosion, and resistance to stress-corrosion cracking. The alloys are extensively used in decorative applications for gift- and tableware (usually silver plated — hence the name electro-plated nickel silver, EPNS), for keys and as a base metal for jewelry; in architecture for handles, door knobs, stair rails; and in engineering applications for springs, instruments, marine fittings, and fasteners.

Nickel silver alloys contain from 10 to 30% nickel, but the most common are the 18% alloys. The alloys have good resistance to corrosion by chloride solutions, but in tests in artificial sweat and in patch tests the copper corrosion products exert an adverse effect, and high nickel release rates and high incidence of patch test

TABLE 9.2
Tests on Copper–Nickel–Zinc Alloys

Alloy Composition (%)			Rate of Nickel Release in Artificial Sweat (μg/cm^2/week)	Patch Test Positives (%)	Reference
Cu	Zn	Ni			
64	24	12	33	81	Menné et al., 1987
61	20	19	33	–	Cavalier, Foussereau, and Massin, 1985
60–65	bal	11–13	20	49	Lidén, Menné, and Burrows, 1996

positives are obtained as shown in Table 9.2. While silver plating will reduce greatly the release of nickel from the nickel silver, it is unlikely to eliminate it completely because of some porosity in the plating.

9.2.3.3 Coinage Alloys

Many alloys used for coinage contain nickel. Indeed wrought nickel itself makes a good coinage material, having the desirable characteristics of resistance to wear, bright appearance, ability to take an impression, magnetic properties, and low nickel-release values in sweat. Wrought nickel has been used for coins for over 100 years. More commonly, copper-based alloys are used for coinage. Typical are those used in the U.K.: the 10p coin, 75 Cu/25 Ni; the 20p coin, 84 Cu/16 Ni; the £1 coin, 70 Cu/24.5 Zn/5.5 Ni.

If tested in artificial sweat, all these alloys will release nickel at a rate greater than the value of 0.5 μg/cm^2/week specified in Directive 94/27/EC for articles in direct and prolonged contact with the skin. However, because of the transient nature of the contact, the handling of coins rarely causes contact dermatitis. In a provocation study by Christensen and Möller (1975), on 12 patients with contact allergy to nickel, intense handling of nickel-contaminated metal objects did not induce any visible eczematous activity. Some cases relating to cashiers are reported in the literature (Husain, 1977; van Ketel, 1985).

Nickel is released from coins washed with artificial sweat (Pedersen et al., 1974). Lidén and Carter (2001) found that the amounts obtained from the U.K., 10p, 20p, and £1 coins in 2 min of washing in 10 ml of artificial sweat, were 1.32, 1.91, and 3.56 μg, respectively. These concentrations of nickel (0.132, 0.191, and 0.356 ppm) were considerably below the minimum eliciting threshold of 100 ppm found by Menné and Calvin (1993) in nonoccluded exposure of nickel-sensitive individuals. Their exposure involved application of nickel chloride solutions to the forearms of 51 nickel-sensitive females for periods of 2 and 3 days. In reviewing the association of hand eczema with nickel allergy, Wilkinson and Wilkinson (1989) concluded that the relevance of nickel sensitivity is often overestimated.

9.2.3.4   Alloys of Iron and Chromium with Nickel

Nickel is frequently added to steel and cast iron in order to improve strength and wear resistance, but amounts used are small and nickel release rates are low (Lidén, 1998). Articles made from low-alloy steels and cast irons rarely come into prolonged contact with the skin. A nickel–iron alloy coating, containing 65% nickel, gives a 79% positive response in patch tests and has a rate of release of nickel in artificial sweat of about 75 µg/cm^2/week (Menné et al., 1987). However, it is unlikely to have applications where it would come into prolonged contact with the skin.

9.2.3.5   Stainless Steels

Iron-base alloys containing more than about 10.5% chromium are termed stainless steels and derive their good resistance to corrosion from the presence of a surface film of chromium oxide (Cr_2O_3). There is a wide range of stainless-steel compositions (grades) and a correspondingly wide variation in resistance to corrosion. Alloying elements considered beneficial to resistance to corrosion are chromium, nickel, molybdenum, and nitrogen, while those detrimental to corrosion performance are sulphur, phosphorus, and carbon if present as carbide. Copper is beneficial in acid environments but is thought to be detrimental to resistance to chlorides. Compositions of some commonly used stainless steels in increasing order of resistance to corrosion are given in Table 9.3.

Stainless steels covered by an intact surface film are termed passive. There is no significant difference in corrosion performance of the various grades of stainless steel when all are in the fully passive condition. The chromium oxide film is not wholly impermeable and a minute passage of metal ions can occur across the metal–solution interface as a result of slow film dissolution or of metal at flaws in the film and healing of such flaws by film growth. Formation of metal ions in this way is usually too small to be detected analytically but can be determined by electrochemical means. Most stainless steels when tested in artificial sweat by the CEN EN 1811:1998 procedure usually show no measurable release of nickel (see below). It is common experience that stainless steels and similar chromium-containing alloys, when in the fully passive condition, do not give rise to contact dermatitis (Fisher, 1987).

If the passive oxide film becomes unstable in a corrosive environment, the stainless steel will become active and may then suffer a high rate of corrosion. Release of metal ions could reach significant levels — but with wide variations between the different grades of steel. The exposure conditions causing such loss of passivity are acidity and presence of chloride ions: in acid conditions the film is dissolved and a uniform corrosive attack occurs; in neutral chloride solutions penetration of the film occurs at isolated points and pitting corrosion develops. The severity of the conditions necessary to cause loss of passivity is a function of the grade of stainless steel.

When stainless-steel articles form a crevice, for example by tight contact with the skin, the solution within the crevice loses oxygen, and acidity can develop by hydrolysis. The fall in pH is dependent on the dimensions of the crevice, the

TABLE 9.3
Compositions of Stainless Steels

	Composition (%)								
	C (max)	Mn (max)	P (max)	S (max)	Si (max)	Cr	Ni	Mo	Other
Steel AISI Type									
430	0.12	1.00	0.040	0.03	1.00	16.0–18.0			
301	0.15	2.00	0.045	0.03	1.00	16.0–18.0	6.0–8.0		
303	0.15	2.00	0.045	0.15 min	1.00	17.0–19.0	8.0–10.0		
304	0.08	2.00	0.045	0.03	1.00	18.0–20.0	8.0–10.5		
316	0.08	2.00	0.045	0.03	1.00	16.0–18.0	10.0–14.0	2.0–3.0	
316L	0.03	2.00	0.045	0.03	1.00	16.0–18.0	10.0–14.0	2.0–3.0	
ISO									
5832 D	0.030	2.0	0.025	0.010	1.0	17.0–19.0	13.0–15.0	2.25–3.5	0.10 max N; 0.50 max Cu
5832 E	0.030	2.0	0.025	0.010	1.0	17.0–19.0	14.0–16.0	2.35–4.2	0.10–0.20 N; 0.50 max Cu

Note: The ISO 5832–1:1997 stainless steels are specified for surgical implants.

compositions of the sweat and of the steel, and the time available to reach equilibrium (Oldfield and Sutton, 1977). Thus a patch test conducted on a specimen tightly bound to the skin without movement for 48 h provides a particularly severe corrosive environment for stainless steels. There are few reports where close contact of stainless steel articles with the skin has apparently caused dermatitis (Fischer et al., 1984a; Oakley, Ive, and Carr, 1987; Kanerva et al. 1994).

The differences in corrosion performance of the various grades of stainless steel lie in their differing abilities to retain passivity when under adverse corrosive conditions, more than in the actual rate of corrosion when passivity is lost. Ability to retain passivity is dependent primarily on composition, but smooth surface finish, absence of impurities — especially sulphide inclusions — and homogeneity of structure also play a part. The chromium content is particularly important in retention of passivity. Thus the low chromium 12 Cr/12 Ni stainless steel, now obsolete but formerly used for manufacture of watch cases, releases more than 0.5 μg/cm^2/week nickel when tested by the CEN EN 1811:1998 procedure.

The corrosion testing of stainless steels in chloride media, such as artificial sweat solution, presents difficulties, since the determination of most interest is measurement of the period before loss of passivity occurs rather than the actual release of metal ions to the solution. Generally measurement of metal release is conducted over a time period sufficiently long to cover the period of usage.

Menné et al. (1987) carried out nickel-release measurements on a 18Cr/9Ni stainless steel using a composition of artificial sweat solution that was subsequently standardized in CEN EN 1811:1998. Test periods of 1, 3, and 6 weeks were used. A nickel-release rate of about 0.03 μg/cm^2/week was measured after one week and lower values for the 3- and 6-week periods. A patch test incidence of 3% positives was observed in previously sensitized individuals.

Haudrechy et al. (1994; 1997) conducted patch tests and nickel-release tests in artificial sweat at pH 6.6 and down to pH 3.0 on 303, 304, 316L, and 430 grade stainless steels. It was found that the release of nickel from steels containing less than 0.03% sulphur was less than 0.5 μg/cm^2/week, while the free-machining 303 grade steel, containing about 0.3% sulphur, released about or more than this level. The patch tests showed that 4% of patients reacted to the 303 grade steel, whereas none reacted to the other grades. It was concluded that use of the resulphurized (S > 0.1%) grades of stainless steel should be avoided for articles coming into contact with the skin.

Lidén, Menné, and Burrows (1996) reported patch test results on 12 mm diameter discs of a 18 Cr/8 Ni steel and a steel to the ISO 5832 composition (steel for surgical implants). Patch tests were made on 111 nickel-sensitive subjects but no positive reactions were observed.

It may be concluded that, apart from the 303 grade, conventional stainless steels such as 304, 316, and 430 grades should not cause contact dermatitis in nickel-sensitized persons (Haudrechy et al., 1994).

9.2.3.6 Nickel–Iron–Chromium and Nickel–Chromium Alloys

Those alloys containing more than 12% Cr behave similarly to stainless steels. They are characterized by excellent heat and corrosion resistance and therefore find considerable use in applications involving exposure to high temperatures, e.g., resistance elements in electric heaters and ovens, components in jet engines, and components handling hot exhaust gases. The alloys are unlikely to be used in applications involving extensive handling. Alloy 600, the nickel-base alloy containing 15% Cr and 8% Fe, has low nickel release in artificial sweat but is subject to crevice corrosion and therefore reacts positively in patch tests (Menné et al., 1987). The alloys that also contain molybdenum have exceptionally good resistance to corrosion and would not be expected to react with sweat.

9.2.3.7 Other Nickel Alloys

Alloys of nickel with aluminium, cobalt, molybdenum, or silicon, while of industrial importance, are unlikely to be handled by the public. The shape memory nickel–titanium alloy (55% Ni) has been used in clothing and specialist medical devices. Its rate of release of nickel in sweat has been measured as 0.8 $\mu g/cm^2/week$ (Haudrechy et al., 1997).

9.2.3.8 Alloys of Noble Metals and Nickel

Nickel occurs, in amounts generally less than 0.5%, in certain gold, silver, and palladium alloys used for electrical contacts. Alloys of platinum with up to 20% nickel have application (although limited) as a result of their good strength at high temperatures.

The most common alloy of a noble metal with nickel is white gold, which is often used in jewelry. Nickel-containing white gold is essentially a gold–copper–nickel alloy, often also containing 5 to 12% zinc. Nickel is present in amounts greater than about 5% in order to effect whitening, and this is aided to some extent by the zinc. Palladium also has a strong whitening effect and if present permits a reduction in nickel content. Copper is an essential constituent necessary to resist cracking of the alloy during heat treatment. White golds vary from 9 to 18 carat. Exposure to nickel-containing white gold is known to cause contact dermatitis in persons hypersensitive to nickel (Fischer et al., 1984b).

Alloys of noble metals with nickel or other electrochemically active metals such as zinc, can suffer corrosion by "de-alloying" when exposed to sweat. The active metal atoms are preferentially dissolved, leaving a porous structure composed of the noble metals (Au, Ag, Pd). It is evident that a certain minimum content of active metals must be present in the alloy if corrosion is to progress beyond the initial surface. By analogy with the "de-zincification" of copper–zinc alloys (brass), which has been extensively studied, that minimum content is about 15 atomic percent. For nickel alloys with gold or platinum that amounts to 5 wt% Ni, i.e., 95 wt% Au and for alloys with silver or palladium about 9 wt% Ni, i.e., 91 wt% Ag. Thus for alloys containing more than 95% Au or 91% Ag or Pd, the balance being nickel or nickel plus other active metals, the rate of release of nickel in sweat at body temperature will be very low and controlled by the rate of diffusion of nickel atoms to the reacting surfaces (Pickering and Wagner, 1967). Examples are the electrolytically deposited, hard gold coatings that contain 0.5 to 2.0% nickel or cobalt.

TABLE 9.4
Nickel Release from White Gold Alloys

White Gold Composition (%)							Nickel Release
Au	Ag	Pd	Cu	Zn	Ni	Au + Ag + Pd	(µg/cm²/week)
37.8			40.0	2.0	6	37.8	4.00
58.5	0.5		27.0	7.0	7	59.0	1.05
76.0			18.0	2.0	6	76.0	0.54
75.0		13.5	7.5	2.0	6	88.5	0.02
58.5	18.0	14.0	6.6	0.9	2	90.5	0.03

Adapted from Bagnoud, P., Nicoud, S., and Ramoni, P., Nickel allergy: the European directive and its consequences on gold coatings and white gold alloys, *Gold Technol.*, 18, 11, 1996.

Noble-metal alloys containing more than the critical amounts of nickel plus other active metals will undergo preferential corrosion in sweat. The rate of release of nickel and other active metal ions will depend on the content of noble metals. For alloys of high noble-metal content the rate of release in artificial sweat can be quite low, as illustrated in Table 9.4.

9.2.4 NICKEL COATINGS

Nickel coatings can be obtained by electro-deposition or chemical reduction from solutions of nickel salts or decomposition of nickel carbonyl vapor or flame spraying. The nickel coatings most commonly encountered are those obtained by electro-deposition from solutions of nickel sulphate or sulphamate and nickel chloride, and which are used to provide a decorative finish to articles made from steel, brass, or zinc alloys. The deposits may also be used to provide protection for engineering components or for repair of worn or mismachined parts. However, deposits for engineering applications are more often obtained by chemical reduction from nickel chloride or chloride plus sulphate solutions using sodium hypophosphite or much less frequently sodium borohydride as the reducing agent. Vapour deposited and flame sprayed coatings are rarely encountered.

Electro-deposited nickel coatings on intricately shaped articles show variation in thickness over the contour, being thin in recesses and thick on protuberances. Bright nickel coatings are obtained from solutions to which organic brightening agents have been added. The use of such brighteners adds sulphur to the coating and consequently causes a reduction in its resistance to corrosion. Semibright and dull nickel coatings contain only minor amounts of sulphur, and their corrosion resistance is similar to that of wrought nickel. The release of nickel in artificial sweat (test procedure CEN EN 1811:1998) is shown in Table 9.5.

TABLE 9.5
Comparison of Release from Wrought
and Electrodeposited Nickel

Form	Release of Nickel (µg/cm²/week)
Wrought nickel	2.5; 3.6
Bright electrodeposited nickel	60; 296

Bright nickel coatings without a top-coat are sometimes used on keys, fasteners, handles, paper clips, toys, and tools. Use of nickel-plated handheld tools may be a risk factor for nickel allergy (Cavalier, Foussereau, and Massin, 1985).

9.2.4.1 Top-Coats on Nickel Substrates

In most applications the bright nickel coating is covered by a top-coat such as chromium, gold, or silver. The latter two coatings sometimes have a further, very thin coating of rhodium. The top-coat can significantly reduce the release of nickel from the undercoat.

The chromic acid solutions used for the deposition of chromium have very poor "throwing power" (the ability of a plating solution to produce a uniform metal distribution on an irregular surface). In consequence there is great variation in thickness of chromium coatings when deposited on intricately shaped articles. Moreover, chromium coatings of the usual thickness of about 0.2 µm are porous, while thicker coatings, say above about 0.6 µm, are cracked. Thus chromium top-coats cannot be relied upon to prevent release of nickel from the undercoat. Similarly, the results from patch tests and nickel-release tests tend to be inconsistent. However, the value of the chromium coating in reducing rate of nickel release is evident from the results shown in Table 9.6 (Lidén, Menné, and Burrows, 1996; Cavalier, Foussereau, and Massin, 1985).

Gold and silver top-coats on nickel substrates are usually electrolytically deposited from cyanide solutions that have good throwing power, so the thickness of the coating does not show great variation over the contour of intricately shaped articles. A coating on a good piece of costume jewelry would have a thickness of about 2

TABLE 9.6
Effect of Chromium Coating on Nickel Release, (Lidén, Menné,
and Burrows, 1996; Cavalier, Foussereau, and Massin, 1985)

Substrate	Chromium Thickness (µm)	Positives in Patch Test (%)	Release of Nickel in Artificial Sweat Test (µg/cm²/week)
Bright nickel plating on brass	0.2	3	0.13
	0.6	21	0.21

to 4 μm, while cheap jewelry may have only sufficient thickness to color the surface. Even at 4 μm thickness the coatings are porous, and it is considered that a thickness of 10 μm is necessary to obtain a pore-free coating. Moreover, the coatings are soft (even the so-called hard deposits) and hence the wear resistance is poor. It may be concluded that gold and silver top-coats at economic thicknesses will not prevent release of nickel from the substrate.

Many gold coatings contain 0.1 to 2% of nickel or cobalt in order to increase hardness and improve resistance to wear. At this content of nickel or cobalt there would be negligible release when such coatings are exposed to sweat (see Section 9.2.3.8).

9.2.4.2 Tin–Nickel Coatings

The tin–nickel alloy coating is deposited from a fluoride solution. It has a pleasing pinkish-silver color and is sometimes used as a decorative finish. The deposit has composition 65 Sn/35 Ni and consists of the intermetallic alloy SnNi, an alloy that can be obtained only by electrodeposition. It has good resistance to corrosion but will nevertheless release a small amount of nickel when exposed to sweat solutions. The results of some tests in artificial sweat are given in Table 9.7.

9.2.4.3 Chemically Reduced (Electroless) Nickel Coatings

These coatings are produced by the reduction of hot nickel chloride or sulphate solutions by sodium hypophosphite. The deposits contain 3 to 12% phosphorus depending upon the operating conditions and are characterized by uniformity of deposit thickness and hardness. The hardness may be increased by heat treatment. The resistance to corrosion is similar to that of wrought nickel. The high phosphorus deposits are superior to low phosphorus deposits in resistance to corrosion by acids, but the opposite is true for alkaline solutions. The uniformity of deposit thickness, corrosion resistance, hardness, and wear resistance make the deposits extremely attractive for engineering applications. It would be exceptional for chemically reduced coatings to be used as a decorative finish on articles involving handling.

TABLE 9.7
Nickel Release from Tin–Nickel Alloy Coatings

Material	Positives in Patch Tests (%)	Release of Nickel in Artificial Sweat ($\mu g/cm^2/week$)	Reference
2 μm thick SnNi on brass	7	0.06	Lidén, Menné, and Burrows, 1996; Cavalier, Foussereau, and Massin, 1985
10 μm thick SnNi on copper	22.5	0.50	Menné et al., 1987

9.3 CONCLUSIONS

Nickel is one of the most versatile of metals. Its corrosion resistance, high temperature properties, and ability to form alloys are responsible for the many important applications of nickel-containing alloys and coatings in use today.

The direct cause of nickel allergic contact dermatitis is reaction to the soluble products resulting from corrosion of a nickel-containing metal by sweat. The corrosion rate of alloys, and hence nickel release rate, is not just a simple function of the nickel content of the alloy. Since the corrosion product must have time to accumulate, transient skin contact is rarely damaging.

The release of nickel from coatings depends on the nature of the entire coating system, particularly of any metallic overcoating that may be present.

While some of the nickel-containing alloys in common use may release nickel when tested according to the CEN EN 1811:1998 procedure at a rate greater than the value of 0.5 $\mu g/cm^2$/week specified in Directive 94/27/EC, many of their applications are such that they are rarely in direct and prolonged contact with the skin. Other nickel-containing alloys that are in widespread use, including for skin contact, are sufficiently corrosion resistant that the nickel-release rate is much less than that. The common grades of stainless steel come into the latter category.

9.4 ACKNOWLEDGMENT

The authors would like to thank their colleagues in the nickel industry for help in preparing this chapter.

REFERENCES

Artik, S. et al., Nickel allergy in mice: enhanced sensitisation capacity of nickel at higher oxidation states, *J. Immunol.*, 163, 1143, 1999.

Bagnoud, P., Nicoud, S., and Ramoni, P., Nickel allergy: the European directive and its consequences on gold coatings and white gold alloys, *Gold Technol.*, 18, 11, 1996.

Cavalier, C., Foussereau, J., and Massin, M., Nickel allergy: analysis of metal clothing objects and patch testing to metal samples, *Contact Dermatitis*, 12, 65, 1985.

Christensen, O.B. and Möller, H., External and internal exposure to the antigen in the hand eczema of nickel allergy, *Contact Dermatitis*, 1, 136, 1975.

Fischer, T. et al., Nickel release from ear piercing kits and earrings, *Contact Dermatitis*, 10, 39, 1984a.

Fischer, T. et al., Contact sensitivity to nickel in white gold, *Contact Dermatitis*, 10, 23, 1984b.

Fisher, A.A., *Contact Dermatitis*, 3rd ed., Lea & Febiger, Philadelphia, 1986.

Flint, G.N., A metallurgical approach to metal contact dermatitis, *Contact Dermatitis*, 39, 213, 1998.

Haudrechy, P. et al., Nickel release from nickel-plated metals and stainless steels, *Contact Dermatitis*, 31, 249, 1994.

Haudrechy, P. et al., Nickel release from stainless steels, *Contact Dermatitis*, 37, 113, 1997.

Husain, S.L., Nickel coin dermatitis, *Br. Med. J.*, 2(6093), 998, 1977.

Kanerva, L. et al., Nickel release from metals and a case of allergic contact dermatitis from stainless steel, *Contact Dermatitis*, 31, 299, 1994.

Lidén, C., Menné, T., and Burrows, D., Nickel-containing alloys and platings and their ability to cause dermatitis, *Br. J. Dermatol.*, 134, 193, 1996.

Lidén, C. et al., Nickel release from tools on the Swedish market, *Contact Dermatitis*, 39, 127, 1998.

Lidén, C. and Carter, S., Nickel release from coins, *Contact Dermatitis*, 44, 160, 2001.

Menné, T. et al., Patch test reactivity to nickel alloys, *Contact Dermatitis*, 16, 255, 1987.

Menné, T. and Calvin, G., Concentration thresholds of non-occluded nickel exposure in nickel sensitive individuals and controls with and without surfactants, *Contact Dermatitis*, 29, 180, 1993.

Oakley, A.M.M., Ive, F.A., and Carr, M.M., Skin clips are contraindicated when there is nickel allergy, *J. R. Soc. Med.*, 80, 290, 1987.

Oldfield, J.W. and Sutton, W.H., Crevice corrosion of stainless steels, *6th Eur. Congress on Corrosion,* Society of Chemical Industry, London, 1977.

Pedersen, B. et al., Release of nickel from silver coins, *Acta Derm. Venerol. (Stockh.)*, 54, 231, 1974.

Pickering, H.W. and Wagner, C., Electrolytic dissolution of binary alloys containing a noble metal, *J. Electrochem. Soc.*, 114, 698, 1967.

van Ketel, W.G., Occupational contact with coins in nickel-allergic patients, *Contact Dermatitis*, 12, 108, 1985.

Wilkinson, D.S. and Wilkinson, J.D., Nickel allergy and hand eczema, in *Nickel and the Skin: Immunology and Toxicology,* Maibach, H.I. and Menné, T., Eds., CRC Press, Boca Raton, FL, 1989, p. 141.

Glossary of Terms

Allergic contact dermatitis (hypersensitivity) A type IV or delayed hypersensitivity — expressed as an eczematous skin reaction in sensitized humans that arises approximately 1 to 7 days after encounter with an antigen, typically reaching a maximum at 48 h. It is mediated by antigen-sensitized T cells. Allergens may be small haptens (e.g., nickel) that react with normal host proteins and, by modifying them, create an antigen.

Antigens Molecules recognized by the immune system and inducing an immune reaction.

B-cell tolerance Immature B cells are more susceptible to tolerance than mature cells and can be tolerized by smaller doses of tolerogen. Conversely, if only B cells are tolerant, then T cells may still be able to produce a cell-mediated immune response.

Desensitization or Hyposensitization (Immunotherapy) Reduction or elimination of allergy in a previously sensitized organism. Traditionally it is used for treating immediate (humoral) hypersensitivity reactions to insect venom, animal dander, and pollen (urticaria, allergic rhinitis, and bronchial asthma). More recently it is used to treat immediate and delayed (cellular) type hypersensitivity by oral (Panzani et al., 1995) or epicutaneous (Boerrigter and Scheper, 1987) hapten application.

Through continuous treatment of an organism with established contact allergy, symptoms can be alleviated with low-dose oral exposure (Bagot et al., 1995; Christensen, 1990; Santucci et al., 1988). Subimmunogenic doses of antigen interact with antibody, thereby preventing cooperation of macrophages, T helper cells and B cells.

Immunologic unresponsiveness can also be achieved with high-dose oral therapy, i.e., exposure to large amounts of antigen leading to activation of T suppressor cells (Sjövall et al., 1987), or development of the blocking antibody IgG.

Haptens/Prohaptens (from the Greek word *haptein*, to fasten) Usually small molecular weight, electrophilic compounds that are not immunogenic but can react with protein (nucleophiles), e.g., with antibodies of appropriate specificity, the immunogenic carrier. Nickel is a hapten that was demonstrated to react specifically with the nucleophilic histidine residue in the major histocompatibility complex (MHC) molecule, a cluster of genes important in immune recognition present in all mammals (Sinigaglia, 1994).

Molecules that are not electrophiles, and therefore cannot function as haptens, may be converted to haptens through metabolic processes, e.g., in the skin. They are referred to as prohaptens.

Hypersensitivity An immune response that occurs in an exaggerated or inappropriate form. Reactions are classified into four types, according to the speed in which they occur and the mechanisms involved:

Type I (immediate) hypersensitivity, manifest in allergic asthma, allergic rhinitis (hay fever), and contact urticaria that develop within minutes of exposure to antigen, is dependent on the release of mediators of acute inflammation.

Type II (antibody-mediated) hypersensitivity is caused by antibody to cell-surface antigens, mostly induced by drugs. These can sensitize the cells for antibody-dependent cell-mediated cytotoxicity by K-cells, or complement mediated lysis. It also becomes manifest in the destruction of red-blood cells in transfusion reactions, and in haemolytic disease in the newborn.

Type III (immune complex mediated) hypersensitivity is due to the deposition of antigen–antibody complexes in tissue and blood vessels. The antigens stem from persistent pathogenic infections (e.g., malaria), from inhaled antigens (e.g., extrinsic allergic alveolitis), or from the host's own tissue (autoimmune diseases).

Type IV (delayed) hypersensitivity arises more than 24 h after contact with the antigen, and is mediated by antigen-sensitized T cells that release lymphokines; these attract T cells and macrophages to the site activating them, leading to tissue damage. This type of hypersensitivity can be in response to skin contact with allergens.

Immunogens/Antigens Molecules that are recognized by the immune system and induce the formation of antibodies are immunogens. Those which react with antibodies are antigens. Only complete antigens, i.e., complex macromolecules, can do both. Substances can be antigenic without being immunogenic. Nickel ion is an antigen, too small to be recognized by the immune system and induce formation of antibodies. Only when bound to a protein (carrier) forming a hapten–carrier conjugate (a complete antigen), nickel becomes an immunogen, able to induce the formation of antibodies.

Lymphocytes Cells controlling the immune response, derived from pluripotent stem cells; they undergo an orderly process of differentiation generating mature B cells or T cells. They specifically recognize "foreign" material and distinguish it from the body's own components. Of two main types, B cells develop in the bone marrow and produce antigen-specific antibodies. T cells develop in the thymus and have a number of different functions helping B cells to make antibody, recognizing and destroying cells infected by virus, activating phagocytes to destroy pathogens, and controlling the nature and degree of the immune response.

Sensitization A general term used in immunology to describe altered reactivity on contact with an antigen or allergen. It encompasses all types of immune reactions. After presentation of the antigen by an antigen presenting cell, specific T cells in the case of type IV (ACD or delayed type) and specific B cells in the case of type I, II, or III hypersensitivity are induced. Immune reactions of the skin, also known as allergic contact dermatitis (ACD) or delayed hypersensitivity, are caused by penetration of the skin by a foreign substance (a hapten or an antigen).

T-cell tolerance T cells (mediators of delayed type hypersensitivity) are more easily tolerized than B cells. Once established, T-cell tolerance is usually longer-lasting than B-cell tolerance.

Tolerance The acquisition of (immediate or delayed) specific nonresponsiveness in a naive subject to a molecule recognized (as foreign) by the immune system. Whether a molecule induces an immune response or tolerance is largely determined by the way it is first presented to the immune system.

Tolerize To administer a molecule in a way that makes an organism or cell population tolerant to it.

Tolerogen A molecule that induces tolerance.

Index

A

Absorption in skin, *See* Skin absorption
Active protective creams, 19–20
Aerosols
    metal, 10–11
    nickel, 4
Allergens, 55
Allergic contact dermatitis
    amino acids role in, 209
    asymptomatic, 13–14
    atopy and, 58
    contributing factors, 204
    delayed-type, 7, 12–13
    description of, 203, 224
    development of, 186
    gender predilection, 40, 203
    genetic predisposition for, 204–205
    immediate-type, 7, 10–12
    incidence of, 204
    literature regarding, 8–9
    metal–metal interactions in, 212
    patch testing
        description of, 41–45, 54–55, 173
        guidelines for, 173–174
        studies of, 58–63
    preventive levels of exposure, 22
    silent, 13–14
    studies of, 67–68
    treatment of, 13–122–23
    triggering of, 12
    zinc sulfate effects, 213
Allergic contact stomatitis, 8–9
Alloys, *See specific alloy*
Angry back syndrome, 54, 122, 173
Antioxidants, 19
Atomic absorption spectrophotometry, 114
Atopy, 13, 41, 57–58, 74

B

Beauticians, 69
Beryllium, 119
Burning mouth syndrome, 129–130

C

Carboxyvinyl polymer gel, 20
Chase-Sulzberger phenomenon, 187
Chelators, 19–20
Coins
    nickel alloys used in, 229
    nickel leaching from, 116, 135
Construction workers, 69
Consumer products
    electron charge of compounds in, 148
    nickel exposure, 72
    stainless steel, 222
Contact dermatitis, *See* Allergic contact dermatitis
Contact urticaria syndrome, 4
Cooking utensils, 134–135
Copper-nickel alloys
    applications for, 223, 228
    properties of, 223, 228
Copper–nickel–zinc alloys, 228–229
Corrosion
    description of, 224
    implant metals, 116
    sweat effects, 94
Corticosteroids, 15
Creams
    active protective, 19–20
    barrier, 18
    passive protective, 18–19
    studies of, 22

D

DDC, 22–23
Delayed-type hypersensitivity, 7, 12–13, 187
Dental materials
    description of, 4, 115
    gold-based, 125
    nickel allergy hypersensitivity and, 137
    nickel in
        description of, 119, 186
        nickel–chromium alloys, 193–195
Dermatitis, *See* Allergic contact dermatitis
Detection methods
    atomic absorption spectrophotometry, 114
    dimethylglyoxime spot test, 112, 117–118

inductively coupled plasma-atomic emission
spectroscopy, 113
inductively coupled plasma-mass
spectroscopy, 113
nitric acid spot test, 112–113
particle induced x-ray emission, 114
Diagnosis, of nickel allergy hypersensitivity,
14–15
Diethylenetriamine, 20
Dimethylglyoxime spot test, 112, 117–118
Disappearance method, for measuring skin
absorption, 156–158

E

Ear piercings, 60, 66, 73, 123–124, 192, 196
Earring studs, 21
Electro-plated nickel silver, 228
Epidermis, 84
Ethylenediamine tetraacetic acid disodium salt,
18, 20
European Dangerous Preparations Directive, 22
European Nickel Directive, 21–22, 120
Excited skin syndrome, 55

F

Ferro-nickel, 220
Fick's concept of permeability, 157
Finn Chambers, 57, 121

G

Galvanic element, 92
Gastrointestinal exposure, 133–135, 188
Genetics, 57, 74, 204–205
Gingivostomatitis, 128
Gloves, 18
Gold-based dental restorations, 125–126
Gut-associated lymphoid tissue, 188

H

Hairdressers, 69
Hand dermatitis, 5
Heredity influences, 57, 74, 204–205
Hypersensitivity
delayed-type, 7, 12–13
immediate-type
description of, 7, 9
etiology of, 11

nickel-releasing orthodontic devices
exposure and, 128
pathophysiology of, 10
signs and symptoms of, 10
T helper cell response, 7, 9
Hyposensitization, *See also* Tolerance
in animals, 189
experimental, 188–189
in humans, 189–190

I

Immediate-type hypersensitivity
description of, 7, 9
etiology of, 11
nickel-releasing orthodontic devices exposure
and, 128
pathophysiology of, 10
signs and symptoms of, 10
Immune response
allergic contact dermatitis, *See* Allergic
contact dermatitis
delayed-type hypersensitivity, 7, 12–13
description of, 101
divergent, 7–10
immediate-type hypersensitivity, *See*
Immediate-type hypersensitivity
immunotoxicity, 15–16
Immunoglobulin E antibodies
description of, 11
testing for, 14–15
Immunologic contact urticaria
description of, 7
literature regarding, 8–9
Immunotoxicity, 15–16
Implant metals
corrosion of, 116
ion release in, 119
orthopedic, 130–133
Inductively coupled plasma-atomic emission
spectroscopy, 113
Inductively coupled plasma-mass spectroscopy,
113
Intercellular diffusion, 85
Interleukins, 210
Intracellular adhesion molecule-1, 210
Iron, 211, 230

J

Jewelry, 123–124, 204, 235

K

Keratinocytes, 210

L

Lactate, 90
Langerhans cell, 12
Lewis acids, 202
L-histidine, 18
Liquefied natural gas, 223
Lymphocyte migration inhibition factor, 131–132
Lymphocyte transformation test
    description of, 167–168
    diagnostic value of, 176
    discussion of, 177–179
    mechanism of, 174–177
    metal sensitivity testing, 175
    methodology for, 174
    nickel allergy hypersensitivity diagnosed
        using, 176–179
    reaction development, 168
    studies of, 175–176
    timing of, 178

M

Macrophage migration inhibition test, 176
Magnesium, 211–212
Major histocompatibility complex class
        molecules, 177, 205
Manganese, 211
Medical workers, 70
Memory lymphocyte immunostimulation assay,
        177
Metal(s)
    exposure to
        immediate-type hypersensitivity caused
            by, 10
        toxic effects caused by, 202
    extracellular reactions with, 202
    nickel interactions with, 211–213
    transition
        electrovalences of, 202
        Lewis acids and, 202
        ligand binding of, 202
        types of, 201–202
Metal aerosols, 10–11
Metal plating, 20–21, 24, 122, 204
MOAHL index, 57
Mucous membranes, 136

N

Nickel
    anodic reactions for, 224–225
    characteristics of, 203, 220, 237
    chelate rings of, 12
    chelation of, 19
    commercial uses of, 2, 5–6
    complexes of, 206–207
    detection methods, See Detection methods
    dietary intake of, 134
    discovery of, 206
    electropositivity of, 136
    fatty acids reactions with, 84
    forms of, 220
    hybridization of, 207
    immunogenic forms of, 16
    immunotoxicity of, 15–16
    metal interactions with, 211–213
    mucous membranes absorption of, 136
    naturally occurring, 6
    oral exposure to, tolerance induced by,
        190–192
    oxidation states of, 207–208, 226
    percent dose absorbed measurements,
        155–156
    properties of, 220
    protein complexing with, 208–211
    pure, 220–221
    skin absorption of, See Skin absorption
    skin contact-induced diffusion of, 92
    solubilization of, 73
    synthetic sweat levels of, 92–93, 102–111,
        114–119
    tolerance to, 16–17, 41
    toxic effects of, 203
Nickel(II)
    description of, 206–207
    sensitizing potential of, 211
    in vivo transportation of, 208
Nickel(III), 206–207
Nickel aerosols, 4
Nickel allergy hypersensitivity
    age-based prevalence of, 48–51
    allergic contact dermatitis
        asymptomatic, 13–14
        delayed-type, 7, 12–13
        immediate-type, 7, 10–12
        literature regarding, 8–9
        silent, 13–14
        triggering of, 12
    asymptomatic, 13–14
    atopy effects, 13, 41, 57–58, 74
    dental materials and, 137
    diagnostic methods, 14–15

ear piercings and, 60, 66, 73
epidemiology of, 3–4
etiology of
    exposure, 6, 100–101
    skin penetration, 6–7
familial disposition for, 57
Finn Chambers, 57
gender predilection
    statistics regarding, 14, 73–74, 101, 186
    studies of, 58–63
genetic predisposition to, 57, 74
heredity of, 57, 74, 204–205
incidence of
    description of, 56
    occupation and, 68–71
    patient age and, 65–68
    studies regarding, 58–63, 65–68
lymphocyte transformation test for
    diagnosing, 176–179
MOAHL index, 57
occupational prevalence of
    description of, 52–53
    studies of, 68–71
oral induction of, 133
orthodontics, 128, 136
overview of, 2–3
patch testing, *See* Patch testing
population studies of, 46–47, 63–64
preexisting, 190
prevalence of
    increases in, 72–73
    occupation and, 68–71
    patient age and, 65–68
    statistics regarding, 24, 40, 56
prevention of
    active protective creams, 19–20
    barrier creams, 18
    gloves, 18
    metal plating, 20–21, 24, 122
    overview of, 16–17
    passive protective creams, 18–19
    personal hygiene practices, 17–18
    regulations, 21–22
    workroom exposure monitoring, 17
prognosis, 5–6
remission of, 5
Repeat Open Application Test, 56
risk factors for, 2–3, 75, 124
skin piercings, 124, 196
studies of
    age-based, 65–68
    description of, 3–4
    gender-based, 58–63
    geographic location-based, 58–63
    leaching experiments, 116–117

limitations, 72, 75
occupation-based, 68–71
population-based, 63–64
suggested types of, 76
variables that affect, 76–77
T cells associated with, 168
Thin Layer Rapid Use Epicutaneous Test,
    56–57
treatment of
    desensitization methods, 23–24
    systemic, 23–24
    tetraethylthiuramdisulfide, 23
    topical agents, 22–23
underreporting of, 72
Nickel alloys, *See* Nickel-containing alloys;
    specific alloy
Nickel chloride
    sensitization potential of, 176, 211
    stratum corneum penetration of, 55
Nickel coatings
    description of, 234
    top-coats, 235–236
Nickel exposure
    consumer products, 72
    safe levels of, 120
    workroom exposure monitoring, 17
Nickel ion
    adhesion molecules expressed by, 211
    alloy release of, 137
    amino-acid ligands and, 209
    antigen response to, 209
    bioavailability of, 117
    biological properties of, 203–204
    in catalyst enzymes, 203
    description of, 100
    immune reactions to, 101
    keratinocytes activation by, 210
    release of, 6
    skin penetration of, 6–7, 85, 101, 159
Nickel powder
    description of, 221
    skin contact with, 226–227
Nickel rash, 85
Nickel release
    blood transport after, 124
    chromium coating effect, 235
    from clothing, 193
    coatings effect on, 235–236
    from cooking utensils, 134–135
    description of, 121
    detection methods for
        atomic absorption spectrophotometry, 114
        dimethylglyoxime spot test, 112, 117–118
        inductively coupled plasma-atomic
            emission spectroscopy, 113

inductively coupled plasma-mass
spectroscopy, 113
nitric acid spot test, 112–113
particle induced x-ray emission, 114
experiments of, 116–119
gastrointestinal exposure, 133–135
intraoral, 126
from jewelry, 123
orthodontics, 124–130, 192–197
orthopedic implants, 130–133
rate of, 121
skin contact, 121–123, 135
skin piercings, 123–124
in synthetic sweat, 92–93, 102–111, 114–119,
204
from tools, 123
water faucets, 133
Nickel salts
inflammatory reaction caused by, 210
irritancy of, 169
patch testing of, 212
skin penetration of, 6, 152–153
skin reactions caused by, 159, 210
sweat formation of, 83
Nickel sheet, 220
Nickel sulfate, 177–178
Nickel–chromium alloys, 193–195, 232–233
Nickel-containing alloys
anodic reactions for, 224–225
coinage, 229
description of, 221
industrial contact with, 224
intermetallic compound, 221
plating of, 21, 24, 122
production of, 221
stainless steel, 222
sweat reactions with, 227–228
Nickel-copper alloys
applications for, 223, 228
properties of, 223, 228
Nickel–copper–zinc alloys, 228–229
Nickel–iron alloys, 223, 230
Nickel–iron–chromium alloys, 232–233
Nickel-removable prosthesis, 127
Nickel-silver alloys, 224, 228–229
Nickel–titanium alloy, 233
Nitric acid spot test, 112–113
Noble metals, 233–234

O

Occupation
nickel aerosol exposure in, 4, 116

nickel allergy hypersensitivity and
description of, 52–53
studies of, 68–71
Orthodontics
blood analysis after receiving, 125, 128, 195
fixed appliances, 127
nickel allergic hypersensitivity symptoms,
128, 136, 186–187
nickel alloys used in, 118–119
nickel release from, 124–130, 192–197
nickel-removable prosthesis, 127
palladium-based alloys, 125
saliva testing, 127
stainless steel use, 129
studies of, 128–130
titanium, 125
tolerance induced by, 190–192
Orthopedic implants, 130–133
Oxidation states, 207–208

P

Palladium-based alloys, 125
Particle induced x-ray emission, 114
Passive protective creams, 18–19
Patch testing
active sensitization caused by, 172
description of, 41–45, 54–55, 121, 168–169,
226
discussion of, 173–174
false-negative reactions, 172–173
false-positive reactions, 72, 168, 172–173
irritant effects, 172
metal–metal interactions evaluated using, 212
nickel compounds, 169
nickel sulfate, 171
sensitivity levels, 172
site for, 171–172
studies of, 58–63, 170–171
technique of, 168–169
test concentrations for, 169–171
vehicle for, 169
Phyto haemagglutinin, 131
Polyethylene glycol, 22
Pompholyx, 5, 121
Prevention, from nickel allergy hypersensitivity
active protective creams, 19–20
barrier creams, 18
gloves, 18
metal plating, 20–21, 24
overview of, 16–17
passive protective creams, 18–19
personal hygiene practices, 17–18
regulations, 21–22

workroom exposure monitoring, 17
Protein complexing, 208–211
Protons, 91
Pyruvate, 90

R

Radioallergosorbent test, 10
Reactive oxygen species, 211
Repeat Open Application Test, 56
Rusters, 115

S

Sebum, 91–92
Sensitization
    development of, 186, 203
    nickel chloride, 176
Silver–nickel alloys, 224, 228–229
Skin
    acid mantle of, 91–92
    cleansing of, 17
    corneocyte layer testing, 17
    defense mechanisms of, 203
    diffusivity, 148
    exudates
        composition of, 85
        description of, 83
    nickel absorption in, *See* Skin absorption
    nickel allergy hypersensitivity prevention
        methods, 17–18
    nickel salts-induced reaction, 159
    patch testing of, 41–45, 54–55
    pH of, 91
Skin absorption
    data regarding, 157–159
    description of, 2, 6–7, 73, 84, 121–123, 135,
        148–149, 204
    diffusion methods, 85, 92, 160
    dissolution, 153
    methods of, 84–85
    qualitative findings, 149–153
    quantitative methods for measuring
        disappearance method, 156–158
        limitations for, 160
        predictive models, 157
        in vitro studies, 154–155
        in vivo percent dose absorbed
            measurements, 155–156
    rates, 152
    studies of, 150–151
Skin piercings, 123–124
Sodium lauryl sulfate, 13

Stainless steel
    classification of, 222
    commercial uses of, 222
    composition of, 230–231
    corrosive performance of, 232
    description of, 112, 117–118
    orthodontics use of, 129
    orthopedic implant use of, 132–133
    passive, 230
    properties of, 222
    sweat reaction to, 230–232
Status allergicus, 178
Stratum corneum
    acid mantle effects, 91
    anatomy of, 84
    barrier creams for, 19
    free acids in, 91
    homeostasis of, 91
    keratin in, 149
    nickel deposition in, 2, 6, 94, 149, 152
    nickel salts permeation in, 159
Sweat
    analysis of, 86
    "cell-rich," 86
    characteristics of, 85–86
    collection methods for, 86
    components of
        amino acids, 89
        chloride, 87
        description of, 86, 94, 115
        lactate, 90
        macro-electrolytes, 87–88, 94
        proteins, 89–90
        pyruvate, 90
        sodium, 87
        trace metals, 90–91
    corrosivity of, 94
    lead levels in, 86
    nickel reaction with
        alloys, 227–233
        copper–nickel–zinc alloys, 228–229
        description of, 224–226
        powder form, 226–227
    noble metal alloys reaction with, 233–234
    osmolality values, 88
    stainless steel reactions, 230–232
    synthetic
        nickel release in, 92–93, 102–111,
            114–119, 149, 204
        types of, 93
Sweat glands, 84
Systemic allergic reactions, literature regarding,
    8–9

T

T cells
    antigen response of, 209
    description of, 168
    experimental hyposensitization, 188–189
T helper cells, 7, 9, 188
TAP1, 205
TAP2, 205
Tetraethylthiuramdisulfide, 23
Thin Layer Rapid Use Epicutaneous Test, 56–57,
        130, 169
Tin–nickel coatings, 236
Titanium, 125
Tolerance, *See also* Hyposensitization
    antigen-specific induction of, 187–188
    description of, 16–17, 41, 196

intraorally placed alloys, 125
orthodontic device-induced, 190–191, 196
Top-coats, 235–236
Trace metals, 90–91
Transepidermal water loss, 15, 22–23

W

White gold, 233–234
Workroom exposure monitoring, 17

Z

Zinc sulfate, 211, 213